Health Services Research

Health Services Research

Key to Health Policy

Edited by Eli Ginzberg

A Report from
The Foundation for Health Services Research

Harvard University Press
Cambridge, Massachusetts
London, England

First Harvard University Press paperback edition, 1993

Library of Congress Cataloging-in-Publication Data

Health services research : key to health policy / edited by Eli Ginzberg.
p.   cm.
Includes bibliographical references.
Includes index.
ISBN 0-674-38575-6 (alk. paper) (cloth)
ISBN 0-674-38576-4 (pbk.)
1. Medical policy.   I. Ginzberg, Eli, 1911–
[DNLM: 1. Health Policy.   2. Health Services Research.
W 84.3 H434]
RA425.RA425   1991
362.1—dc20
DNLM/DLC   90-4955
for Library of Congress   CIP

Contributors

Stuart H. Altman, Ph.D.
Dean and Sol C. Chaikin Professor of National Health Policy, Heller
School, Brandeis University

Robert H. Brook, M.D., Sc.D.
Chief, Division of Geriatrics and Professor of Medicine and Public
Health, UCLA Center for the Health Sciences, and Corporate Fellow
and Deputy Director, Health Sciences Program, The RAND
Corporation, Santa Monica, California

Lawrence D. Brown, Ph.D.
Professor, Division of Health Administration, Columbia University

Karen Davis, Ph.D.
Professor and Chair, Department of Health Policy and Management,
School of Hygiene and Public Health, Johns Hopkins University

Paul B. Ginsburg, Ph.D.
Executive Director, Physician Payment Review Commission,
Washington, D.C.

Eli Ginzberg, Ph.D.
Director, Conservation of Human Resources, Columbia University

Philip R. Lee, M.D.
Chair, Physician Payment Review Commission, and Director, Institute
for Health Policy Studies, University of California, San Francisco

Harold S. Luft, Ph.D.
Professor of Health Economics, Institute for Health Policy Studies,
School of Medicine, University of California, San Francisco

Elizabeth McGlynn, Ph.D.
Health Policy Analyst, The RAND Corporation, Santa Monica,
California

Ellen M. Morrison, Ph.D.
Postdoctoral Fellow, Institute for Health Policy Studies, School of
Medicine, University of California, San Francisco

Joseph P. Newhouse, Ph.D.
John D. and Catherine T. MacArthur Professor of Health Policy and
Management, John F. Kennedy School of Government, Harvard
University

Ellen K. Ostby, M.M.H.S.
Heller School, Brandeis University

Uwe Reinhardt, Ph.D.
James Madison Professor of Political Economy, Woodrow Wilson
School of Public and International Affairs, Princeton University

Diane Rowland, Sc.D.
Brookdale National Fellow, and Assistant Professor, Department of
Health Policy and Management, School of Hygiene and Public Health,
Johns Hopkins University

Contents

Foreword

New ideas conceived through health services research are crucial to the evolution of national health policy. How those ideas are developed, debated, and made the cornerstones of new policies is the major theme of this story, untold until now.

Previous writings about health policy have focused on the later stages of the legislative process, on times when political opportunity and personal entrepreneurship take center stage. In those periods, ideas have already been absorbed into the fabric of policies under negotiation and thus go unrecognized and unreported. The result is that most accounts overlook the manner and extent to which new ideas have been an independent and influential force in shaping national health policy.

This book puts health policy development in broader perspective. In so doing, it is true to John Maynard Keynes's observation that "ideas . . . both when they are right and when they are wrong, are more powerful than is commonly understood . . . I am sure that the power of vested interests is vastly exaggerated compared with the gradual encroachment of ideas." How are new ideas formulated, tested, challenged, verified, and improved through health services research? These questions are addressed in this volume, primarily through historical considerations of major health policy issues written by the nation's leading practitioners of health services research. Their chapters underscore the continuing contributions of thousands of researchers nationwide who produce new knowledge about health services for the purpose of improving them.

Special recognition goes to the members of the board and staff of the Foundation for Health Services Research, under whose leadership this project came into being. Alice Hersh, founding executive director of the Foundation, brought her exceptional skills and tenacity to directing the project. Eli Ginzberg developed the intellectual enterprise into the rich resource you have before you. Anna Dutka, as editor, worked with great precision to make each chapter clear and accessible.

Thomas W. Moloney
The Commonwealth Fund

Preface

The first chapter contains important background information about how this book came to be written. But such information must be supplemented by my calling attention to those who helped turn the idea into a reality.

My first debt is to the authors of the various chapters, who, despite their heavy schedules, made time to deal comprehensively with their assignments and to do so within a very tight publication schedule.

My next acknowledgment goes to my long-term colleague, Anna B. Dutka, who identified many of the materials presented in the two chapters that I wrote, and who further took over much of the arduous editorial work required to turn the work of fourteen authors into a useful whole. I am greatly in her debt.

Although advances in technology with duplicate disks contributed greatly to the preparation of the final manuscript, Shoshana Vasheetz was in charge of transcribing all of the chapters and seeing that all of the additions and corrections were made. This was no small task, but one that she carried out with her usual skill and good nature.

Alice Hersh was a source of strength and support from the first day to the last.

Eli Ginzberg
Columbia University

Abbreviations

AAMC	Association of American Medical Colleges
AAPCC	Adjusted Average Per Capita Cost
AARP	American Association of Retired People
ADAMHA	Alcohol, Drug Abuse, and Mental Health Administration
ADL	Activities of Daily Living
ADS	Alternative Delivery Systems
AFDC	Aid to Families with Dependent Children
AHA	American Hospital Association
AHC	Academic Health Center
AHCCCS	Arizona Health Care Cost Containment System
AHCPR	Agency for Health Care Policy and Research
AHSR	Association for Health Services Research
AMA	American Medical Association
BLS	Bureau of Labor Statistics
CBO	Congressional Budget Office
CCMC	Committee on the Costs of Medical Care
CDF	Children's Defense Fund
CHAP	Child Health Assurance Program
CHER	Center for Health Economics Research
COBRA	Consolidated Budget Reconciliation Act
COGME	Council on Graduate Medical Education
CON	Certificate of Need
CPR	Customary, Prevailing, and Reasonable (fees)
CPT	Current Procedure Terminology
CREDOC	Centre de Recherche pour l'Etude et l'Observation des Conditions de Vie
CRS	Congressional Research Service
DEFRA	Deficit Reduction Act
DHEW	Department of Health, Education, and Welfare

DHHS	Department of Health and Human Services
DRGs	Diagnosis-Related Groups
DSM	Diagnostic and Statistical Manual
ECF	Extended Care Facility
EPO	Exclusive Provider Organization
EPSDT	Early and Periodic Screening, Diagnosis, and Treatment
ESP	Economic Stabilization Program
ESRD	End Stage Renal Disease
FFS	Fee for Service
FHSR	Foundation for Health Services Research
FMG	Foreign Medical Graduate
GAO	General Accounting Office
GDP	Gross Domestic Product
GHAA	Group Health Association of America
GHC	Group Health Cooperative
GNP	Gross National Product
GMENAC	Graduate Medical Education National Advisory Committee
HCFA	Health Care Financing Administration
HHS	See DHHS
HIAA	Health Insurance Association of America
HIE	Health Insurance Experiment
HIO	Health Insuring Organization
HIP	Health Insurance Plan
HIS	Health Interview Survey
HMO	Health Maintenance Organization
HPDP	Health Promotion and Disease Prevention
HPEAA	Health Professions Educational Assistance Act
HSUS	Health Services Utilization Study
IADL	Instrumental Activities of Daily Living
IMC	International Medical Centers, Inc.
IPA	Independent Practice Association
LTC	Long-Term Care
MDE	Maximum Dollar Expenditure
MediCal	California Medicaid Program
MEI	Medicare Economic Index
MMPS	Medicare Mortality Predictor System
MOS	Medical Outcomes Study
MVPS	Medicare Volume Performance Studies
NACHM	National Advisory Commission on Health Manpower
NCHS	National Center for Health Statistics

NCHSR	National Center for Health Services Research
NHPRDA	National Health Planning and Resources Development Act
NHSC	National Health Services Corps
NICHMOD	National Industry Council for HMO Development
NIH	National Institutes of Health
NIT	Negative Income Tax
NLT	National Long Term Care
NMCES	National Medical Care Expenditures Survey
NMCUES	National Medical Care Utilization and Expenditures Survey
NMES	National Medical Expenditure Survey
NNHS	National Nursing Home Survey
NRSA	National Research Service Awards
OBRA	Omnibus Budget Reconciliation Act
OEO	Office of Economic Opportunity
OTA	Office of Technology Assessment
PGP	Prepaid Group Practice
PHP	Prepaid Health Plan
PHS	Public Health Service
PPO	Preferred Provider Organization
PPRC	Physician Payment Review Commission
PPS	Prospective Payment System
ProPac	Prospective Payment Assessment Commission
PSRO	Professional Standards Review Organization
RAPs	Radiologists, Anesthesiologists, and Pathologists
RBRVS	Resource-based Relative Value Scale
SGA	Southern Governor's Association
SHMO	Social Health Maintenance Organization
SNF	Skilled Nursing Facility
SOA	Supplement on Aging
SRI	Stanford Research Institute
SSI	Supplemental Security Income
TEFRA	Tax Equity and Fiscal Responsibility Act
UI	Urban Institute
VE	Voluntary Effort

Health Services Research

Health Services Research
and Health Policy

Eli Ginzberg

This introductory chapter has a number of distinct objectives. The first is an explanation of how this volume came to be written and a description of its sponsorship and contributors, as well as the principal objectives that the participants hope to achieve. To furnish perspective and balance, I next provide a brief, highly selective review of efforts that were precursors to the emerging discipline of health services research (HSR). Finally, I present a summary of the points of departure and the principal lines of analysis that the authors pursue.

The Commonwealth Fund, through the initiative of its senior vice-president, Thomas Moloney, a long-time member of the board of the Foundation for Health Services Research (FHSR), an adjunct to the Association for Health Services Research (AHSR), both of which were established in 1981, made a grant in 1988 to the Foundation for the purpose of sponsoring the writing and publication of a basic introductory volume. This volume would have the threefold purpose of serving as an introduction for graduate students entering the field; of demonstrating to federal and state legislators and policymakers, and to members of their staffs, the potential of health services research in the hope and expectation that information about its past achievements and prospective accomplishments would increase the appropriations for the training of researchers and for the broadening of funding of research; and finally of publishing a readable volume about major trends in health services research with a strong economics orientation that would inform the growing number of citizens who are increasingly perplexed by the relentless increase in health care expenditures, which in 1989 came to about $620 billion, or about 11.2 percent of GNP.

The leadership of the AHSR together with the Commonwealth Fund decided on the researchers who would be asked to participate in this collaborative venture. Each prospective author who was approached agreed to participate. The request that I serve as editor was surely influenced by the fact that I belong to the older generation of health policy researchers, with roots going back to World War II, many decades before the term *health services research,* but not the endeavor, first came into use. This provides me with an elongated perspective.

The year 1990 marked the twenty-fifth anniversary of the passage of Medicare and Medicaid, which fundamentally altered the role of the federal government in the financing of the nation's health care system. In 1965 total federal expenditures for health amounted to $5.6 billion; in 1989 the total was in excess of $150 billion, which corrected for inflation still amounted to almost a fivefold increase.

There is a direct and close relationship between the passage of Medicare and Medicaid and the explosive growth of health services research as a rapidly growing field of scholarly endeavor. Confronted with steeply rising expenditures for health care, federal officials through in-house efforts and contractual arrangements have sought to learn more about the complex forces affecting the demand for services, the production and delivery of services, alternative ways of reimbursing providers, and the impact of services on the health of vulnerable population groups.

In 1968 Congress appropriated funds to establish the National Center for Health Services Research and Development, including the National Center for Health Statistics (the latter was incorporated into the Centers for Disease Control in June 1987). The establishment of these new federal instrumentalities reflected a belief among members of the Congress that improving the information base about mortality and morbidity as well as collecting new data about how the American people made use of health care services were necessary and desirable additions to the knowledge pool. This would supplement the scientific advances in the biomedical arena that were forthcoming as a result of large-scale congressional appropriations for biomedical research and development. It would take me too far afield to provide even a summary sketch of the forces that led Congress to legislate these new centers into existence, and more particularly to explore the reasons for Congress's early disenchantment; to put it simply, the legislators and their staffs did not find the early research directly helpful to them as they explored policy alternatives.

The relationship between the passage of Medicare and Medicaid and health services research assessed in the chapters that follow can best be illustrated by considering how many of the chapters are directly linked either to the legislation passed in 1965, or to the recently expanded role of the federal government in the national health policy area. The first substantive chapter establishes the dimensions of the political arena within which health policy has been fashioned and refashioned. Let me quickly add that one chapter on the political discussion of health services research versus eight others on the economic aspects of various innovations in health care delivery does not provide a balanced view of the field; rather, it reflects the dominant orientation of the researchers who were invited to contribute to this volume.

Five chapters related to the passage of Medicaid and Medicare deal with hospital reimbursement, physician payment, the poor, the elderly, and the role of the health insurance experiment (HIE) in influencing the demand for medical care. The remaining three chapters, on alternative delivery systems, physician personnel, and the appropriateness of medical interventions, are but one stage removed. Small wonder that many graduate students first starting their studies believe that health services research emerged as a new discipline a quarter of a century ago. But they are mistaken. Even without searching for the earliest traces of health services research, which would surely lead to identification of contributions as early as the middle of the nineteenth century, one would find that the field has a respectable set of accomplishments dating from the first decades of the twentieth century.

One could assert that the field investigation carried out by Abraham Flexner in the 1909–10 academic year of the 150 medical schools in the United States and Canada, and his ensuing report as to their strengths and weaknesses (including a strong recommendation that all but 31 be closed), was the single most important piece of health services research carried out in this century. I make this judgment despite the fact that more than twice the number of schools designated for closure continued to operate, although many were eventually upgraded. The Flexner Report accelerated by many years the antecedent and concurrent efforts of the American Medical Association to raise the quality of medical education, thereby improving by an order of magnitude the quality of medical care available to the American people.

Also dating from the pre–World War I era were the several efforts of a small but deeply committed group of students of social legislation, among whom Abraham Epstein was a leader. These advocates were in the forefront of studying European efforts to establish workmen's compensation with a view to its introduction in the United States and of exploring the potentials of national health insurance. In the presidential election of 1912 Theodore Roosevelt endorsed national health insurance, a reminder of how long the issue has been on and off the nation's health agenda.

It is worth noting that the American Medical Association in 1916 supported compulsory health insurance, only to withdraw its endorsement four years later. Since that time the AMA has been in the forefront initially of opposition to all health insurance programs, and, since the passage of Medicare, to a governmental system of universal coverage.

In the mid-1920s a distinguished commission with funding from the major health foundations under the chairmanship of President A. Lawrence Lowell of Harvard University, with Willard C. Rappleye of Columbia University serving as director, explored the quantitative and qualitative adjustments that should be undertaken in the education of medical students in light of the advances in biology and other sciences. Reporting in 1932, the commission, among its other recommendations, urged a reduction in the number of admissions to medical schools, a policy that most schools followed in the ensuing years.

But the major national effort to assess the strengths and shortcomings of the U.S. health care system took place under the aegis of the Committee on the Costs of Medical Care (CCMC), which got under way in 1927 and issued its final report in 1932. During the long period of its deliberations it published no fewer than 27 volumes of data and analysis on all facets of our health care system. Never before nor since has there been a research-assessment effort of comparable breadth and depth. The final report of the CCMC dealt with a number of critical issues including group medical practice, hospital planning, strengthening public health, improving professional medical education, and the financing of medical care. The committee split on the last issue, with a few favoring a system of governmental insurance, the plurality favoring voluntary health insurance, and a significant minority consisting mostly of physician members firmly opposed to any insurance initiative.

Some of the most important contributors to health services research in the pre– and post–World War II years gained experience and prominence as a result of their involvement in the CCMC, including Michael M. Davis, C. Rufus Rurem, I. S. Falk, Louis B. Reed, Milton Roemer, Cecil Sheps, and many more.

Brief mention, at the very least, should be made of another important strand of research that had more of a clinical than an economic focus. Early in the century, Ernest A. Codman and Elmer L. Henderson of Boston (Massachusetts General Hospital and Harvard University) raised fundamental issues about the quality of medical care and its value to patients, the same issue that in the post–World War II era engaged Paul A. Lembcke (Johns Hopkins University) and Avedis Donabedian (University of Michigan), the father of modern quality assessment.

In 1962 the first Conference on the Economics of Health and Medical Care was held at the University of Michigan. The Conference Planning Committee was chaired by Selma J. Mushkin and included among others Agnes Brewster, Rashi Fein, and Herbert Klarman. A review of the eighty or so participants reveals that many were subsequently major contributors to health policy analysis, and about twenty are still active. But it is also worth pointing out that not one of the contributors to the present volume, the editor alone excepted, was an active participant at the Ann Arbor conference.

There is no need to marshal additional evidence to underscore my contention that although health services research is a new and rapidly growing discipline, there has been a long and distinguished group of predecessors who made important contributions to health care policy. If one seeks to differentiate health services research before and after Medicare, emphasis must be focused on the change in methodology: the earlier investigators were "institutionalists" who made use of simple statistical and economic tools, while the present generation of researchers uses far more sophisticated methodologies, reflecting advances in econometrics and computerization.

But if health services research has had, as noted above, a long and distinguished group of predecessors who have made important contributions to analyzing and assessing the strong and weak points of different types of health care systems, something new and important has been added in the last quarter-century. The U.S. health care system is now vastly larger, constitutes a much larger percentage of the GNP, and involves many more people both as users and providers. With increased scale has come increased complexity and, in turn, increased challenges to health services research to assess what is working well and what needs improvement. All concerned groups—providers, users, payors— have come to appreciate that good intentions and good values do not suffice for modifying and improving the health care system.

These recent developments have created an environment more conducive to health services research, for without the benefit of new data, new knowledge, and new understanding it is not possible for politicians, acting on instinct alone, to refashion and reform the extant health care system. For better or worse they need, in fact are dependent on, the establishment of a foundation based on facts and figures and a growing body of knowledge. Scale and complexity in health care delivery have created the preconditions for the expansion of health services research.

The remainder of this chapter is devoted to summarizing the three basic dimensions of each of the nine substantive chapters that constitute this volume: the central theme that is addressed, the lines of analysis, and the principal conclusions for health care policy.

Lawrence Brown, a political scientist by training, addresses in Chapter 2 the important question of the relationship between new and improved knowledge (research) and power (health care policy). Brown selects two initial cases, the prospective payment system for reimbursing hospitals for treating Medicare patients and a new system for fee control of physicians treating Medicare patients, to demonstrate the interactions among documentation, analysis, and prescription. These three dimensions encompass the points of interaction between health services research and health policy.

There is no question in Brown's view that health services research can and does make a considerable contribution to improving the level of debate about health policy by adding new knowledge. The trouble comes when the research community confronts the politicians who are responsible for deciding whether and how to change the status quo. Brown makes the important point that the three subgroups of health services researchers—economists, technocrats, and planners—are seldom in a position to provide the political leadership with directly useful advice, first because of disagreements among themselves and second because they cannot sketch out the likely consequences that will follow upon the enactment of their recommendations.

More and better documentation and analysis have added much to understanding the critical issues in the ongoing debate about health policy. But Brown observes that the accommodation of an ever-larger body of knowledge can burden, as well as facilitate, health reforms. Significant reforms in a modern democratic society with multiple interest groups are in the last analysis heavily dependent on historical and cultural factors that are perhaps beyond the cognizance of most health services researchers. Such reforms depend heavily on a congruence between changing public expectations and the ability of leading politicians to envision at least the near-term results of the reforms that they may be willing to support.

The senior author of "Paying for Hospital Care" (Chapter 3), Stuart H. Altman, has long divided his time between government service and academic life. An economist by training and profession, Altman serves as dean of the Heller School of Brandeis University as well as the chair of the Prospective Payment Assessment Commission (ProPAC) since its establishment. This oversight body advises the Health Care Financing Administration (HCFA) and Congress on the Medicare prospective payment system that was passed and implemented in 1983 to slow the rise in federal hospital reimbursement expenditures for Medicare beneficiaries.

Altman and Ostby's chapter moves back and forth between health services research and policy challenges and responses and is strengthened by its sensitivity to the role of the past in setting limits on current policy and even more on limiting choices for the future. The authors start their account by reminding us of the input of health services research in the pre-Medicare era when hospital costs and health care costs generally were advancing rapidly but when, in the view of most analysts, the cost reimbursement system had at best only minor responsibility for health care inflation.

The authors go on to explain how the Economic Stabilization Program (ESP) in the early 1970s precipitated a host of operational issues involved in cost reimbursement, such as the nature of hospital prices and output. They then continue their review of various innovations by different payors to moderate the rise in hospital reimbursements and pay close attention to the more ambitious undertakings by a number of states directed at regulating all hospital rates. Among their more interesting conclusions is the fragile nature of health services research when it is directed to assessing events over a short time span. They point out that the preliminary conclusion of the researchers that hospital rate regulation was not effective had to be modified once the period of assessment was lengthened. The revised findings demonstrated that the states that had enacted rate control experienced over a longer period of time a lower rate of hospital cost inflation.

The failure of the Certificate of Need (CON) approach contained in federal legislation of 1974, the rejection by the Congress of President Carter's plan to set budgetary limits on hospital outlays in 1978–1979, and the eventual collapse in 1981 of the Voluntary Effort (VE) at cost containment designed and supported by the American Hospital Association (AHA) and its allies, all set the stage for the rapid design and passage of the Prospective Payment System (PPS) based on the diagnosis-related groups (DRGs), a methodology developed at Yale in the 1970s that was the basis for an experiment in the state of New Jersey in the early 1980s.

In assessing the six-year experience with PPS, Altman and Ostby are careful not to claim too much for it. They note that Susan Horn and other researchers have criticized the system's insensitivity to "severity of illness." They point out that the providers' ability to upgrade the diagnostic codes has led to large additional expenditures. They also take note of the 1989 study of Russell and Manning which points to large overall savings for the new system, on the order of 20 percent, but go on to remind the reader that these savings might be considerably smaller if full account could be taken of secondary costs in nursing homes and home care as a result of patients' being discharged earlier from the hospital.

Altman and Ostby conclude their informative chapter by pointing to the fact that much of the health services research involved in hospital reimbursement was "reactive" in the sense that solutions were devised to handle past problems. By finding many of the solutions wanting, health services research in their view helps to set the stage for further policy innovations. And so the point-counterpoint between research and policy continues.

The chapter by Paul Ginsburg and Philip Lee entitled "Physician Payment" has many parallels to the preceding chapter by Altman and Ostby. What they have in common is a major operational problem affecting the Medicare payment system, in the one case payments to hospitals, in the other payments to physicians. The authors of Chapter 4, like Altman and Ostby, are also situated in two camps—the research community and a prominent advisory role to the federal government. Lee is the chairman of the Physician Payment Review Commission (PPRC), and Ginsburg is the executive director. Their chapter is focused specifically on five critical problem areas that the Physician Payment Review Commission explored during the past several years and that provided the basis for its proposal to the Congress for a reform of the Medicare payment system for physicians (Medicare B), which was approved with only minor changes in November 1989.

The first problem area was centered on efforts to develop a resource-based relative value scale (RBRVS). The major research was carried out by Professor W. C. Hsiao and his colleagues at Harvard University under a grant from the Health Care Financing Administration. The unique aspect of this research investigation was the active cooperation of the American Medical Association and many of the specialty societies. Hsiao's policy findings (1988) went a fair distance to suggest how a physician fee schedule could be related to physician time, effort, and practice costs.

The PPRC submitted the Hsiao study to in-depth reviews in which the representatives of the medical community had ample opportunity to submit their criticisms and countersuggestions, many of which were incorporated by the commission into the proposals which it forwarded to the Congress. The PPRC modified the treatment of practice costs in the relative-value-scale component of the fee schedule, an action that had significant impact on the proposed Hsiao fee adjustments. With respect to the debate on assignment and balance billing, the PPRC recommended a limit on balance billing because the simulations showed that such action would reduce the aggregate by a substantial amount.

The authors set the stage for a discussion of the policy reforms by calling attention to the very rapid increases in health care expenditures in the United States compared to many other advanced countries in the 1980s, particularly the runaway increases in physician expenditures. On the policy front, Ginsburg and Lee start by pointing out that a fee schedule is not the only approach to containing expenditures for physician services. Another approach would look to alternative delivery systems (ADS) in which payments to physicians would be incorporated in a more comprehensive purchase of health care services through an HMO or a Preferred Provider Organization (PPO).

The PPRC recommended to the Congress the desirability of adopting expenditure targets, renamed by the latter Medicare Volume Performance Standards. This proposal sought to forewarn physicians that they should not resort to increased services to outfox fee controls because if the total billings exceeded the target figure, the following year would see a fee reduction to bring the two back into line, although any individual physician breaking ranks would be better off. Building on the work of Brook, Wennberg, and their colleagues, the PPRC also recommended that Congress fund research on medical appropriateness and outcome measures more liberally, a recommendation that was accepted.

In their conclusions the authors stress that health services research made two critical contributions to public policy, shaping the alternatives facing the political leadership as it sought to introduce reforms and providing critical information to give substance and direction to the reforms that Congress settled on.

In Chapter 5 Karen Davis, a long-time senior federal governmental health expert, currently on the Johns Hopkins faculty, together with her colleague, Diane Rowland, has provided an extended critical review of the passage of Medicaid, with special attention to the contribution of health services research to this critical dimension of the nation's health care system that is the primary provider of care to the poor. The authors begin by reminding us that although Medicaid was less debated than Medicare when it was passed in 1965, the former had its roots in two earlier pieces of legislation—the medical vendor payments for people on welfare of 1950 and the Kerr-Mills legislation of 1960 for the "medically needy" aged. The authors also note the role of advisory groups in lobbying for the passage and later the expansion of Medicaid, and the impact that the health services research data and analysis had on the legislators who had to be convinced to pass the original legislation and expand it in subsequent years. The authors note in passing that the original estimates of Medicaid's cost were grossly underestimated.

Medicaid has been from the outset a joint program between the federal government and the states, with Washington covering a minimum of 50 percent of the cost (up to 78 percent for the lower-income states) and establishing the eligibility requirements for single-parent families on AFDC and SSI while providing flexibility to the states to cover different groups of "medically needy" up to a specified limit. Responsibility for administering the program rests with the states, and from the outset they have differed greatly in the breadth and depth of the coverage that they provide. About one-third of the states have failed to cover half of their poor who fall below 50 percent of the federal poverty level.

By the second half of the 1970s (1976–1980), the program was under increasing strain, as reflected in a decline in the number of eligibles and steeply rising total expenditures. President Reagan sought to cap the federal contribution to Medicaid in 1981, but the Congress refused to go along, although it agreed to three years of budgetary cutbacks. Despite this effort, total outlays for Medicaid increased between 1980 and 1985 from $23 to $37 billion with no net increase in enrollments.

The authors note that starting in 1984 Congress changed tack and by mandates and financial persuasion encouraged the states to improve coverage for pregnant women, children, the poor elderly, and the disabled, actions that Davis and Rowland relate specifically to health services research studies of the value of prenatal care, which showed a cost/benefit ratio of 3 : 1. The researchers also called attention to the sizable numbers of the near-poor elderly who were forced into poverty because of high outlays for their uncovered medical expenditures. In 1988 Congress required the states to use Medicaid to fill Medicare coverage gaps for their poor elderly.

Although the authors were able to demonstrate many constructive interactions between health services research and the Medicaid program, they stress the slippage between the two largely because of the following: the weakness of standardized data across states; the absence of an ongoing sample of users; lack of information about health status; inadequate financing of research on the Medicaid population by HCFA, which has concentrated its research support on analyzing Medicare; and the lack of studies aimed at assessing the cost/benefits of alternative approaches to enlarged coverage. They conclude their chapter with several pages of important research questions that have not been addressed and that call out for study.

In Chapter 6 Diane Rowland, drawing on her policy experience both in HHS and as a congressional staffer, begins her analysis of financing health care for elderly Americans by identifying two primary issues: closing the gaps in Medicare, an acute care system for the elderly; and addressing the lack of public/private insurance coverage for long-term care (LTC). She indicates the considerable number of good data sets that have been developed that permit the analyst to determine how effective Medicare has been in responding to the acute needs of the elderly and the gaps that remain to be filled. According to Rowland, health services research demonstrated that Medicare had contributed a great deal to broadening access of the elderly to physician and hospital services; to reducing the initial discrepancies based on income, race, and location; and to documenting the residual problems affecting the rural population. Researchers have also pointed out the serious financial problems that the poor elderly faced because of coinsurance requirements and incomplete coverage, particularly for drugs, which led Congress over time to amend Medicaid and even attempt to provide catastrophic coverage under Medicare to reduce the vulnerability of elderly patients. Researchers uncovered the important fact that 80 percent of the catastrophic health burden of the elderly (exceeding $2000 a year) was due to spending for nursing home care.

The author provides a brief discussion of how health services research helped to focus attention on benefit areas severely constrained or absent from Medicare relating to home health, hospice care, preventive services, prescription drugs, and mental health. Although these studies led Congress to make modest changes, it was not until the amendments for catastrophic coverage of 1988, now repealed, that Congress was willing to take a big step forward in extending entitlements. Rowland shows how, despite the lack of a consensus about the scale and scope of needs for LTC, health services research has contributed to estimating by basic demographic characteristics the size of the population in need and the sources of formal and informal support. By developing a scale based on the need for assistance with activities of daily living (ADL), researchers were able to establish a common framework for analysis.

Reviewing the different demonstrations and waivers directed at enabling more of the sick and infirm elderly to be cared for at home, Rowland concludes that most of the results as to costs are equivocal, either because of lack of random assignment, insufficient time to assess the results of the demonstrations, or for other reasons. There is little reason to believe that total costs will decline if more of the sick and disabled elderly are kept at home, although that is the preference of most of them.

In her review of the nursing home population Rowland notes that the last decade has been marked by relative stability, with about 1.3 million persons (5 percent of the elderly), half of them over 85, on the rolls. Relatively few among the elderly can cover the average $25,000 or more annual charge out of their savings, with the result that patients relatively quickly spend down their assets to a point where they are eligible for Medicaid. However, one of the provisions of the catastrophic amendments that survived the 1989 repeal was the protection of some assets for the spouse living in the community.

Rowland concludes her broad analysis by pointing out that the repeal of catastrophic coverage suggests that the services that need to be covered to improve the health and well-being of the elderly must be assessed with greater care and that the costs of coverage must be more carefully calculated. The repeal spoke primarily to the resistance of affluent elderly taxpayers to the use of progressive taxation to finance costly benefits for the elderly in need of LTC.

Chapter 7, entitled "Controlled Experimentation as Research Policy," tells the story of the Health Insurance Experiment (HIE) carried out by The RAND Corporation for the federal government in the 1970s and 1980s, the results of which are still being published although the major findings have been available since the early 1980s. The author of the chapter, Joseph P. Newhouse, was the director of the HIE, and the story that he tells is both authentic and authoritative.

Newhouse begins by remarking on how little health services research at the beginning of the 1970s was able to speak definitively about the interactions between people's ability to pay for health care services and their demand for services, and even less about the consequences of their different patterns of utilization on the buyer's health status. Specifically, the HIE had the following principal objectives: to estimate how the use of various services responded to insurance plans that varied cost sharing; to estimate the consequences of such variations for health status; to determine whether the answers to the foregoing varied by income group; to determine the effects of covering outpatient as well as inpatient services; and to estimate the reduction in use, if any, and the resulting health status outcomes, in a well-established staff HMO.

Newhouse summarizes the findings of the experiment, which proved that the type of insurance plan (cost sharing) had a significant effect on use. Patients who received free care used about 50 percent more services, including more hospital admissions, than those with the highest cost sharing. But hospital care among those hospitalized differed little among those on any plan, among other reasons because 70 percent exceeded the $1000 Maximum Dollar Expenditure (MDE), so that any additional expenditure was fully paid for. In terms of health status, there was little measurable effect of the type of plan on outcome other than dental care. However, those who were hypertensive at the outset of the plan, or who had correctable vision problems, encountered adverse effects, which were concentrated among the poor. The key findings for the single HMO site pointed to a 40 percent lower use of inpatient hospital treatment, which translated into a 25 percent lower overall cost. But once again the sick poor apparently were not as well off in an HMO, although the average member was satisfied.

Newhouse suggests that the publication of the early findings from the HIE in 1981 and 1983 contributed not only to the growth of deductibles and coinsurance in private insurance, but also to the expansion of insurance coverage at the "back-end." The author acknowledges that he cannot present definite proof of the impact of HIE on these changes, although the coincidence in timing is surely suggestive; but he goes on to point out that in the period since 1983 the results of the HIE have had little to contribute to the attempts to reform Medicare.

In his concluding pages Newhouse stands back to ask some basic questions about the rationale for spending the considerable sums that controlled experimental studies require. He decides that such studies surely have a claim on governmental support because they are in the best position to develop "hard" findings that will carry conviction to a public whose opinions are firmer than its knowledge of how the costly health care system operates. Newhouse recognizes that the long time period necessary to plan and carry out a controlled experimental study yields dividends beyond the dollar costs. He concludes that even if the political environment changes so that many questions that were asked may lose some or much of their salience and others that should have been asked will not have been included, any serious long-term health services research effort must make room for controlled experimental studies.

The senior author of Chapter 8, Harold Luft, is one of the country's leading experts on health maintenance organizations (HMOs) and a faculty member at the University of California, San Francisco. He and his colleague, Ellen M. Morrison, have written about alternative delivery systems (ADS). Their principal goal is to identify and assess the changes that have occurred in the financing and delivery of health care in the United States, primarily during the last two decades, as background for assessing what can be determined about the relative cost and quality of care provided under differing delivery systems from classic fee-for-service (FFS) arrangements to staff model health maintenance organizations (HMOs) and preferred provider organizations (PPOs).

In pursuing their historical-comparative analysis, the authors have noted both the strengths and weaknesses of health services research in providing the data bases and the analyses required for valid judgments and particularly how the results of health services research can be used to guide new developments in health policy. In their view, the growth of ADS really dates from the end of World War II with the establishment and growth of selected prepaid group practices (PGP) plans in California, Washington, D.C., and New York City. They note that the Health Insurance Plan (HIP) in New York City had on its staff three prominent health services researchers—Sam Shapiro, Paul Densen, and Marilyn

Einhorn—whose investigations added significantly to the knowledge pool about ADS and their impact on their members' health and well-being.

The authors note that prior to the federal legislation of 1973, "health enhancement" was the center of interest for advocates of HMOs. Congress however was willing to appropriate funds for the establishment of new HMOs in the belief that more competition, on a level playing field, might help to contain the rise in expenditures of the dominant system of FFS medicine.

Luft and Morrison call attention to major structural changes in the health care environment of the 1980s which have made it much more difficult to compare the performance records with respect to costs or quality among different ADS. They note in particular the shift in hospital reimbursement from cost reimbursement to prospective payments; the blurring of lines between inpatient and outpatient services; the growing concerns about entrepreneurial behavior of physicians; the substantial growth of members in both HMOs and PPOs; and the many different types of restrictions within FFS systems as well as widening choices and more copayments among many HMOs.

Against the background of these substantial changes in the larger health care environment, the authors look at the evidence with respect to whether HMOs contribute to health promotion, provide improved services to the poor, are effective in containing costs, and contribute to more competition. They note that critics have argued that HMOs, because of fixed budgets, are likely to lead to poor quality of care and to other negative results. To choose among these contradictory views is not easy for, as the authors stress, there is often a lag of six years between the announcement of an innovation and the availability of sufficient data to evaluate it. After a careful analysis, the authors conclude that with respect to health promotion and disease prevention, HMO enrollees may receive more preventive services than persons enrolled in FFS plans, but once account is taken of self-selection factors and other variables such as differences in coverage, the results are not clear-cut.

Despite the federal government's encouraging the states to use HMOs to provide health care for the poor, particularly those on Medicaid, a great number of difficulties, from clinic locations to methods of payment, have resulted in few successes. Moreover, many Medicaid patients place a high value on their existing freedom of choice. Regarding cost containment, the authors conclude that HMOs *can* contain costs relative to open-ended FFS systems with minimal copayments, but they go on to point out that during the past decade most FFS plans have adopted more "utilization management" with preadmission requirements, second opinions, and so on. The authors also point out the need to differentiate between the various aspects of the contrasting systems of delivering care, particularly in regard to the cost burden on the plan, the enrollee, and the employer.

On the issue of promotion of increased competition, the evidence fails to prove that HMOs have made much, if any contribution, in part because of their limited membership, with few areas having reached an enrollment level above 20 percent. Moreover, local markets often restrict outright competition between FFS and HMOs.

As regards quality, the authors are very cautious, emphasizing that with freedom on the part of enrollees (if they are dissatisfied) to withdraw from an HMO and the relatively muted complaints of poor quality, a balanced judgment suggests that there are no gross differences in quality between HMOs and FFS systems. The authors also explore some interesting issues regarding HMOs and payor responsibility as well as related questions growing out of biased selection and equitable payment. The burden of their analysis is to remind the reader once again that in an open, pluralistic system such as that in the United States, it is difficult to find data and studies that present simple, clear-cut answers regarding the differences among plans based on costs or quality.

In their concluding section, entitled "A Policy-Oriented Research Agenda," the authors stress that the question of whether HMOs could save money without jeopardizing quality is no longer relevant because of the environmental and structural changes that have affected both HMO and FFS medicine. They call for better measures of benefits among different types of health plans; for improved measures of quality of care; for understanding differences in HMO performance; for additional improvements bearing on incentives for health promotion; for the avoidance of biased selection; and for the establishment of "fair" rates and improved marketplace rules for viable competition. Their concluding sentences are pertinent: "The medical care system is a moving target composed of man-made systems and incentives which adapt to changing social, economic, and policy factors. This means that it will probably be impossible to design a set of policy measures that will always be optimal. However, if we increase our understanding of how the medical care system and its components work, then it will be easier to identify policy changes to continually improve the system."

Uwe Reinhardt, professor of economics at Princeton, has long been interested in the supply of physicians from both a theoretical and a policy perspective. In Chapter 9 he discusses the difficulties of forecasting the physician supply, makes some suggestions about improving the methodology, examines the relations between forecasts and health policy, and ends with some suggestions for future health services research.

In his initial section Reinhardt points to the difficulties of developing a "population needs" basis for health care services. He reminds the reader about the substitution problem between physicians and other health care providers, and suggests that we know less than we need to about the health production function other than that more inputs lead to reduced morbidity, although with rapidly diminishing marginal effect. Reinhardt then calls attention to important changes in the settings in which health services are provided—from inpatient to outpatient, from FFS to HMO, with corresponding implications for manpower use. He notes further the absence of detailed information and studies of different production functions that would point the way to the most economical use of manpower resources to provide a desired level of services. He points out however that such studies are likely to be forthcoming in the years ahead as hospitals confront serious and possibly long-term shortages of nurses and other critical personnel.

After setting out briefly the two contrasting approaches to forecasting future demand for health care services—the needs-based and demand-based approaches—Reinhardt finds them both lacking, if on different grounds. He then shifts attention to the policy realm. In the pre–World War II decades the medical leadership was absorbed with the "oversupply" of physicians. But in the postwar decades, the continuing assumption, based on some normative physician-population ratio, pointed to a present and prospective shortage which led to federal action to expand our medical school capacity. Later on policymakers began to wonder whether they had overshot the mark, and researchers took a closer look at productivity and other variables that might affect their supply projections.

In his concluding section Reinhardt emphasizes that it is a mistake to analyze the production of health care services in terms of fixed production coefficients. There are many alternative ways of producing needed health care services. Since all projections are likely to be off, possibly seriously off, because of the difficulties that the researcher faces in estimating not only demand but also flexibility on the supply side, health services research is confronted with a dilemma: will a policy of excess supply be better or worse than a policy that results in a shortfall of physicians?

Robert H. Brook, a member of the medical school and public health faculty at the University of California, Los Angeles, and a senior member of the RAND staff, and his colleague from RAND, Elizabeth A. McGlynn, are the authors of Chapter 10, which discusses the public's role in maintaining the quality of care. They introduce their chapter by reviewing a series of basic questions about what health is: how is health measured? how is quality assured? and is there evidence that a problem with quality exists? They also explore in their introduction a conceptual definition of health and conclude that it is multidimensional and may be viewed differently by patient, family, physician, and society.

The authors note that good measures are available for most biological and clinical aspects of health, as well as functional and self-assessed health status. What is more equivocal is the role that medical care can play in changing a person's functional status. After summarizing the measurement of and mechanisms for improving health status, the authors go on to discuss the relationships between quality and health status: high quality produces positive changes in a person's health, low quality accelerates a decline. Finally the authors note that identifying who is responsible for improving the health of a group is a critical but unanswered question.

Brook and McGlynn point out that the quality of health care has both a technical and an "art of care" dimension and that both are important in defining quality. But they emphasize that the public needs help in assessing the technical aspects, since the "art of care" may be in the eye of the beholder.

The authors note that a restriction in the dollars spent on health care can and often does affect quality adversely, but they go on to point out that the existence of too many services may also impair health status. They then examine the striking variations in the utilization of health care even among large areas, a phenomenon better described than understood. Variations in complex procedures show ranges of twofold to fourfold. A related issue is the appropriateness of care, which is defined as the potential of services producing benefits to patients that exceed the risks of treatments. Studies of appropriateness disclose both overuse and underuse of medical interventions.

A critical concern of the authors is to define and illustrate the public's role in assessing quality. They distinguish between continuous "internal" improvement in which the providers are the center of the action, and external monitoring where the public has the lead role. To date, little information has been released to the public, but the authors advocate the public's involvement through the release of critical information. Brook and McGlynn go on to outline what a public quality information system would look like, focusing on data bearing on "appropriateness" as well as on "patient outcomes."

In their concluding section the authors emphasize that data already exist that shed light on both appropriateness and outcomes, although a substantial public investment in further data collection and evaluation would be required to assess in more breadth and depth the quality of current medical treatment, including both overuse and underuse. The related question that they raise is how such information could be tapped by the public to lead to improved choices so that the health care which they sought could contribute more to improving their health status. The authors recognize that the program they outline will not be easy to implement, but without the public's active involvement the quality of medical care is not likely to be significantly improved.

In the closing chapter of this volume, I examine the potential for health services research in light of its past accomplishments and the challenges that it confronts.

· 2 ·

Knowledge and Power: Health Services Research as a Political Resource

Lawrence D. Brown

It probably strikes most health services researchers as obvious that knowledge ought to be a primary basis, perhaps *the* primary basis, of health care policy. What can "good" policy mean if not "informed" policy? But it probably strikes most health services researchers as equally and disappointingly evident that a wide range of intervening variables extraneous to the merits of issues—constituency demands, partisan promises, ideological biases, interest group preferences—invade and generally conquer the policy process. On a good day, ideas may gain a hearing amidst the swirl of political considerations, but it must be a very good and rare day indeed when policymakers take their cues mainly from scientific knowledge about the state of the world they hope to change or protect.

Unfortunately, such large generalizations about the "role" of health services research (or other forms of ideas) in the policy process are close to useless. The outcomes that policy generates and the behavior and actors it recognizes and rewards differ widely from case to case. Accordingly, health services research as a political resource has not one role but rather several that shift with time, place, and circumstance. In this chapter I try to map a middle ground between the agnostic view that "it all depends" and facile generalities that decry the disjunction between knowledge and politics. I begin with two brief recent case studies that spotlight the contribution of health services research to political change; I then sketch a simple typology of forces for change and use that typology to speculate about knowledge as power and health services research as a political resource in the policy process.

An Opening Case: Prospective Payment Comes to Medicare

By 1977 Medicare had run for more than a decade without significant change in the methods, based on the retrospective payment of actual costs, by which it reimbursed hospitals. By 1977 that system was under increasing attack as a "blank check" that invited soaring annual rates of increase in hospital spending and that gave Medicare, and its hospital component in particular, pride of place within the notorious ranks of "uncontrollable" federal programs. By 1977 the federal government had begun nibbling at the edges of the problem by means of health maintenance organizations, professional standards review organizations, certificate-of-need laws, health systems agencies, and the Economic Stabilization Program, but to little avail. In 1977, therefore, the Carter administration proposed to attack the heart of the matter: after less than four months in office, the President sought enactment of a national hospital cost containment plan that would set annual limits on both the revenues most hospitals could accrue and the capital spending they could undertake (Abernathy and Pearson, 1979, pp. 73–94).

The plan was instantly and angrily denounced by the hospital industry and anti-regulatory conservatives. The industry proclaimed its own "Voluntary Effort" to hold down costs without government's heavy helping hand; meanwhile conservatives paraded before the media shopping carts overflowing with documents purporting to portray the new burden of red tape hospitals would face if the Carter plan passed.[1] Deliberations stalled; the administration amended and softened its bill. The drumbeat of opposition from industry and conservative forces increased. And the VE seemed to be working: annual rates of increase in the average cost per day for nonfederal short-term hospitals, which stood at 14.2 percent in 1976 and 13.9 percent in 1977, slowed to 11.7 percent in 1978 and 11.8 percent in 1979 (U.S. Bureau of the Census, 1989, table 162). Simultaneously, a growing national infatuation with deregulation of airlines, trucking, telecommunications, banking, and other industries made it seem ever less likely that Congress would accept firm new regulation of the hospital sector. In November 1979 the Carter plan, which had earlier passed the Senate, died by a lopsided vote in the House.[2]

With the failure of the Carter plan, hospitals found themselves liberated for the first time in a decade from any credible threat of new federal regulation as a penalty for financial indiscipline. In November 1980 the election of Ronald Reagan put regulation further on the defensive: the new administration pledged to devise market-based, competitive cost containment strategies that would purge the health care system of most federal regulatory impositions. By 1981 most political observers agreed that hospital regulation was an idea whose time had gone.

In 1982, however, trends reversed abruptly. Hospitals, which had slowed their increases in per diem costs in 1977 and 1978, greeted the demise of the Carter plan, as if on cue, by registering sizable increases in 1980 (12.8 percent), 1981 (16.0 percent), and 1982 (15.1 percent). Reagan's fabled pro-competitive replacement for regulation was not forthcoming. Senator Robert Dole (Republican–Kansas), a leading opponent of the Carter plan, began warning hospitals publicly that they must change their ways or face new federal controls. Richard Schweiker, Reagan's Secretary of Health and Human Services, had heatedly criticized the Carter bill as a Republican senator from Pennsylvania and ranking minority member of the Health Subcommittee of the Labor and Human Resources Committee; now, however, he set staff at the Health Care Financing Administration to work designing a new system of prospective Medicare payments for hospitals. Suddenly regulation—federal regulation that set hospital prices—stood high on the health policy agenda.

In 1982 the Tax Equity and Fiscal Responsibility Act (TEFRA) set some prospective limits on hospital prices and instructed HHS to deliver to Congress a full-blown prospective payment plan by year's end. Under Schweiker's strong leadership, the department complied. With little discussion and less controversy, both House and Senate cleared the prospective payment measure and attached it to amendments to the Social Security Act, which Reagan signed in April 1983 (Menges, 1986). In 1979 the hospitals had buried the Carter bill; in 1982–1983 they pleaded for a place at the bargaining table in Washington. Chastened by the tough TEFRA provisions (themselves an expression of the legislators' sense of betrayal by the propagators of the voluntary effort) and convinced that they could no longer block significant change, the hospitals had within a mere three years won a battle and lost a war.

If one tries to explain why the federal government so obligingly adopted PPS only three years after it had firmly rejected Carter's cost containment plan, three factors stand out. First, between 1979 and 1982 there emerged a clear, widely acknowledged call to arms. In 1977, high and rising rates of hospital spending were worrisome; after another five years had passed and the huge Reagan budget deficits had arrived, they were insupportable. In 1977, doing something serious about the problem was a debatable (and much debated) option; in 1982 it was widely viewed as imperative, unavoidable. What had been a problem was now perceived as a "crisis."

A call to arms, even if widely recognized, is not in itself, however, a guarantee of action. In the United States it is possible, indeed usual, for "crises" to be declared and decried and yet linger on unsolved for years, perhaps decades. (The health care cost "crisis" and the growing plight of the uninsured are cases in point.) A major sticking point is often disagreement about who—the public or the private sector, one level of government or another—should take the lead in problem solving. Policy action requires, therefore, a second facilitating condition, evident in the PPS case, namely the authoritative discrediting of nonfederal solutions, especially market solutions. Prospective payment sailed through the Congress in part because the market (reliance on the hospital industry itself) had been granted a sincere and conspicuous test and had failed it badly. The Reagan administration had also promised to use the market in innovative ways but had likewise failed to deliver. Nor was federalism—deference to the fifty states—a plausible means of containing hospital costs in Medicare. By 1982 even those who instinctively recoiled from expanding the federal role had concluded, under the persuasive tutelage of trial and error, that there was simply no available, workable alternative to firm new federal intervention.

Policymakers may agree on the urgency of a problem and the implausibility of nonfederal correctives and still reach a deadlock if they cannot decide precisely what the federal government should do, if they do not feel confident that they themselves know what to do. A third condition for change, therefore, must usually be present—a widely appealing strategic model. In the PPS case the model was rate-setting as implemented by a half-dozen states in the 1970s. In the early 1980s, as evidence on the cost-containing effects of HMOs and such regulatory programs as PSROs seemed to offer little hope, and as policymakers began to stir from their short-lived dogmatic competitive slumbers, a growing body of research showed that something—rate-setting—did work after all. Brian Biles and others demonstrated that in six states with mature, rigorous rate-setting programs, the annual rate of increase in hospital spending ran about 3 percent below the national average (Biles et al., 1980). Reports by Abt Associates and other researchers reinforced this finding (Coelan and Sullivan, 1981; Eby and Cohodes, 1985). The supply of research findings coincided nicely in timing and tenor with the policymakers' demand for something sensible to do now that they had concluded that federal action had to be taken. Still, rate-setting raised questions about controls for case mix. Luckily, one of the six pioneering rate-setting states had addressed precisely this problem by means of diagnosis-related groups (DRGs), the icing on the cake as it were. Equipped with an attractive strategic model, policymakers answered the call to arms with a significant reform—a new federal price-setting system for Medicare.

An Exception That Proves the "Rule": Reform of Physician Payment in Medicare

Soon after PPS was enacted, some influential legislators (notably Robert Dole) predicted that 1984 could well be "the year of the physician." Hospitals had been put on a shorter fiscal leash; now it was the physicians' turn to sacrifice for the greater good. But 1984 saw no major extension of payment reforms to doctors, and at the beginning of 1989 the year of the physician had still not arrived, although it was very much at hand.

One explanation is that until the end of the decade the three preconditions of change found in the PPS case had not converged in the case of physician payment reform. The call to arms was comparatively muted: payments to doctors were a much smaller share of Medicare's total budget, and had been rising more slowly, than those to hospitals. Measured by the index of medical care prices (a component of the consumer price index), annual increases in the price of a hospital room outstripped increases in physician prices by 2 to 3 percent between 1977 and 1980. The differences rose dramatically in the early 1980s—3.9 percent in 1981, 6.3 percent in 1982, and 3.5 percent in 1983, the year that saw enactment of the prospective payment system. In 1984 the difference narrowed (8.3 percent for hospitals, 6.9 percent for physicians), and in 1985 it vanished (5.9 percent for both sectors) (U.S. Bureau of the Census, 1989, table 144), but a vague sense of intersectoral equity was not enough to induce policymakers to renew hostilities with organized medicine on such a basic bread-and-butter issue. Moreover, policymakers had not agreed on the implausibility of nonfederal solutions. In the mid-1980s some observers argued that the combined growth of the physician surplus and of alternative delivery systems was bound eventually to force doctors into price-reducing competition. The market might work after all. This was not a universally shared view, of course, but even critics of market solutions were deterred from activism by the third factor—no one knew exactly what to do; no broadly appealing strategic model was at hand.

As the 1980s ended, however, all three variables changed in ways strikingly analogous to the politics of PPS. In 1986, the rate of increase in physician prices surpassed the rate for hospitals and then continued to do so. Standing out like the proverbial sore thumb (as did hospital growth rates in the early 1980s), physician services increasingly triggered a general call to arms.

Moreover, five years (1984–1989) of waiting for the physician surplus and the spread of alternative delivery systems (ADS) to slow the rate of growth of spending for physician services proved to play the same role as did five years of deference to voluntarism between 1977 and 1982. Even the firmest believers in the merits of revitalized markets grew disappointed, their pleas discredited. Finally, by 1989 policymakers had available what was lacking in 1984, a strategic analogue to New Jersey's DRG-based rate-setting program. The Resource-Based Relative Value Scale (RBRVS) developed at Harvard by William Hsiao and his associates (1988) was widely heralded as a sensible, workable approach to improving the equity and efficiency of physician reimbursement.[3] Later in 1989 the pieces of the political puzzle fell into place, and as with PPS, years of discussion, delay, and deadlock gave way to quick and little disputed adoption of major payment reforms that will, effective January 1, 1992, employ resource-based fees and "volume performance standards" in setting Medicare reimbursements for physicians (McIlrath, 1989).

The Roles of Research as Agent of Change

Two mini-cases are not sufficient in themselves to validate a "theory" of policy change; they do, however, offer a reasonable working framework for exploring the roles of knowledge (in this case, health services research) in promoting (or retarding) policy change. The framework constructed from the two cases isolates three key variables in the explanation of policy change; each variable implies a distinct political role for research.

(1) Documentation. The first role is documentation, that is, gathering, cataloguing, and correlating facts that depict the state of the world that policymakers hope to change. Such measures can be indispensable in winning broad agreement among policymakers on a call to arms. In the PPS case the simple annual movement of statistical indicators, captured in graphs showing rates of growth of hospital spending over time, gave policymakers their motivation: spending growth was high in 1977, diminished a bit in 1978 and 1979 under the threat of federal regulation, and then, when the threat had disappeared, moved sharply upward again. This simple statistical picture was worth a thousand words. Likewise, when increases in Medicare spending for physicians' services claimed the booby prize in 1988, simmering interest in payment reform began to boil.

Such statistical indicators are perhaps not so much specimens of health services research as they are the raw materials from which such research is fashioned, but they are nonetheless important for that. As Daniel P. Moynihan (following Galbraith) observed years ago, society cannot act on social problems until it knows it has them, and it often does not know it has them until it can *count* them (Moynihan, 1970, p. 30). Crime in the streets became a salient issue not only because rates of crime increased dramatically over time but also because improved reporting and record keeping in the 1960s gave a more reliable picture of how much crime occurs. The supposed policy returns from refining and deploying such descriptive statistical information inspired the "social indicators" movement of the late 1960s (U.S. Department of Health, Education, and Welfare, 1989; Bell, 1969; Olson, 1969).

Beyond—and perhaps above—the compilation of statistical *facts* lies the documentation of statistical associations, that is, *correlations*. Probably the best early modern example of the influence of such research on health policy is Roemer's law. In the late 1950s Milton Roemer, examining the relation between the supply of hospital beds and occupancy rates, concluded that supply generates demand, that availability promotes use (Roemer and Shain, 1959). The explanation for the association was not Roemer's main concern and is debated to this day: perhaps hospital administrators pressure medical staffs to fill empty beds, perhaps physicians relax their standards for admission and length of stay when beds are plentiful, perhaps other dynamics are at work. Whatever the reason, Roemer's documentation of the correlation has had a sizable impact on policy: if overuse of inpatient services is a prime source of rising health care costs, and if Roemer's law holds good, then payors should save money by enacting such regulatory measures as certificate-of-need laws to restrict hospitals' freedom to enlarge bed supply.

New and better documentation can sound a convincing call to arms by teaching policymakers about problems which they did not know they had, or the gravity of which they may have underestimated. For many decades, child abuse was of concern mainly to social workers in the federal Children's Bureau, which lacked the resources to do more than convene conferences and encourage "a network of researchers" to investigate the problem. In 1962, however, Dr. C. Henry Kempe and colleagues published an article entitled "The Battered Child Syndrome" in the *Journal of the American Medical Association,* whereupon the popular media embraced and broadcast the issue. Documentation soon generated interest in additional information, analysis, and prescription. "Medicine, law, education, social work, and the social sciences created a demand for scholarly research on how to define, treat, and prevent child abuse. The professions then set about to fill the demand they themselves created." As the literature proliferated, state and federal politicians proved to be attentive consumers of professional findings (Nelson, 1984, pp. 47, 63).

Surely the best recent example of such influence in the health arena is the diffuse but powerful impact of small area analysis as developed by John Wennberg and others in the 1970s and 1980s. In essence, Wennberg and his colleagues showed that contiguous small areas such as rural counties in Maine and Vermont display widely varying rates for common surgical procedures (Paul-Shaheen et al., 1987). The researchers did not *explain* these remarkable variations—indeed their inability to explain them by reference to such obvious variables as demography is one of their most striking findings. Yet their thorough documentation of these differences has had a powerful corrosive effect on a payment system that reimbursed actual costs and usual and customary charges on the assumption that these sums captured the true, fair value of medical acts that reflected the considered professional judgment of highly trained practitioners. The small area studies show that these judgments about kindred cases vary widely and inexplicably, and thereby call into question the normative foundations of the payment system. The practical policy implications are that any plausible leveling scheme deserves a respectful hearing, that some reasonable, if crude, version of average costs or charges (perhaps defined in a fee schedule or relative value scale) may be tolerably accurate and acceptably fair. In this case documentation of major differences in rates of treatment, even without—indeed especially without—a convincing explanation, influenced policy by shaping policy-makers' perceptions of the system's workings and its legitimacy. It is difficult to link small area studies directly with specific policy changes, but one can hardly overestimate their impact on the intellectual climate that incubated and nourished change.

Documentation is not always a step toward action; sometimes it stultifies it. It is widely reported that more than 30 million Americans—about 17 percent of the non-aged population—have no health insurance. Some observers—many Europeans and Canadians, for example—believe that this brute fact should per se constitute a clear call to arms. Policymakers, however, want to know more about these people: Is the true number 37 million or "only" 31 million? How many work? How many have coverage through spouses or parents? How many lost insurance because they lost a job and are likely to regain the former with the latter? How many are dependents whose breadwinner declined, or was denied, family coverage? How many work part-time, how many for small firms, and so on? Researchers have worked diligently to answer these questions, but the data are often sparse and the methods unreliable. Knowing that all major options are likely to be expensive to the federal government (new subsidies or entitlements), business (mandates), the states (expansion of Medicaid), or the hospitals (revenue assessments), and lacking confidence and coalition support to make choices from the menu, federal policymakers plead the need for fuller, more definitive information. In the case of the uninsured, policymaking has succumbed to an information-indignation trade-off; strange to say, the more of the former we collect, the less of the latter we seem able to sustain. Information can be a highly potent force in moving policy from talk to action when the underlying predisposition is (for whatever reason) lively, but it cannot by itself create that predisposition.

(2) Analysis. A second role that health services research plays in shaping policy is analytical, that is, showing what does and does not work and explaining why. In the context of a strong call to arms, research shedding doubt on the omnipresent list of alternatives to governmental intervention can nudge policymakers toward action. But analytical research is a double-edged sword, capable of discrediting current policy as well as the alternatives.

Perhaps the best example of the influence of analytical research on policy is the massive report, entitled *Equality of Educational Opportunity,* prepared in the mid-1960s by the sociologist James Coleman and his colleagues (Coleman et al., 1966). Coleman was commissioned by the federal government to investigate the correlates of scholastic achievement among elementary and secondary school pupils. To almost everyone's surprise, the findings seemed to rebut the traditional model that equated better schools with more resources (more and better paid teachers, bigger and more modern facilities, and so on). The most compelling correlates of achievement were (in most cases) subjective, psychological variables, such as the pupil's sense of causal efficacy, which were closely linked in turn to family background. The Coleman report implied that the most salient influences on pupil achievement left their mark before the student ever passed through the school's portals. The findings caused boundless consternation within the educational establishment and encouraged federal policymakers to move slowly in expanding federal commitments and budgets for education (Harvard Educational Review, 1969). Similarly, in the 1960s and 1970s implementation studies became a growth industry among political scientists and policy analysts. Purporting to show that federal domestic programs rarely achieved their declared goals and made life miserable for the state, local, and private actors who had to manage them, these studies filled the pages of such journals as *The Public Interest,* provided copious polemical ammunition for the neo-conservative movement, and ridiculed the alleged federal propensity to "throw money at problems."

Conversely, however, sound analytical studies can show the implausibility or unreliability of nonpublic solutions based on markets, the professions, or the voluntary sector. Because the political culture and structure of the United States favor private decision making, such clearing of the conceptual underbrush is crucial in narrowing and shaping the policy agenda and persuading policymakers that an enlarged public role is necessary, albeit a necessary evil. American political sensibilities are at once deeply principled ("ideological" is the more common, but less accurate term) and highly pragmatic—stubbornly devoted to markets, states' rights, and small government, but prepared to temper these values and embrace big government when nothing else seems to work. Analytical research can energize the transition (usually gradual) from principle to pragmatism by showing that cherished institutions are, alas, not up to the jobs everyone agrees need to be done.

Oftentimes the corrosive effects of analysis are implicit in documentary research—that is, they lie latent, waiting to be imputed by policy-makers with a critical bent. Roemer's law does not prove that the higher use associated with increased bed levels is excessive and wasteful, but policymakers who believe that the system is too large and inefficient seldom shrink from that analytical leap. Since the 1960s many studies have shown the importance of personal preventive practices—diet, exercise, smoking, driving habits, stress, and more—to health outcomes. These findings do not establish that the money society spends on the treatment of diseases that might have been prevented or deferred is not "worth it," but the thought will suggest itself to the efficiency-minded. Wennberg's small area studies do not demonstrate that areas with higher procedural rates harbor "too much" care, but they have created a lively curiosity among policymakers as to whether that might not be so. In the early 1980s, the graphs plotting the upward drift of hospital spending after the death of the Carter plan did not precisely speak for themselves—*something* new might have been happening to justify those climbing rates—but what policymakers chose to hear was a damning indictment of the hospital industry.

Sometimes, however, analytical research challenges market strategies (or other nongovernmental strategies) directly. One reason why policymakers have remained skeptical of predictions that growth in the number of physicians and ADS will inevitably produce price-constraining competition is a well-founded body of research supporting the "target income hypothesis" (Feldman and Sloan, 1988; Rice and Labelle, 1989; Wedig et al., 1989; Feldman and Sloan, 1989). That theory holds that under many conditions physicians can largely define the demand they then meet, which allows them to manipulate volume and price in order to realize income they think appropriate to their lofty status and long training.

Some of the most germane analytical research derives from demonstrations—which by definition try to implement in the real world problem-solving hypotheses that are thereby tested for all to see. One reason why the problems of the uninsured linger on despite rising concern about the 31 to 37 million is that consensus on the necessity (and therefore the legitimacy) of a governmental solution has yet to form. About three-fourths of the uninsured, after all, are workers or their dependents. If the market (that is, workplace-based private health insurance) covers most of the non-aged population, why cannot American ingenuity find the means to extend it to the rest? The reply—that the lower-income workers who constitute the majority of the uninsured, and their (usually small) employers, generally cannot afford adequate coverage at today's market prices—is not universally accepted. Therefore such demonstrations as the Robert Wood Johnson Foundation's Program for the Medically Uninsured, which funds the development and marketing of innovative insurance products aimed at uninsured workers in small firms in fifteen sites, could offer valuable analytical evidence to assist the second step toward change, "proving" that the market is not the answer. If fifteen sites labor heroically to design and sell market products that are supposedly both affordable and acceptable, and largely fail, policymakers and interest group advocates lose the argument that private-sector solutions must be exhausted before the states or the federal government are enlisted.

The institutional character of most foundations—they are prohibited from lobbying and leery of working directly with a governmental "partner" that seldom needs their money and rarely accepts their direction, but are burning to launch demonstrations with large, visible, positive results—makes them particularly fruitful sources of instruction on the limits of solutions anchored in the market, the professions, and the voluntary sector. There is, of course, a certain irony here: foundations usually proclaim an ambitious prescriptive mission, to fund demonstrations that will yield lessons and models for national acclaim and emulation. The positive lessons that do emerge, however, are often rather obvious—talented people supported by foundation funds may, under favorable circumstances, create fruitful projects that less talented people without external support (or in refractory circumstances) cannot produce. The negative lessons, the familiar dissections of how millions of foundation dollars got spent with little to show for them, can be highly educative, by contrast, for they are real-world rebuttals to the hope, which springs forth eternally in the United States, that government intervention is dispensable. Foundations intend not to understand the world but to change it by showing what works. In practice they contribute to change mainly by refining policymakers' insights into the unworkable (Brown and McLaughlin, 1988).

(3) Prescription. Policymakers may agree that they face urgent problems that nongovernmental approaches cannot solve yet still fail to act because they do not know what to do or do not feel confident that available strategies will not boomerang or embarrass them. The unveiling of an appealing strategic model, therefore, can be one of the most significant contributions of research to policy.

In the PPS case, the research depicting the success of state rate-setting programs in slowing the growth of hospital spending coincided in political time with the policymakers' quest for promising solutions. The studies in question carefully evaluated state programs that the federal government had encouraged since the early 1970s. Empirical evaluations are not the sole source of appealing strategic models, however: the DRGS developed at Yale in the 1970s and the RBRVS fashioned at Harvard in the 1980s are analytical inventions that use data to build more "rational" (efficient and equitable) approaches to paying providers. Without the rate-setting evaluations, policymakers might have been slow to embrace DRGs; without DRGs, they might have hesitated to adopt rate-setting strategies that took little explicit account of case mix. Whether working together or separately, however, both empirical evaluations and analytical constructs carry political force because they give the blessing of "science" to proposals that take policymakers in directions they already favor, given an insistent call to arms and a depletion of nongovernmental alternatives.

If the urge to act is sufficiently strong, models can be quickly adopted with little or no empirical or analytical foundation. In the early 1970s many congressmen believed that some form of regulation of physician behavior in Medicare and Medicaid was desirable, but professional self-regulation was the only approach then deemed tolerable. As it happened, Utah, home of Wallace Bennett, ranking minority member of the Senate Finance Committee, was trying out a prototype of what came to be called professional standards review organizations (PSROs). In 1972 Utah's wish became Congress's command (Winsten, 1976).

In 1970 the Nixon administration embraced health maintenance organizations as a national cost containment strategy because such plans allowed it to avoid political and ideological pitfalls (cutbacks in health benefits, national health insurance, regulation), could be sold in terms it approved (markets, competition, incentives, choice), and called to mind prepaid group practices such as Kaiser-Permanente, which the Californians who ran the Nixon White House and HEW knew worked. There was a sizable research literature on PGPs, and advocacy documents repeated the refrain that HMOs deliver care for "10 to 40 percent less" than the cost of traditional plans; but few if any of those pushing them knew whether the claim was true, or understood what it meant, or cared. All that mattered was that the two key elements of Kaiser-type PGPs—group practice and prepayment—could allegedly be plugged into a host of management and ownership structures with efficiency-enhancing results (Brown, 1983a, pp. 195–275). The advent of PSROs and HMOs derived not from the empirical findings or analytical modeling of researchers (though both programs were much studied after their adoption) but rather from the speculative musings and vigorous salesmanship of policy entrepreneurs appealing to desperate "clients."

Despite their different origins and aims, the four strategies mentioned here—rate-setting, relative value scales, PSROs, and HMOs—share one politically important property: the basic idea behind each can, for better or worse, be explained to policymakers in (so to speak) 25 words or less. All four involve enormous conceptual and practical complications, of course, but in each the strategic "bottom line"—rationalizing the relation between hospital costs and charges (rate-setting), paying physicians sums that more closely reflect the true value of their efforts (RVS), encouraging doctors to review the necessity and appropriateness of one another's use of hospital care (PSROs), redesigning providers' incentives so as to reward frugality (HMOs)—could be sold as straightforward and unexceptionable. Equally important, the seeming simplicity and flexibility of the strategies encouraged various "perfecting" refinements that policymakers thought to be politically desirable.

A conceptually attractive strategic model that lacks the appearance of simplification and flexibility is unlikely to survive political natural selection even if—perhaps especially if—it is highly ingenious. A vivid example, indeed now something of a hardy perennial, is Alain Enthoven's Consumer Choice Health Plan. The proposal is a compelling piece of policy logic—*if* one elects to accept all the "ifs" and "thens" that constitute it (Enthoven, 1980a, 1980b; Enthoven and Kronick, 1989). Alas, explaining the complex connections among the rules governing benefit levels, premium setting, enrollment practices, brokering functions, competitive dynamics, and the rest requires many more than 25 succinct words, and the "Swiss watch" nature of the plan irritates policymakers, who have no objection to complicated legislation so long as they themselves create the complexity. Similar problems may defeat predictions that sophisticated schemes of quality assessment and assurance will emerge on the front lines of policy action in the 1990s.

The Political Evolution of Knowledge as Power

The roles that health services research has played in the policy process are for the most part recent developments—scarcely more than two decades old. To understand the present and future strengths and limits of these roles, one should explore their political origins and evolution—that is, one needs to examine not only what researchers supply but also what policymakers have been demanding, and why.

Until the end of World War II, the federal government intervened very little in the delivery and financing of health care in the United States, and health services research did not constitute a recognized discipline. The political side of the equation began to change in the late 1940s as the federal government debated and enacted subsidies that encouraged providers of health care services to expand the stock of technology and biomedical knowledge (National Institutes of Health), hospitals (Hill-Burton program), and personnel (programs to advance the education of nurses, ancillary personnel, and, later, physicians). These programs took little inspiration from health services studies, drawing rather on the conventional wisdom of the day. Everyone knew that biomedical research had produced striking breakthroughs during the war; given federal stimulus and funding, surely it could find peacetime cures for cancer, stroke, and other dread diseases. Everyone knew that the hospital was increasingly the technical center of community care, the repository of advancing medical science; reasonable and timely access required that most if not all counties have a hospital. One should be able to get a doctor when one needed one, but everyone knew that physicians were in short supply; obviously the federal government should increase the supply of physicians and other health personnel. Political reality reinforced policy intuition: national health insurance, the strategy at the top of Harry Truman's agenda, was not about to be enacted (and so the recommendations of the most impressive prewar venture in health services research—the multiple volumes issued by the Committee on the Costs of Medical Care—gathered dust on the shelf). Federal policy leaders who wanted to address the health system's problems were obliged to detour around financing reforms in favor of supply-enhancing measures based on the notion that more is better.

For two decades these supply-side subsidy programs dominated federal health care policy. By 1965, however, sufficient consensus had developed to enact limited financing reforms, Medicare and Medicaid. Like the subsidy programs, Medicare was a product not of research or analysis but rather of political crafting and fine-tuning. New Dealers who had been seeking national health insurance unsuccessfully for thirty years had pondered the reasons for their failure and designed Medicare to address them (Marmor, 1973). Although a financing program limited to one age group (in this case the elderly) was by comparative standards odd, such targeting would tap the perceived legitimacy of a deserving group, reduce the stigma of a "welfare giveaway," and lift financial burdens from the beneficiaries' grateful children. Compulsory participation by the elderly in the hospital component alone might neutralize physicians' cries about socialized medicine. Organized medicine would go right on protesting, of course, but legislators might be less inclined to respond if the program had an obligatory Part A and a voluntary Part B. Tying the program's financing to the Social Security system let it be sold (and defended over the years) as contributory social insurance, not a welfare handout. Making its eligibility provisions and benefits universal instead of income-related traded off economic efficiency for political durability—poor people's programs were poor programs, Medicare's creators believed, so engaging the political might of the middle class was essential. Thus sculpted, the Medicare proposal sat in HEW until its time finally came. And its time finally came not because research or analysis on the needs of the elderly or the likely efficacy of the program finally proved irrefutable, but rather because in 1964 the electorate overwhelmingly endorsed Lyndon Johnson and dozens of new liberal Democrats for reasons that had little direct relation to Medicare or health policy.

Although research had little to do with the enactment of Medicare and Medicaid, experience with these programs had everything to do with the rise and growth of health services research. Within five years of their start the federal government and many states concluded that they faced a significant health cost crisis. They knew this because their basic statistical and budgetary indicators told them so; to learn more, in hopes of controlling costs, they began gathering additional and more refined measures of utilization, pricing patterns, provider supply and distribution, and still other dimensions. New centers (for instance, the National Center for Health Services Research and Health Care Technology Assessment established in 1968) and surveys proliferated, and the documentary capabilities of health services research expanded rapidly.[4]

The growing concern about rising costs also encouraged scholars (increasingly well armed with government and foundation grants) to explore analytically the causes of the problem, and in particular to identify objects of spending that failed to yield fair value for the money. By the middle and late 1970s policymakers discussed with increasing fluency such challenges to the market, the profession, and the voluntary sector as the target income hypothesis, small area analysis, cost/benefit analyses of prevention versus treatment of various diseases, Roemer's law, the Institute of Medicine report on excess hospital capacity, and the findings and projections of the Graduate Medical Education National Advisory Committee. In the 1940s and 1950s, more had been equated with better. In the 1960s policymakers began to suspect that, at least as far as costs were concerned, more might be worse, and in the 1970s health services researchers handed them evidence that often confirmed their fears.

Government's demand for ever more documentation and analytical knowledge powerfully spurred researchers to augment the supply. By 1980 knowledge about the system's workings was far greater than it had been in 1970. More abundant knowledge is not necessarily more usable knowledge, however. As a source of prescriptive guidance, health services research has been highly erratic. The prescriptive *task* differs markedly from documentation and analysis: showing how the system works and why it works that way is of itself a "contribution to knowledge," but such contributions do not (of themselves) tell policymakers how to *fix* the system. Recall the Coleman Report, which discredited widely accepted notions about good educational practice but pointed in causal directions—pupil self-image, family background—that are not, at least in American society, reparable by government. Prescription demands understanding not only of how actors and institutions in the health care system behave under existing conditions and why, but also (or rather) how their behavior might change under *new* conditions; on this question even the most plentiful body of facts never speaks for itself. Prescription, therefore, requires that health services researchers play entrepreneur as well as expert, that they confidently offer predictive leaps of faith and recommendations that draw only partly or little on the solid base of their scholarly knowledge. Moreover, that knowledge may saddle them with a "trained incapacity" (Veblen's phrase) to give due weight to variables beyond those viewed as most serviceable within their chosen disciplinary and theoretical frameworks.

In their prescriptive endeavors, health services researchers tend to divide into three camps. The first contains *economists,* who apply to every issue the measuring rod of money and seek in the tenets of supply and demand, and more broadly in market theory, reforms that will make the health care system more efficient and otherwise better behaved. The second camp may be termed *technocrats;* these try to invent categories and systems, usually based on the technical properties of medical work, that can be used for reimbursement or other system-steering purposes. The third group, *planners,* advocate broad, integrated macro-level system reforms, generally envisioning a large directive role for government; these reforms aim to reconcile needs and resources so as to strike desirable trade-offs among such social values as equity, efficiency, and effectiveness.

Each camp has its distinctive strengths and weaknesses as a source of policy advice. Economists rightly emphasize the great motivational power of money but often give short shrift to professional, ethical, political, social, psychological, organizational, and cultural factors that also shape the behavior of consumers, providers, purchasers, and others. Moreover, even the economists' sharpest micro-level insights can rarely inform macro policy without being obscured—and perhaps lost—in the translation. A rigorous demonstration that making people pay more money for their health care will induce many of them to consume less of it will be useful to policymakers only if they accept that consumers tend to be overinsured, that cost sharing deters the "right" people from over-using the "wrong" types of care, that quality does not suffer, and so on—none of them peripheral issues. Policymakers embraced a decentralized and helter-skelter promotion of HMOs as an overdue victory for competition but have consistently refused to buy Enthoven's system-transforming consumer choice health plan, which appears to carry economic logic too far. Congress has even declined to alter federal provisions that exclude employer-purchased health insurance from the taxable income of employees despite near-universal consensus among economists that doing so would promote equity, efficiency, and fiscal responsibility. Liberals deplored a new "tax on working Americans," conservatives feared that deterrents to generous private insurance might encourage national health insurance, and all shades of opinion shrank from antagonizing millions of voters. In general, the purer the economic logic, the poorer are the political prospects.[5]

Even if the economists' style of reasoning were widely shared by policymakers, however, its practical utility would be limited by the camp's tendency to fall to quarreling about basics. Since the early 1970s, for example, many economists have extolled the virtues of competition as a cost containment policy. But by this some mean markets revitalized by increased consumer cost sharing, others mean rivalry among alternative delivery systems seeking customers by any legal means (including selling "bad" cheap insurance to good risks, leaving the bad risks to "good" plans such as HMOs), while still others mean a disciplined, structured, price-conscious system like Enthoven's plan. If after twenty years of advocacy economists themselves cannot agree what competition means and what forms of it are desirable, it is not surprising that policymakers have not embraced broad pro-competitive legislation (Brown, 1988). Though perhaps the first, Truman was surely not the last political leader to plead for one-handed economic advisers.

Unlike economists, technocrats do occasionally invent full-blown strategic systems that policymakers accept and refine (or deform) in concrete legislation. The DRGs and RBRVS are two dramatic examples. In the nature of the case, however, technocrats are not trained to "think big." Their solutions are usually devised for, and applicable to, limited sectors of the system—payment of hospitals, physicians, psychiatrists, nursing homes, or whatever—and may destabilize one sector by the very act of rationalizing another. As noted earlier, policymakers are now attracted to the RBRVS for physician payment in Medicare partly because their earlier adoption of DRGs for hospital payment encouraged doctors to shift activities from inpatient to outpatient settings.

The planner's virtues correct the technocrats's vices: the former's forte is to sketch new, improved systems that coherently link the parts to each other and to the larger whole. Sophisticated examples include William Glaser's extensive quest for foreign lessons for Americans and Howard Hiatt's musings on a system to ensure Health for the Year 2000 (Glaser, 1970; Glaser, 1978; Glaser, 1987; Hiatt, 1987). But the planner also typically exhibits the vices of his virtues: his macro reforms may require technical tools as yet unavailable, may stand at odds with deeply rooted economic interests and organizational norms, may presuppose more government intervention and bureaucracy than Americans prefer, or may otherwise fail to fit American constraints. Like the economist's insistence that money matters, however, the planner's Big Thinking can have a significant, if diffuse, impact on policy. The United States is not about to ignore all values but the economic, yet repeated analytical revisiting of the incentive effects of payment systems and other policy choices may forestall facile but costly political compromises. Likewise, the United States is not about to imitate Canada or Europe, but policymakers who think carefully about the achievements of the Canadian and European systems may make choices different from and better than those they would otherwise have made.

In theory, an intellectual coalition of the three camps could fashion an encompassing systematic plan founded on suitable technologies and appropriate economic incentives. In practice, however, the three orientations work within largely distinct conceptual universes and are more devoted to demonstrating the superiority of their own world views than to building on cross-disciplinary strengths. Nor has any of the three camps adequately integrated insights from such disciplines as sociology, psychology, history, and anthropology, whose prescription-minded practitioners in the health field tend to be comparatively self-effacing and too few to constitute a "camp" unto themselves.

Ideas and Interests, Government and Groups

The effectiveness of health services research in influencing policy tends to vary inversely with the complexity of the task. Research is most directly of value in describing (documenting) the system; more erratically useful in analyzing its workings and explaining to policymakers what works, what does not, and why; and most limited (though not unimportant) in prescribing solutions to concrete policy problems. Research assists policy less by offering definitive answers to questions under debate than by improving the quality of debate, less by inventing the elusive idea whose time has come than by shaping the temper of the time in which policymakers review the long parade of ideas proffered by proponents of various intellectual persuasions (Weiss, 1977; Majone, 1989).

Some may disparage such a "shaping" role as but one further example of the talk that so often befogs the American policy landscape when clear-sighted action is needed, merely another arcane footnote appended by the history of ideas to the coarse realities of interest group politics. Changing the character of public (and for that matter private) debate is, however, a far more important form of power than is often recognized; an "either/or" counterpositioning of ideas and interests, government and groups fails to fit the facts of post-Medicare health politics. Ideas are not a poorer, weaker alternative to groups, but rather an increasingly potent force for changing the balance of power within group struggles in which government itself is increasingly a preeminent contender.

The conventional wisdom of pluralist political science paints government as an umpire of group differences, likely to move only under the stimulus of exogenous social forces and then only when prodded by powerful groups whose preferences for policy action are not checked by countervailing counterparts with different or opposed aims. Post-Medicare health care politics stands this image completely on its head. None of the major federal health policy innovations of the past twenty years percolated up from "social forces"; most were devised and promoted within the government itself. None depended on heavyweight interest-group supporters to make their way onto the federal agenda and into public law; most passed over the objections of strong provider groups. The explanation is evident: by thrusting the federal and state governments into a major purchasing role, Medicare and Medicaid broke the traditional pluralist pattern that made of government a largely passive reflector of the balance of power among interests in society. With billions of its dollars newly on the line each year, government itself soon became an "interest" with an increasingly "corporate" sense of self and the commanding presence of the proverbial 800-pound gorilla. As the public health care budget grows, government is ever more the reality that keeps breaking in to upset the settled expectations of providers (Brown, 1983b; Tierney, 1987). The continuing, cumulative force of government as "group" is all the more remarkable because for 16 of the last 20 years the federal executive branch has played the activist *malgré lui;* the Nixon, Ford, Reagan, and Bush administrations have all expanded federal intervention in the health sphere despite ideologies that honor deregulation and reprivatization. The new public purchaser-driven politics has, of course, not eliminated the power of provider groups in policymaking, but it has reconfigured the raw materials of power and the terms on which it may effectively be exercised. The new realities of power require that groups struggle to prevent government from cornering the market on ideas.

Over the last twenty years government has invested vast sums in the health care system and has increased its capacity to document its sources and patterns of spending. This documentary information is a constant, growing source of questions—nagging, irritating, impolite—that throws provider groups onto the defensive, renders them (as they sometimes protest) guilty—of waste, excess, and inappropriateness—until they prove themselves innocent. Bereft of the trust, legitimacy, and deference they once enjoyed, provider groups must now augment their own documentary resources—data bases, computers, in-house staff, contracts with academics and consultants—if they are to answer back persuasively. Seeking to make sense of statistical trends, the government has also invested heavily in analytical research—small area studies, demonstrations, large-scale data sets, surveys, and more—whose findings have often challenged existing practice patterns and payment levels and methods. The provider group that cannot either discredit such research conceptually or methodologically, or offer sophisticated explanations that restore the rationale for the status quo, risks ceding the debate to the critics. Finally, as government has repeatedly called for new prescriptive proposals that might ease its burdens, implicated interest groups have learned that one cannot beat something with nothing, that the best defense may be a good offense. Once confident of their power to persuade policymakers that the status quo is the best of all possible worlds, these ex-veto groups now recognize that they must be "pro-active," must contribute "constructively" to the debate about change, must stay at the bargaining table "in good faith" on pain of being shut out. Like government, the groups have been drawn by the logic of public purchasing into a self-fueling dynamic of change in spite of themselves.

Argumentation has always been important to an effective self-interested appeal, of course—in the debate over Medicare, for instance, policymakers and the public might have scoffed at the American Medical Association's frantic incantations about "socialized medicine" had the group not labored to link the slogan to all the darker possibilities facing American medicine. Today, however, the force of argument is more than window dressing and cynical syllogisms are more easily deflated. Today the group that cannot skillfully deploy its own arsenal of documentation, analysis, and prescription may not keep pace politically with government change agents secure in their command of the findings and recommendations of health services research and devoted to ideas whose time they want to hurry along. One can sympathize with the lobbyist who, at a recent conference of the National Academy of State Health Policy, noted the dominance on the program of researchers and program managers, "people doing things, on the cutting edge," and added forlornly: "Maybe that's why people rarely want a lobbyist on these programs anymore; they seem to know the least."

Policy Knowledge and Political Wisdom

Practitioners and admirers of health services research may see in the progress depicted here the dawning of a new age of enlightenment in health care policy. The infiltration of research into policy deliberations may be gradually producing better-informed, and therefore better, policy outcomes. Such optimism should, however, be constrained, for no matter how large the demand for and supply of research may grow, three wide disjunctions between the worlds of research and policy are likely to remain unbridgeable.

One disjunction, discussed at some length earlier, lies between the respective "technologies" (or task structures) of doing research and making policy. Extensive information on the incidence and nature of problems may move policymakers to action (payment reforms in Medicare), or it may confuse and inhibit them (covering the uninsured). Sophisticated analytical work can inform policymakers about the futility or limits of existing efforts and then leave them at sea: how, for example, can policymakers get their hands around local physician practice norms? When analytical arguments lead (as they often do and should) to cultural variables, policymakers may conclude that their search for the actionable is over. Nor is most prescriptive research well suited to address these issues: the dominant persuasions (economist, technocrat, planner) generally make little room for cultural nebulas; the disciplines that do (sociology, anthropology, history) tend to stand on the sidelines of the policy game.

The troublesome world of cultural questions aside, however, the dominant prescriptive camps are often ineffective on their own turf. Economists tend to disagree with each other over recommendations that are highly concrete but politically impractical. Technocrats present convincing suggestions for repairing individual rooms in a huge edifice that goes on crumbling around them. Planners weigh in with broad systemic reforms (global budgets, structured negotiations) generally unaccompanied by an instruction sheet explaining how the United States might assemble and use the contents of such a package.

These disagreements in theory and practice within and between research disciplines and camps can be very confusing to practical people who look to the experts for answers. The unhappy, counterintuitive fact is that the more academic knowledge we amass about policy problems, the less we know how to solve them. In the early 1980s the business community, hit with rapidly rising health insurance premiums in the midst of a recession, talked of an "employer revolution" and looked to policy analysts for strategic advice. The experts—mainly economists, with whom business felt comfortable—informed them that they had a choice between competition and regulation and must by all means choose the former. For much of the decade business leaders joined local community coalitions, increased employee cost sharing, touted and encouraged alternative delivery systems, and listened with befuddled admiration to Walter McClure's thoughts on "buying right." At the end of the 1980s the business community again found itself hit with rapidly rising health insurance premiums: its leaders had followed the experts' advice, but nothing had worked.

Meanwhile, the federal government had accumulated regulatory leverage as a prudent purchaser of hospital services in Medicare. The Prospective Payment System is, within its own terms, a success, but unfortunately the system as a whole does not play on those terms. Providers recouped DRG and Medicaid "shortfalls" by boosting prices for other payors—especially business firms—and shifted activities from the price-regulated inpatient care sector to the more weakly regulated ambulatory setting. Economists and technocrats had exercised hitherto undreamed-of influence over the private and public sectors, but at the end of the 1980s system costs were no better controlled than they had been a decade before. Theory had promised cost containment but health care institutions preferred cost shifting—from the public to the private sector, among private purchasers, and among service settings. The larger and more flourishing the world of health services research becomes, the more extensive is its menu of findings, explanations, arguments, and recommendations—and the more chaotic and inchoate the research appears to be to policymakers who try to learn from it. A larger research community doubtless generates better policy debates; better policy outcomes do not necessarily follow. The more abundant the research outpourings, the more policymaking consumers of research are obliged to choose from its offerings arbitrarily—on the strength of ideology, intuition, or politics. Research-based recommendations may make a sensible series of small repairs to discrete parts of the system and yet fail to fix—indeed may aggravate the weaknesses of—the system as a whole.

Even if health services research were single-minded, concrete, and addressed directly to variables that policymakers could manipulate, its impact would be limited by a second disjunction, that between the specialization that drives research and the breadth of view that policy generalists seek (or should seek) to maintain. Health research can effectively enlighten policymakers about the trade-offs and opportunity costs of spending within the health sector, but it seldom encourages them to ponder the claims of health in the context of other policy arenas. For example, health research may illuminate the health needs of the homeless and the trials of treating them in hospital emergency rooms, but policymakers also need help in viewing the homeless within multiple policy settings—housing, nutrition, employment, mental health, and more. Today's policy agenda overflows with the problems of a long list of disadvantaged groups—the elderly in need of long-term care, children, the hungry, the homeless, people with AIDS, drug addicts, the mentally ill, the disabled, and others whose needs demand a range of social services in addition to health care. These needs should not be unduly "medicalized," but they are often squeezed into the framework of Medicare and (especially) Medicaid for want of creative and eclectic combinations of health, education, housing, transportation, law enforcement, and nutrition programs. Because thriving research communities tend to accompany big-spending policy arenas (health, defense), there is a significant risk that unbalanced growth in one specialized sector may drive others out of sight and therefore out of policy generalists' minds.

Even if health services research helped policymakers to apportion resources rationally among policy arenas, to each according to its need, its power to steer the system would be limited by a third enduring disjunction between the deliberated nature of the changes it recommends and the accidental character of political change in the health care system. "Accidental" here means that major transformations imposed on the system by government generally follow in the wake of (and therefore must wait upon) larger political developments that have little to do with health, or the merits of health policy options, per se. As noted earlier, Medicare passed in 1965 because in 1964 the electorate decided for a mix of reasons—the trauma of Kennedy's assassination, fears about the Republican presidential candidate, a general if temporary leftward shift of opinion on urban and racial problems—to elect a liberal Democratic president and an unusually liberal Congress on whose agendas Medicare happened to stand high.

Arguably the social indicators most pertinent to the prospects for national health insurance are not the number of uninsured, the percentage of gross national product spent on health care, or related variables, but rather crime and unemployment rates. Unless crime (and the "social issue" more broadly) is tamed, a liberal Democrat is likely to win the White House only if unemployment (or inflation) soars. But until a liberal Democrat occupies the White House, national health insurance is unlikely to pass. *If* such a figure wins the presidency, and *if* the electorate supplies him or her with a sizable ideological majority in both houses of Congress, and *if* NHI is high on his or her list of priorities, and *if* he or she encounters no major disagreements with congressional leaders on what NHI should look like, *then* NHI might emerge.

In health services research, as in other pursuits, those who play the game in hopes of enjoying the tangible fruits of victory may be disappointed by the severe limits of short-term policy influence. Many are called, but those with a chance of being chosen must usually be in for the long haul, endowed (like Wilbur Cohen, a major architect of Medicare) with the commitment and tenacity to wait for years, possibly decades, for the (brief) opening of a political window of opportunity through which their policy proposals may be pushed. Health services research can no more shape the large macro political changes that transform and reform the health care system than it can generate from within its own ranks clear strategic blueprints for policymakers or a judicious delimitation of the claims of health programs within multiple policy arenas. The most important policy choices depend on public sensibilities that are beyond the power of research to shape. Policy knowledge can carry a society only so far toward political wisdom.

3

Paying for Hospital Care:
The Impact on Federal Policy

Stuart H. Altman and Ellen K. Ostby

In this chapter we focus on the findings of health services research and how this research has influenced the federal payment system for inpatient hospital services and the availability of those services to Medicare recipients. Although it is not possible to reference all the research that has transformed the federal hospital payment system, this chapter highlights many projects that influenced the political and economic climate since the passage of Medicare in 1965.

We begin with a discussion of the cost-based hospital reimbursement system, and the opposing views of its impact on inflation in the health care industry. An analysis of the Economic Stabilization Program (ESP) follows. ESP was designed to reduce general inflation in the economy, and it led to important discoveries about the nature of hospital inpatient costs and related expenditures. The chapter then focuses on a series of amendments to the Medicare reimbursement system. Section 223 of the 1971 Social Security Amendments attempted to limit Medicare payments for routine hospital costs. We next discuss four state demonstration rate-setting programs authorized under Section 222 of the same 1971 amendments and what was learned from them regarding national policy. The chapter continues with an analysis of the justification for health services planning and certificate-of-need (CON) legislation and the resulting negative evaluation of their efficacy.

We next describe the unsuccessful attempt by the Carter administration to extend federal efforts to control overall hospital spending and then return to the discussion of changes in the Medicare hospital reimbursement system. The Tax Equity and Fiscal Responsibility Act (TEFRA) of 1982 substantially toughened Section 223 and led to the creation of the Prospective Payment System (PPS). The development and application of Diagnosis Related Groups (DRGs) under PPS are covered next, along with criticisms of the design and application of PPS. Our goal throughout the chapter is to link the research findings of the period to the actual federal policies they affected.

The Structure of the Hospital System and Its Impact on Hospital Inflation

When Medicare was passed in 1965, it consisted of an inpatient hospital care program (Part A) and physician and outpatient services (Part B). The Part A hospital payment system was modeled after the cost-based system used by Blue Cross plans, particularly those in the northeastern United States. Thus, hospitals were to be paid only for the costs of the services they provided to Medicare beneficiaries, and only if those costs could be documented by a retrospective audit. The 1965 Medicare law, however, explicitly prohibited government officials from questioning the medical appropriateness of those expenditures or whether it was possible to provide those services in a more economical manner. In essence, if funds were spent by hospitals for Medicare patients, they were paid. Although some suggested that a reimbursement system that paid whatever was billed lacked any incentive to control spending, the majority view was that such a cost-based system was fair, simple, and unlikely to have a differential impact on hospital inflation.

Anderson and Neuhauser (1969) argued that inflation was inherent in modern health care systems, and not necessarily caused by the cost-based reimbursement of third-party payors. They compared health care systems in England and Wales and in Sweden with those in the United States and found that all were experiencing dramatic increases in expenditures (see Table 3–1). The authors attributed these increases to factors other than the escalation of the price of services based on cost-based charges.

At the same time, Anderson and Hull (1969) were comparing utilization and expenditure patterns in Canada with patterns in the United States. They found that even the Canadian reimbursement system, with its tighter utilization controls, made little appreciable impact on health care cost inflation. The authors concluded that the Canadian reimbursement system was no more effective at containing hospital costs than the

Table 3-1. Index of total expenditures for all hospitals (1955 = 100)

Year	U.S.A.	England and Wales	Sweden
1955	100	100	100
1956	108	110	114
1957	116	118	128
1958	128	127	140
1959	139	137	149
1960	151	146	159
1961	168	160	180
1962	181	174	206
1963	196	189	235
1964	215	206	273
1965	231	228	323

Source: Anderson and Neuhauser, 1969.

cost-based system in the United States. In hindsight, this conclusion was premature, given the much higher United States spending experience of the last 20 years (see Figure 3–1).

Hospital size and service capacity were considered far more important variables in generating the cost escalation. Carr and Feldstein (1967) reviewed the independent effect of hospital size on the per diem cost of providing care in voluntary, short-term acute care hospitals. Their study focused on those economic variables that affected cost. The authors determined that there were eight economic factors that had an independent impact on per diem costs: (1) hospital size as measured by average daily census; (2) the number of capabilities and services available (particularly as they reflected specialized services); (3) the number of outpatient visits per patient day; (4) the existence of hospital-controlled nursing programs/schools; (5) the number of student nurses in the hospital; (6) the number of different residency and internship programs; (7) the number of residents and interns; and (8) whether the hospital had an affiliation with a medical school.

A study by Klarman (1969) supported the importance of several of these eight variables, in particular wage rate structure differences.

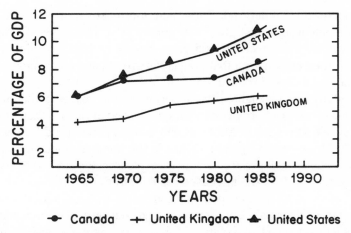

Figure 3-1. Total health expenditures, percentage of GDP, 1965–1986. (From Financing and Delivering Health Care: A Comparative Analysis of OECD Countries, 1987.)

Klarman suggested that increases in hospital unit cost were due to several factors, only one of which was cost-based reimbursement. His research showed that constant lags in productivity gains between the hospital industry and the general economy, the additional cost of education and training in the hospital, technological advances, and catching up periodically with wage levels of competing industries caused most of the inflation. This study was one of the first to highlight the fact that the economics of the hospital industry often operates differently from the rest of the economy. But it was not until the early 1970s that cost-based reimbursement was identified as a primary contributor to the escalation in health care utilization and cost and thus as worthy of congressional interest and legislative action.

Cost-Based Reimbursement: An Inflationary Incentive

Earlier studies of escalating health care costs and utilization focused on supply elements such as hospital structure and provider behavior. In their review of inflation in the health care industry, Altman and Eichenholz (1976) focused on the payment system and attributed a large proportion of the inflation in hospital costs to improper incentives for constant increases in demand. First and foremost, they believed that reimbursement on a cost-plus basis generated a "blank check" environment with no incentives for utilization control or cost containment. In addition, they emphasized that population growth and concomitant price increases contributed to inflation.

The study also highlighted the importance of increases in the number and kinds of services provided to patients as one of the key factors leading to accelerating costs. Although this burgeoning demand for services was in part generated by the increase in the number of individuals covered by public and private health care insurance plans, the authors believed that most of the increases resulted from the provision of more costly services to insured patients compared with uninsured patients with a similar diagnosis. As they observed, out-of-pocket expenditures decreased as a result of expanded third-party coverage, and therefore neither the patient nor the physician had any financial incentive to question the amount or cost of care received.

Altman and Eichenholz outlined the following reasons for the higher inflationary tendencies of the health care industry:

1. Large segments of the industry are nonprofit and respond to financial incentives differently from profit-making firms.
2. The health care industry is labor-intensive, with payroll costs accounting for around 60 percent of total hospital expenses.
3. Restrictive laws and practices have limited the utilization of new forms of health services manpower and delivery systems.
4. Technological advances, expansion of services, and the addition of specialized services encourage unchecked spending.
5. There are no incentives for hospitals to curb the increase in costs because more than 50 percent of hospital revenue is generated through costs incurred.
6. Third-party payor insurance coverage provides no inducement or incentive for patients to use fewer or unnecessary services.
7. Physicians have the ultimate decision about how many and what services a patient receives. Because of fee-for-service reimbursement, the physician has no incentive to curb the use of unnecessary services.

Criticisms of the cost-based hospital inpatient reimbursement system and an understanding of the uniqueness of the health care industry highlighted the fact that future policy decisions about the provision of health care services must focus on those components of the system that pay for these services.

Control of Hospital Expenditures

The Economic Stabilization Program

The creation of the Economic Stabilization Program (ESP) of 1971, and the consequent wage and price controls in the health care industry, were triggered by concern about general inflation throughout the economy. However, once the Nixon administration focused on health care, it realized that health care inflation was being fueled by factors other than general inflation (see Table 3–2).

The ESP began with a freeze on all wages and prices. One of the first obstacles in implementing the program in the health sector was the vague definition of what a price was for in the case of hospital care. Although hospital charges were frozen under ESP, most hospital revenue, particularly for inpatient care, was generated through reimbursement for costs incurred. Initially, third-party payors continued to pay for increasing levels of costs. In 1972, however, the Price Commission decreed that for all third-party payments which were cost-based, per

Table 3-2. Public and private hospital expenditures, 1965–1985 (in billions of dollars)

Year	Personal health care	Direct patient	Third party	Total government	Medicare	Other government	Total
1965	$ 36.0	$ 2.4	$ 11.5	$ 5.4	$—	$—	$ 13.9
1970	65.4	2.8	24.9	14.6	5.0	9.6	27.8
1975	116.5	4.0	40.2	28.9	11.6	17.3	52.1
1980	219.7	7.9	93.7	53.9	25.9	28.0	101.6
1983	314.7	13.3	133.6	76.8	40.5	36.3	146.8
1984	340.1	14.1	142.0	83.9	44.5	39.4	156.1
1985	368.3	15.4	151.4	90.5	48.2	42.3	166.7
1986	401.6	16.7	161.7	95.4	50.4	45.0	178.4
1987	442.6	18.5	176.2	102.2	53.3	48.9	194.7

Source: Letsch, Levit, and Waldo, 1988; Gibson, 1980.

diem costs were to be the hospital prices and therefore were under the control of ESP regulation.

In 1973, under Phase III of the ESP, the unit of output of hospital care to be regulated became the second operational obstacle. As Ginsburg (1976) noted, a crucial issue was whether the determination of the regulated unit of output was to be a single hospital service, an aggregate of all services included in a day of care, or all services used during a total hospital admission. The proposed 6 percent limitation on increases in hospital prices would be much more stringent if imposed on all services used per day or per admission as opposed to the same limit on the price per service. The Health Services Advisory Committee (which had been appointed to recommend what special health care provisions should be included in the ESP regulations) concluded that the more aggregative unit of per-day expenses was the correct price of hospital care. Two years later the follow-up agency to ESP, the Cost of Living Council, ruled that the price to be regulated was the cost of *all* services provided per admission. Such a ruling focused hospital payment regulation on both escalation in the prices per unit of services and in the number of services used per admission. These two decisions of ESP, that the price of hospital care was its costs and that it was appropriate to use all expenses per admission as the unit of hospital care, were critical ones that affected all future hospital payment control systems. As explained below, these decisions were in part derived from research findings of the period.

Much controversy still exists on just what impact the ESP controls had on the hospital sector. In a study following the end of ESP, Ginsburg (1976) concluded that ESP did not have a significant impact on the underlying structure of hospitals and therefore had little impact on their costs of care. In a later summary analysis, Sloan and Steinwald (1980) determined that ESP did have a moderating influence on hospital cost inflation. Less controversial was the conclusion that the techniques used under ESP helped to shape several future federal and state efforts to control hospital spending. It was also evident that the analysis of the research community concerning the causes of inflation in the health sector generated many of the mechanisms used by the ESP commission. For example, ESP was the first regulatory program to differentiate explicitly between a hospital's fixed costs and its marginal costs and to use the findings of health services research to determine the appropriate differentiation. The findings of research were also used to define the effective price of hospital services and to explain why controls on the price (cost) of each service alone could not control hospital spending increases (Lipscomb, Raskin, and Eichenholz, 1978).

At the same time as the Nixon administration was creating its Economic Stabilization Program, Congress was attempting to control the continued spiral of hospital costs and utilization under Medicare.

The Medicare Reimbursement Limitations

The increasing costs of the Medicare program prompted the Committee on Ways and Means of the 92nd Session of Congress (1971) to comment on the pros and cons of the hospital payment system.

> Under present law, institutional providers furnishing covered services to Medicare beneficiaries are paid on the basis of the reasonable cost of such services. Payment on this basis, with retroactive corrective adjustments, is consistent with the long history of public and private third party agency reimbursement for institutional health care on a cost basis. However, as experience under the Medicare, Medicaid, Maternal and Child Health, and other third party programs has clearly demonstrated there is little incentive to contain costs or to produce the services in the most efficient and effective manner. (United States Congress, House of Representatives, 1971, p. 80)

These conclusions led to the passage of Section 223 of the Social Security Amendments of 1971 ([PL 92-603] United States Congress, 1971). Under Section 223, the Secretary of the DHEW was charged with ensuring that Medicare would reimburse hospitals for only "costs that would be incurred by a reasonably prudent and cost-conscious management" (United States Congress, House of Representatives, 1971, p. 80). In creating these amendments, Congress acknowledged that the original cost-based reimbursement method used by Medicare could generate excess spending and that some restrictions on the discretion of hospitals to provide services to hospitalized Medicare patients were needed. Congress was reluctant, however, to interfere with the amount of medical care of hospitalized patients and therefore limited the controls to excess spending for routine hospital services.

Hellinger (1979) indicated in his review of Section 223 that the determination of what constitutes a routine cost is arbitrary and differs from hospital to hospital. As a result, he suggested that the impact of regulations that cover only routine costs would be erratic at best and unlikely to be effective. The study made several recommendations to remedy the problems associated with Section 223. First, he suggested a uniform accounting system with specific transaction and records-keeping protocols to create a consistent definition of a "routine" cost. Second, he noted that even if per diem routine costs were equal across comparable hospitals, 15 percent annual increases in overall hospital costs would continue to occur. Hellinger wanted future government regulations to provide mandatory programs with incentives for hospitals to increase output, cut the level of costs, and approve rates for all payors. The author concluded that, while Section 223 had lofty goals to limit the growth of hospital costs, its implementation was timid and restrictive. By focusing on controlling only "routine" hospital costs, it permitted hospitals to shift most of their costs to the uncontrolled ancillary cost side of their budget. Hellinger's observations proved prophetic, and his and other research findings about the limitations of Section 223 directly influenced the debate leading to the passage of the Medicare Prospective Payment System in 1983.

Much of what Hellinger proposed was a result of his observations of the rate-setting demonstration projects authorized under Section 222 of the same Social Security Amendments of 1971. The efficacy of these voluntary rate-setting (demonstration) programs was limited, but they did provide the nation with much-needed knowledge about how to operate a hospital payment control system.

State Rate Setting

Many suggestions for reform of the hospital payment system appeared in the research journals in the 1970s. The health services research community advocated different systems to provide hospitals with incentives to control their costs under either an incentive reimbursement plan or a prospective rate-setting system.

A study by Pauly and Drake (1970) discussed the merits of the growing belief that by rewarding excellence and discouraging inefficiency, hospitals would be induced to make efforts to lower their per diem cost. The authors' work illustrated how different methods of payment for hospital services could affect the short-run operational behavior of hospitals differently from the long-run structure. They reviewed four different reimbursement methods used by Blue Cross in Wisconsin, Illinois, Michigan, and Indiana. These four demonstrations and their subsequent evaluation set the tone for much of the research on prospective payment later in the decade.

Blue Cross used different reimbursement schemes in the four states: Charges only, Cost/Charges-Plus, Cost/Charges-Plus as tied to area-wide planning, and Approved Charges only. Wisconsin Blue Cross paid 97 percent of billed charges to member hospitals and 100 percent of charges to nonmember hospitals. Member hospitals, however, received an add-on for quantity and regularity of payment. (The regularity and certainty of payment offset the 3 percent difference in payment to non-member hospitals.) Wisconsin was considered a case in which the third-party reimbursement scheme exerted no controls, indirect or direct, over hospital operations.

In Illinois, Blue Cross paid 105 percent of actual hospital costs or charges, whichever was the lower. Costs were based upon patient days. The 5 percent excess over full cost was to provide for capital investment, community services, and uncompensated care. Blue Cross of Michigan paid 102 percent of costs or charges, whichever was the lower. The payment was apportioned on a per diem basis. As in Illinois, the 2 percent excess was to be used for community services, improvement, and capital investment. The hospital members had their cost and balance sheets audited. Proprietary hospitals and those which did not meet planning recommendations were not eligible for participation.

The Indiana Blue Cross plan paid 100 percent of approved charges only. These approved charge rates had to be the same for Blue Cross and non–Blue Cross patients. Any services not approved were not reimbursed. The charge systems of each hospital were carefully reviewed. The Indiana Blue Cross plan appeared to have greater control over hospital investment and growth than in the other states studied.

The results of the Pauly and Drake study indicated that when hospitals were reimbursed on the basis of costs or charges alone, as in Wisconsin, the cost per patient day was not affected. When reimbursement was based on a cost-plus method, as in Illinois or Michigan, costs per admission actually increased slightly. The Indiana model of restricted allowable cost had a slight restraining effect on increases in hospital costs, but the reduction was not statistically significant.

The authors concluded that the main difference between the four reimbursement systems studied was the long-run performance of the hospitals. The Indiana model, which involved the most direct control of allowable costs, affected the pattern of allocation of capital to hospitals.

As a result, large hospitals grew more than proportionately and may have increased their occupancy rates as well. The authors further suggested that for the future, efforts to monitor hospital performance and to improve reimbursement policy must focus on both the short-run and the long-run impacts. They argued that unless long-run effects were included in the evaluation, the overall configuration of hospital performance could not be fully captured (Pauly and Drake, 1970).

In their 1973 proposal for incentive reimbursement for hospitals, Lave, Lave, and Silverman (1973) reviewed one existing and two potential incentive reimbursement systems. The first potential system, advocated by the American Hospital Association (AHA), was based on a reimbursement formula to be negotiated in advance. The authors argued that in order for a prospective reimbursement system to be viable, differences in hospital case-mix and the varying rates of inflation in the economy had to be taken into account. The AHA proposal also included a mechanism to set the target rates of cost increases for groups of hospitals, and to reward with cash those facilities whose costs were below the targeted rate. Hospitals which incurred costs above the target rate would not be fully reimbursed for the extra costs. The second potential system evaluated called for forming groups of hospitals with similar case-mix populations and reimbursing them on the basis of the mean average cost for all hospitals in the group. As in the AHA prospective reimbursement system, those hospitals whose average costs were less than the mean average would be rewarded and the others penalized.

Because these two "cluster" reimbursement plans had not yet been implemented, the authors reviewed the only incentive reimbursement plan in operation, that of western Pennsylvania. Blue Cross of Western Pennsylvania had created nine "groups" of hospitals, where group membership was based on location and the extent of teaching programs available in each area. Hospitals were reimbursed based on incurred costs, but within a targeted limit which equaled the mean cost of all hospitals in their group. The Lave et al. study indicated that hospitals under the Blue Cross reimbursement system in western Pennsylvania whose costs were below the group mean had a higher than average cost increase, while the reverse was true for those hospitals with costs above the group mean. When these figures were adjusted for case mix, costs still tended toward the mean. Therefore, the authors concluded that this western Pennsylvania reimbursement system seemed to have little or no effect on slowing the overall increase of hospital costs.

One of the most comprehensive reviews of the state prospective rate-setting systems was by Dowling (1976). His study provided an extensive discussion of the differences between retrospective and prospective rate setting for hospital services. He outlined what program components must be included, as well as how the program should be managed, implemented, and monitored. The Dowling study discussed the many hospital management issues to be covered under prospective rates. He argued that hospitals should demonstrate the need for new facilities and services and provide detailed capital and program cost studies. Dowling made a strong case for understanding the cost implications of the quantity, quality, intensity, and scope of services offered, and for monitoring closely changes in these aspects of hospital operations.

The Dowling study also presented conclusions about expected changes in hospital performance under different plans. Even though Dowling presented strong arguments for the use of prospective rate setting, he did not view this type of rate setting alone as a panacea for cost containment. He argued that any rate-setting system must be linked with system-wide controls over facilities, services, and utilization. In addition, the linkage must include mechanisms designed to encourage consumers and physicians to use hospitals more prudently. This conclusion is in contrast to our current environment, where the federal government has dismantled all system-wide facility controls because of a belief that the incentives under the Medicare Prospective Payment System and the use of HMOs and PPOs are sufficient to assure the appropriate use of facilities and services.

Another important study of the state demonstration models was conducted by Gaus and Hellinger (1976). Their report explained how state prospective payment systems came into being with the help of federal funding authorized through Section 222 of the Social Security Amendments of 1971. The Gaus-Hellinger study critiqued the methods used to evaluate each of the systems, the specific results of each of the four completed evaluations, and the policy considerations that resulted from those evaluations. The four state programs reviewed were those in Western Pennsylvania, New Jersey, Rhode Island, and New York.

The evaluators determined that the five hospitals in Western Pennsylvania that participated in the per diem rate program for fiscal years 1971–1974 registered smaller cost increases than the control hospitals. In New Jersey, the results showed that costs per patient day were 2 to 3 percent lower as a result of the prospective payment system. The

Rhode Island experience, however, clearly demonstrated the problems of separating the experiment from the ESP program. And in upstate New York, prospective payment had a positive but insignificant impact. In downstate New York, the program lowered the average cost per patient day by about 4 percent per year and the average cost per case by 2 percent per year. The authors concluded that the four prospective reimbursement programs were successful in controlling hospital cost inflation, but less than had been expected. Political and legal restrictions were cited as important factors that limited the success of the experiment.

During the 1970s, studies like those by Lave et al. (1973) and Gaus and Hellinger (1976) reported discouraging results from state programs designed to control hospital costs. The negative results of these research reports were to play an important part in defeating the cost containment proposal of the Carter administration and in ending many of the state payment control systems. Interestingly, a later study by Biles, Schramm, and Atkinson (1980) showed that the previous reimbursement program evaluations were incorrect because they were limited to the period they evaluated, stopping at 1975. In contrast, the study by Biles et al. reported substantial reductions in the rate of increase in the cost of a community hospital stay in those rate-controlled states in comparison to non-rate-controlled states based upon performance through 1978.

Using AHA data, Biles et al. compared the 6 states that had comprehensive, legally mandated rate-setting programs to the 44 non-rate-setting states, and to Washington, D.C., for the period 1970–1978. Connecticut, Maryland, Massachusetts, New Jersey, New York, and Washington determined hospital rates on a prospective basis, through a legislatively established public agency. Compliance by hospitals was mandatory, and a majority of non-Medicare hospital costs were subject to regulation. In addition, each of the rate-setting programs had been in operation since 1970 or earlier.

Each of the state rate-setting programs established rates on a per diem basis, as well as a schedule of rates for other services and "revenue centers" (for example, laboratory, operating room, radiology) in each hospital. The study used "expense per equivalent inpatient admission" as the index to compare average hospital costs. Per diem costs were not considered, as they had been in many previous studies, because hospitals could show a decrease in per diem costs by extending the average length of stay per episode of care. The expense per equivalent admission (EPEA) was compared for the rate-setting and non-rate-setting states. No difference could be seen until 1976, when the costs began to diverge. Between 1976 and 1978 the six rate-setting states had statistically smaller annual rates of increase (11.2 percent) than the non-rate-setting states (14.6 percent).

The authors believed that the different findings of their study as compared to previous studies could be explained by four factors. First, the start-up time involved in each program made the measurement of effectiveness in 1975 premature. The early reviews did not reflect the programs at 100 percent operation. Second, in the years between 1976 and 1978, public concern about the high rates of increase in hospital costs heightened, and this may have given state officials additional incentive and perhaps political support to reduce the rate of increase. Third, the Carter administration's hospital cost-containment proposal in 1977 reflected this public concern and may have aided the states in their ability to restrain cost increases. Finally, the Economic Stabilization Program of the Nixon administration, which limited hospital cost increases nationwide, was in effect from August 1971 to April 1974. Its impact on the non-rate-setting states may have masked the effect of the state rate-setting programs during the early period.

Feder and Spitz (1980) presented a new focus on the state prospective rate-setting programs: they discussed the reimbursement system's development and implementation in terms of the political process. The authors recognized that although over time there have been many government programs implemented to alter payment policy for hospital services, few have been successful. Feder and Spitz stated that programs failed because they did not recognize that creating the best policy is a political process involving many public and private groups, and that each of these groups has different interests and agendas that must be coordinated.

Past unsuccessful attempts to control hospital costs, the authors argued, had failed because of the resilience of provider influence in the payment process. Despite changes in payment methods, the authors suggested that professional "judgment" and interests continued to dominate the determination of appropriate levels of government expenditure. Public payment policy and private commitment supported this arrangement. Hospital expenditures skyrocketed because government was primarily concerned with achieving patient equity, while continuing to allow providers to determine utilization levels and quality of care.

If government alters its objectives for equity of care, Feder and Spitz argued, then it must also alter the way it pays for hospital care. Reimbursement based on autonomous hospital expenditures must be replaced by controls over the rate of increase of aggregate hospital expenditures. A revenue ceiling and allowable rates of increase must be based on an independent measure of expenditure increase, such as the non–health care Consumer Price Index. If the ceiling is to contain costs and expenditures, then payments must be tied to the number of admissions, not days of care. A range for the number of admissions must also be specified.

The final recommendation of the authors (which is at the center of much of the cost containment debate of today) was that in order to discourage provider cost shifting, the public revenue ceiling must apply to all purchasers of care, both public and private, and to all types of routine and ancillary services.

Controls On the Supply of Services

Certificate-of-Need Regulation and the Use of Health Services Planning

The Feder and Spitz article highlighted the belief held during the 1970s by many analysts that without system-wide planning the United States health system would generate too many expensive services and facilities. As early as 1959, Roemer and Shain (1959) were investigating the failure of market forces to regulate the optimal number of beds. They believed that excess beds would generate additional demand. This linkage between the number of available beds and the ultimate use of hospital care became known as "Roemer's Law" and was a major impetus for health planning legislation to control hospital construction.

In other sectors of the economy, the power of the market could be counted on to limit such overcapacity. But in the health sector in general and in hospital services in particular, extensive third-party insurance coverage and a system in which payment was based on the cost of the service incurred prevented the generation of the right incentives for efficiency and the penalization of those institutions which overbuilt. It

was therefore concluded that any hospital rate-setting system must be linked with system-wide controls over facilities, services, and utilization (Dowling, 1976).

The most comprehensive national attempt to control capital formation in hospitals was created in 1974 as part of the National Health Planning and Resources Development Act (Public Law 93–641). Each state was required to create a Certificate-of-Need (CON) program and to seek approval for all capital expenditures that exceeded $150,000. These regulations were designed to limit the availability of inpatient beds and specialized equipment. The goal of the program was to balance the overall needs of the community with the wishes of individual institutions and to develop plans consistent with those community needs.

But no sooner had the ink dried on the new legislation than articles began to appear criticizing this form of regulation. A paper by Salkever and Bice (1978) argued that CON regulations actually contributed to increased hospital costs during their initial implementation phase. The authors stated that total hospital investment increased as a result of the lack of clear information and standards to guide CON agencies in the determination of hospital needs for new equipment and facilities.

The studies of CON programs that followed the Salkever and Bice report often echoed their conclusions. In their analysis, Sloan and Steinwald (1980) divided CON programs into two categories: comprehensive (those programs that include service-expansion and equipment purchase review) and noncomprehensive (those programs that do neither, thereby allowing for some inflationary effects.) They also distinguished between newly operational CON programs and those that had matured during the period 1970–1975. They concluded that the comprehensive CON programs had essentially no impact upon hospital costs, while the mature, noncomprehensive CON programs had the opposite effect and *raised* per diem expenses by nearly 5 percent in the short run and over 10 percent in the long run. In addition, their analysis showed that there was a positive anticipatory response to the development of CON. The noncomprehensive programs made little or no impact on reducing or controlling excess beds.

Throughout the late 1970s, researchers continued to evaluate the efficacy of certificate-of-need regulation and the general value of health planning and to make recommendations for better programs. According to research by Pearson and Abernethy (1980), the implementation barriers faced by the National Health Planning and Resources Development

Act of 1974 were substantial. They believed the act was problematic from the beginning because of the delay in providing review standards and criteria for the planning agencies to use in their evaluation. The power of these criticisms, combined with the self-interest of the many who wanted uncontrolled growth of hospital facilities, was strong enough to lead to repeal of the Federal Health Planning legislation in 1984.

The Carter Years

One of the first pieces of health care legislation that President Carter proposed in 1977 was a comprehensive hospital cost containment program built around many of the principles used during the Economic Stabilization period (Davis, 1981). But the hospital industry together with those in Congress who opposed any expansion of the federal government's involvement in health care were able to defeat the Carter proposal. Instead, the various health provider groups told the Congress and the American people that they would develop a new approach to hospital cost containment called the Voluntary Effort (VE).

Hospital cost inflation was continuing to outrace prices in other industries, but rather than adding more top-down regulation, the VE stressed cooperation. But this was not just any type of cooperation. The VE was sponsored by the American Hospital Association, the American Medical Association, the Blue Cross and Blue Shield Associations, and the Federation of American Hospitals. It promoted cost containment at the state and local levels whereby each hospital was asked to voluntarily keep its expenditures at the lowest rate possible and to refrain from service and plant expansion.

Newman, Gibbs, and Gift (1979) evaluated the VE program and noted that because the program was voluntary, some hospitals could choose not to comply and would benefit from the lack of regulation (the "free rider" problem). It was hoped that peer pressure would prevent this behavior and would be a major component in the program's success. During the VE's first year of operation, the rate of growth of hospital expenditures dropped from 15.6 percent in 1977 to 12.8 percent in 1978. This success continued until the early 1980s, when a strong inflation cycle throughout the economy led to a complete breakdown in the voluntary control system.

As the decade of the 1970s closed, there was much confusion in the research community about how to reduce hospital cost inflation, and whether this should be a primary goal of national and state policy. Those who wanted government action believed that some form of prospective reimbursement system based on financial incentives to the provider and the patient was required. Others argued that only through more extensive use of the "market" could health care spending be brought into line with other segments of the economy.

Several new trends in the early 1980s led to a major turning point in the payment systems of hospital services. On the private side, the economic recession of 1981–1983 and the continued escalation in private health care spending led to much more proactive behavior on the part of corporations and private insurance companies. Private payors are for the most part "price-takers" for hospital services; they individually lack the necessary clout to influence the pricing behavior of hospitals. Therefore, their main avenue for controlling hospital expenses rests with reducing the use of services. For the first time, the private sector made extensive use of research results which showed that health maintenance organizations (HMOs) and other forms of managed care could reduce the rate of hospitalization and overall health care spending (Newman et al., 1979). Other research findings supported the use of second-opinion reviews for elective surgery and preadmission certification of most proposed hospitalizations.

Congress repeatedly tried to modify the inflationary tendencies of the cost-based hospital payment system of Medicare. Its first attempt in 1971 was the passage of Section 223, which focused on constraining the growth in routine inpatient hospital expenses. As government tightened the implementing regulations, hospitals restructured their accounting systems, shifting more and more routine expenses onto their ancillary care budgets. The net result was that hospital inpatient expenditures under Medicare continued to grow at an alarming rate (Wallack and Handler, 1983).

During the period 1979–1981, the rate of increase of Medicare spending for hospital care was almost 50 percent. This seemingly uncontrolled growth in spending prompted Congress to include a much tougher Medicare hospital payment control system in the 1982 Tax Equity and Fiscal Responsibility Act (TEFRA). Henceforth, all hospital inpatient expenses—routine and ancillary—were to be reviewed and a total inpatient hospital cost control system was to be put in place. Those hospitals whose inpatient operating costs per case grew at less than a target rate of growth were to receive a small incentive payment, while those which exceeded the target rate were to be penalized. In no case, however, would Medicare reimburse a hospital for more than 120 percent of the mean cost per case for hospitals of the same type. (Each hospital was grouped according to its bed size and location.) In addition, TEFRA included the first use of a Diagnosis Related Group (DRG)–based index of the case-mix of each hospital, which permitted a further adjustment in a hospital's minimum Medicare reimbursable limit. Finally, TEFRA called for the Reagan administration to consider creating a new Medicare hospital reimbursement system which would do away with cost-based reimbursement altogether and would rely instead on a prospectively determined payment approach. It was expected that a crucial component of this new prospective payment system would be the grouping of hospital inpatients into DRGs so that a prospectively determined payment amount per group could be constructed that had both clinical and economic coherence (Fetter et al., 1980).

The Medicare Prospective Payment System

The Health Care Financing Administration (HCFA) in the Department of Health and Human Services was directed by Congress to propose a plan to reimburse hospitals for Medicare services on a prospective basis, including incentives to reward hospital management efficiency. The report was presented to Congress in 1982, and the Prospective Payment System was legislated in April of 1983 and implemented in October of the same year.

The proposed system was based on methodology developed by Mills, Fetter, Riedel, and Averill (1976) of Yale University. Variations of the DRG system had been used in three states before becoming the centerpiece of the federal law. The initial research of Mills et al. had created an interactive computer system called AUTOGRP which allowed a user to define groups of customers based upon independent attributes. Control was enhanced by grouping processes in that manner (Mills et al., 1976, p. 604). The AUTOGRP system was concerned about cost containment as well as quality assurance. The authors believed that the classification of patients according to their patterns of resource consumption was an aid in cost control because it assured that such classes were medically meaningful. The process of classification was applied to

66,402 patients discharged from Yale-New Haven Hospital in the period of April 1971 to September 1973. The AUTOGRP system resulted in the creation of 330 patient groups (the precursors of the Diagnosis Related Groups).

By 1980 Fetter et al. (1980) had developed the DRG classification scheme as a means for hospital administrators to evaluate hospital performance and to assist regulatory agencies in making comparisons across institutions. Each of the initial 383 DRGs were based upon classes of patients with the same clinical, demographic, diagnostic, and therapeutic attributes. This method of classification was based on a procedure called the "significant attribute method." The first division of diagnostic codes created major categories of diseases, which were then subdivided into the final set of groups. The final groupings were based on values for those variables that demonstrated an effect in predicting output as measured by length of hospital stay.

The Health Care Financing Administration specified several objectives which were met by the 383 DRGs. These included the provision that the classification system must provide a definition of cases with the following properties: (1) the variables used to define a case must be limited to primary and secondary diagnosis and surgical procedures, and age; (2) the number of DRGs must be manageable, mutually exclusive, and exhaustive; (3) each DRG must be clinically interpretable; and (4) the patients within a DRG must have similar patterns of utilization (Fetter et al., 1980).

Based on the results of the research by Fetter et al. and the early experience of the New Jersey DRG Demonstration Project, the plan adopted by Congress in 1983 called for Medicare to pay for hospital inpatient care based on the specific DRG category of each patient. By establishing a predetermined amount per admission, this new payment system created incentives for hospitals to minimize the cost of treating each patient. The Prospective Payment System, (PPS), as it was called, was built upon many of the lessons learned during the 1970s, particularly from the Economic Stabilization Program (the cost of admission as the unit of payment) and the state prospective payment demonstration programs (the need to provide hospitals with predetermined budgets and to create positive incentives for efficiency).

The goal of PPS was to keep the plan as simple as possible by minimizing the number of DRG categories and the number of special exceptions. It was also felt that too many exceptions would undermine the cost containment incentives of the system. The plan did, however, include a number of adjustments, several of which resulted from special-interest pleading and the findings of independent research studies. These adjustments included added payments to hospitals which operated graduate medical education programs or treated disproportionately large numbers of low-income patients.

Since the passage of PPS, a large number of research studies have reviewed the operation of the program and have suggested improvements. One of the least understood aspects of the DRG pricing policy was the impact of the patient classification system on payments to hospitals and how hospitals would respond to a system that paid for services based on coding of a patient's diagnosis. This was especially important because the DRG coding system collapsed thousands of diagnoses into 467 categories, and thus each category included a wide distribution of diagnoses, sometimes spanning several thousand dollars in treatment costs.

From the very beginning of PPS, several health services researchers, led by Susan Horn, questioned the appropriateness of the DRG categorization techniques (Horn, Cachich, and Clopton, 1983). She and others argued that there was a systemic bias in the way patients were categorized because of the failure of the DRG system to take proper account of the "severity-of-illness" of a patient within a diagnosis category. Because patients with more severe illnesses are likely to be hospitalized in urban tertiary care centers, analysts argued that the DRG payment system would be biased against certain hospitals. Scores of studies have been done to document this bias and several alternative approaches have been proposed. Unfortunately, although the problem appears to be real, no clear-cut, improved alternative system to DRGs has emerged. While reassuring the federal government that the DRG system in use is not grossly inaccurate, these studies did leave a lingering problem unanswered. HCFA, therefore, has asked the original designers of the DRG system to review their technique and recommend a modified DRG approach.

A possible problem not fully anticipated by the designers of PPS concerns the ability of hospitals to manipulate the coding of patient diagnoses to maximize Medicare payments. Although HCFA did anticipate some "upcoding" in the initial years of PPS, recent reports by ProPAC suggest that the magnitude has far exceeded earlier estimates (Steinwald and Dummit, 1989). According to their estimates, whereas increases in hospital payment to account for inflation and new technology amounted to less than 8.0 percent during the first five years of PPS, the cumulative increases in payments due to case-mix change were over 20 percent. Since a 1.0 percent change in Medicare inpatient hospital spending equals more than 400 million dollars, this represents a differential of more than 5 billion dollars. The key research question with major policy significance is how much the case-mix changes reflected sicker patients and how much resulted from a manipulation of the diagnosis codes. Research has been funded by HCFA and ProPAC to identify the relative importance of each component and to develop techniques to disentangle the two in future years.

In contrast to DRG upcoding, an expected outcome of PPS was the reduction in length of stay of Medicare hospital patients. This outcome was one of the major justifications for PPS. In one of the first studies published on this subject, Morrisey, Sloan, and Valvona (1988) reported that the average length of stay for Medicare patients declined quite substantially after the introduction of PPS. They also determined that the proportion of Medicare patients transferred to post-hospital care has doubled since PPS was implemented. The rate of growth of transfers, however, appears to be declining as PPS continues. Their study did suggest that patients who were ultimately transferred to post-hospital care did use hospital services more intensively. Two questions about utilization of inpatient services were left unanswered: (1) Did total resources used, hospital and post-hospital, change with the introduction of PPS? (2) What impact did these changes have on the quality of patient care? Answers to these questions could determine whether PPS will continue to be the hospital payment system used by Medicare.

In the end, the issue that could determine the fate of PPS is whether it can reduce total Medicare expenditures while maintaining an adequate level of quality of care. The first macro review of Medicare expenditures under PPS was completed by Russell and Manning (1989). The authors concluded that PPS reduced Medicare hospital expenditures substantially and led to a minor increase in out-of-hospital spending. They estimated that the Hospital Insurance Trust Funds for 1990 are expected to be $18 billion less than projected before the advent of PPS. This would represent a saving of almost 20 percent. While most analysts are likely to agree with the direction, if not the magnitude, of these estimated reductions, much more controversy is sure to be generated about whether this is a true saving or simply a shifting of expenses to outpatient and home care or to other payors. The authors acknowledge that they have much less information on this issue but state that some preliminary data suggest that the degree of shifting is small in comparison to the amounts of in-hospital saving. The nature of Russell and Manning's study did not permit an assessment of what changes, if any, occurred in the quality of medical care. For those who have looked at the quality-of-care issue since PPS, the conclusion thus far is positive. For example, ProPAC has concluded that through 1988 "the Commission has not found evidence of systematic quality problems with inpatient care since the implementation of PPS" (Prospective Payment Assessment Commission, 1989). Whether PPS or any other payment reform system has an impact on the quality of patient care is likely to continue as a subject of intense interest to the research and policy community in the years ahead.

Concluding Comments

This chapter provides a history of the findings of health services research about the system used by the federal government to pay for inpatient hospital care, the attempts to limit the availability of that care, and the link between these findings and changes in federal policy. Some might question whether we have overstated the importance of research on these policy changes. Surely other components of the system play important roles and often a dominant role in the shaping of federal policy. Congress and the executive branch often must react to perceived problems that have been brought to their attention by those directly affected by the system, be they patients, providers of care, or those who pay the bill. Even in such situations, however, federal policy will rarely change without some legitimation of these concerns by research findings.

Much of the research of the 1970s and 1980s that we described could be considered reactive because it evaluated the effects of solutions devised to handle past problems. These evaluations were often negative and led to the ending of past programs and the creation of new ones. But such solutions bring new problems and therefore issues for future research. So the process continues, with the impact of research and its effects on the policy process often difficult to determine.

4

Physician Payment

Paul B. Ginsburg and Philip R. Lee

The United States will soon begin an important reform in its methods of physician payment. In November 1989 Congress passed significant legislation to alter patterns of payment in Medicare. There is sufficient interest among private payors to indicate that reform will likely not be limited to Medicare.

Much of the focus of payment reform has been on fee-for-service medicine. This does not imply that its proponents are opposed to alternative payment mechanisms or have less interest in them. Rather, whatever the prospects for other payment mechanisms, fee-for-service is likely to play a major role for the foreseeable future, especially for the Medicare program, which has lagged behind employment-based health plans in the use of alternative financing and delivery systems such as health maintenance organizations (HMOs) and preferred provider organizations (PPOs).

Health services research has played a significant role in the consideration of reforms in Medicare physician payment. Much of it has been communicated to policymakers and has helped shape policy decisions. But some types of studies have been more influential than others. For example, we sense that research that is more oriented to measurement has played a more important role than that oriented toward hypothesis-testing with regression models. Also, in recent years, the speed of change in the health care system often has overwhelmed research, making older research less relevant and new research incomplete at the point where decisions are made.

In this chapter we will review the role of health services research in policy toward payment of physicians. In our review we emphasize the experience of the Physician Payment Review Commission (PPRC), which developed a comprehensive proposal for reform in the mechanism by which Medicare pays physicians (PPRC, 1989). The legislation recently enacted by Congress follows this proposal very closely. We will discuss how health services research affected the deliberations of the commission, those that the commission advises (members of Congress and their staffs), and the administration.

The chapter is divided into two sections. The first reviews the problems that physician payment policy attempts to address, beginning with a discussion of the differences in the approach to these issues by different payors. The problems discussed are the following: relative value issues, geographic variation in fees, overall fee levels, assignment and balance billing, and rising expenditures for physicians' services. The second section of the chapter reviews the policy initiatives that are the focus at this time. This includes the recent payment reform legislation—fee schedule, balance billing limits, expenditure targets (renamed "Medicare volume performance standards"), and federal support of effectiveness research and practice guidelines—as well as departures from fee-for-service payments and contracting mechanisms between HMOs and physicians.

Policy Problems

Although discussions of policy must focus on the options available to *governmental* decision makers, changes in practices on the part of private payors, either in response to public policy changes or independent of them, are important to consider. With this chapter having an inevitable focus on policies of public payors such as Medicare, it is important to begin with a discussion of distinctions in orientation among the various payors.

Objectives of Different Payors

The objective of all payors should be to obtain access to physician services for their subscribers at the lowest possible price. Prior to the 1980s, the options open to most payors were limited. When commercial insurers and Medicare decided how much to pay for physicians' services, they confronted a trade-off: the higher the fees paid, the higher were the premiums for the insurance but the smaller the balance bills faced by beneficiaries.[1] Some Blue Shield plans had an additional option. With large market shares, they developed participating physician programs in which physicians were offered the option of direct payment and notification to subscribers of this special status in return for agreeing not to balance-bill the subscribers. These plans thus gained the ability to pay less than billed charges without having most of the difference shifted to beneficiaries.

In the mid-1980s, Medicare as well began to use its market power. It developed a participating physician program resembling those of some Blue Shield plans, and then went one step further by restricting the amounts that nonparticipating physicians could charge Medicare beneficiaries. With these two steps, Medicare has been able to change the terms of the trade-off between the amount paid and balance billing. The proportion of claims taken on assignment (where the physician bills Medicare and agrees to accept the Medicare approved amount as payment in full) has increased steadily since 1983. More recently, the aggregate balance billing liability of beneficiaries has declined.

Through PPOs, private insurers have found additional ways to use market power. Like participating physician programs, PPOs offer physicians increased numbers of patients in return for discounts on fees and compliance with utilization review standards.

Differences in perspective could lead to different attitudes toward the payment reform issues discussed in this chapter. For example, by having the most extensive market power (Medicare patients account for 32 percent of revenues of physicians in specialties relevant to the elderly [Sunshine and Swartzman, 1989]), Medicare is in the best position to change its pattern of payment and avoid having the changes offset by changes in balance billing by physicians. Blue Shield plans with large market shares, PPOs, and HMOs are in the best position to make parallel changes in their own payment systems.

Another difference is found in the broader objectives of public programs. Federal policymakers' interests need to go beyond that of paying as little as possible without increasing balance billing by an unacceptable degree. The federal government has interests in issues such as equity among physicians in different specialties and in different geographic areas. It also has interests that affect individuals other than Medicare beneficiaries. For example, the federal government has taken steps to increase Medicare payments in rural underserved areas in order not only to increase access for Medicare beneficiaries living in those areas but to encourage a larger supply of physicians for other citizens as well. In addition, physicians in general are an important political constituency, so that concerns over what is a "fair" level of fees in Medicare need to be addressed.[2]

Relative Value Issues

Research has indicated that relative payments for various services do not track closely with estimates of either relative costs or other variables that might be relevant. As background for this topic, we first discuss the mechanism for determining payment that is used by Medicare and most private payors.

Medicare determines what it will pay physicians on the basis of subjecting billed charges to two screens. First, charges are compared to the median charge made by the physician for that service during the previous year (customary charge). Second, the billed charge is compared to the prevailing charge in the locality. The prevailing charge is the 75th percentile of customary charges. However, the prevailing charge screen is also subject to a limit on its percentage increase from a base period. The rationale behind this "customary, prevailing, and reasonable" (CPR) mechanism for determining payment is a linkage to the local market. By paying physicians according to what they normally charged, subject to some constraint based on what others in the community were charging, Medicare would not interfere with the market.

But Medicare proved to be too large and influential for its payment policies not to affect the market. After Medicare initiated its policy, many Blue Shield plans adopted a similar payment mechanism;[3] then commercial insurers adopted the mechanism as well. This led to a situation where too large a proportion of the market was basing payment on what others were paying, and the result was an inflationary mechanism (Frech and Ginsburg, 1978). Physicians who raised charges found that many payors would allow the higher amounts.

In response to fee increases larger than anticipated, Medicare in the late 1960s and early 1970s added constraints to the "reasonable charge" mechanism. The percentile used to determine prevailing charge levels was reduced in the late 1960s to the 75th percentile, and a "Medicare Economic Index" was developed to limit rates of increase in prevailing charge screens to growth in overall practice costs (including the opportunity costs of the self-employed physician's time). These constraints removed much of the inflationary tendency of the reasonable charge methodology. The result was an evolution to a series of *de facto* fee schedules that reflected fee patterns from an earlier period.

Health services research has documented the distortions in both the relative values of different services and the geographic pattern of payment. The work of William Hsiao and his colleagues has been instrumental in making the case that relative values are distorted. An early attempt, published in 1979, drew enormous attention to the issue (Hsiao and Stason, 1979). The current "resource-based relative value study" (RBRVS), which is much more elaborate, has played a large role in stimulating policies to change relative values.[4]

Assessments of distortions in relative values are based on comparisons of current charges to estimates of relative costs. Measurement of the latter is challenging because roughly one-half of physician revenues is retained by the physician as net income, and most of the other costs ("practice costs") are common to most of the services provided by a physician. Thus there is a serious measurement problem for one half of the costs and an insoluble allocation problem for the other half. Hsiao has measured the physician costs of services through a survey asking physicians to rate the relative "work" involved in different hypothetical services. "Work" includes not only time but mental effort and judgment, technical skill and physical effort, and stress.

The Hsiao study documents the serious distortions in relative payments across broad categories of services. For example, it estimates that a general surgeon spends 3.4 times as long performing gallbladder surgery as performing a comprehensive office visit and devotes 1.8 times as much work per minute. But the Medicare payment is 24 times as much.[5]

Cromwell, Mitchell, and colleagues performed a similar study that was recently published (Cromwell et al., 1989). The results are broadly similar, but the authors have interpreted them as showing that relative charges are not significantly distorted. Using procedure code as the unit of observation, they regressed charges on estimates of work from their own survey of physicians. Using a criterion of the predicted charge differing from the actual charge by more than two standard deviations, they identified relatively few services as "mispriced." They also suggest that the values of R-squared in these regressions demonstrate that charges explain variations in physician work adequately. But the specification is unlikely to detect distortions among broad categories of services, and we have doubts that such statistics are the appropriate criteria with which to judge if a procedure is "mispriced."[6] We have more confidence in comparisons of total work and charges for broad categories of services. In our opinion, the Cromwell work does not undermine the evidence from the Hsiao study on distortions in relative payments.

Less research is available on the likely impacts of changes in relative values on the use of services. Theory has not provided clear predictions, principally because of continued dispute between proponents of classical versus target income models.[7] It seems likely, however, that in the long run, the proportion of physician effort that goes into the production of a particular service would move in the same direction as the change in its relative fee, since specialty choice would be affected by changes in relative values.

In a statement to the PPRC, Thomas Rice, one of the investigators most familiar with research on physician behavioral response to prices, documented a virtual absence of empirical research on this issue (Rice, 1988). In a subsequent research project funded by PPRC, Labelle, Hurley, and Rice (1989) studied responses over time to changes in relative values of services in Ontario. Their results were mixed, with some services having statistically significant responses, but others not. The significant responses were not all in the same direction, though negative relationships (utilization changing in the opposite direction from the change in price) were more numerous than positive relationships. The researchers suggest, however, that responses to a Medicare fee schedule could be larger, since changes in physicians' incomes will be larger. With funding from the Canadian government, these researchers are now studying cross-sectional variation in relative values across provinces. PPRC is pursuing similar work using U.S. data from Medicare.

Geographic Variation in Fees

Physician fees vary substantially from one part of the country to another. The phenomenon, long known to practicing physicians attending regional and national meetings, began to be recognized by policymakers as a result of research by Burney, Schieber, et al. (1978). Their study documents three- and fourfold variation in charges for particular services. Large portions of this variation were not explained by crude indexes of costs of living and costs of practice. With the development of more accessible claims data by HCFA, additional research has been completed by PPRC (1988, 1989) and by others (Pope, Welch, Zuckerman, and Henderson, 1989).

The research literature has shown marked variation in fees among individual localities but much smaller differences among broad types of geographic areas. Many have been surprised by how small the differences are between urban and rural areas. For example, Medicare-allowed charges in metropolitan areas with population between one and five million are only 4 percent above the national average, and charges in the smallest rural counties (population under 25,000) are only 13 percent under the national average (PPRC, 1989, table 6–1). When deflated by costs of practice, the differences are even smaller. For example, after adjustment for differences in costs of practice but not cost of living, the above differences are reduced, respectively, to 2 percent above and 7 percent below the national average.

Researchers have been less successful at understanding what is behind the variation in fees than in describing it. Estimates of the cost of practice do explain some of the variation, but—in the minds of at least some researchers—much less of the variation than one would expect. A recent study of Medicare prevailing charges for 16 common physicians' services found that an index of practice costs that included costs of living explained between 5 and 37 percent of the variation in charges and 44 percent of the variation on the average charge for the bundle of services (Pope, Welch, Zuckerman, and Henderson, 1989).

The critical question for policy is whether this pattern of geographic variation is a reflection of an efficiently functioning market, inducing physicians to locate in areas where demand for their services is high (and inducing patients in those areas to demand fewer services), or whether the pattern of fees is not serving this function and perhaps is even impeding it. Many suspect that the pattern has impeded access to care in certain rural areas (for example, National Rural Health Care Association, 1988). Others see the pattern as an issue of equity. With Medicare attempting to keep outlays down by paying substantially less than physicians charge, those physicians whose payments are relatively low even after adjustment for differences in costs of practice feel that they are subsidizing their colleagues in other areas. To the degree that physicians offset low Medicare payments through balance billing, the geographic pattern becomes an equity issue for beneficiaries as well.[8]

Overall Fee Levels

Discussion of the issue of the overall level of fees differs according to the perspective from which one approaches it. When discussed from the perspective of society, physician fees must be high enough to attract a sufficient number of qualified people into the profession but not so high that returns to medical education exceed the returns to other investments in postgraduate education. But studies by economists have shown that rates of return to both undergraduate medical education and specialty training are very high (Burstein and Cromwell, 1985).

When fee levels are considered by a payor, the issue tends instead to concern access to care by patients. In Medicare, for example, if fee levels are to be frozen or increased less than the increase in physicians' billed charges, one is concerned not so much with the broad issue of whether or not physicians earn too much but with what will be the impact on out-of-pocket costs to beneficiaries. As described in the following section on assignment and balance billing, research does show that a reduction in payments relative to charges tends to lower the assignment rate. But the recent experience of Medicare shows how this relationship can be swamped by other factors. During the 1983–1988 period, when Medicare payment increases lagged physician charges by a substantial margin, the assignment rate increased sharply, presumably because of the implementation of the participating provider and supplier program.

A more controversial question among researchers concerns the response of the quantity of services provided by physicians to changes in overall fee levels. Whereas classical models of physician behavior suggest that physicians would provide fewer services in response to a reduction in fees (this assumes that extensive insurance coverage limits any substantial demand effect so that the supply curve is the relevant predictor of response and, in the case of unassigned claims, the patient's demand would result in fewer services),[9] many researchers suspect that the opposite response is indeed the case. They assume that, at least in the short run, physicians will attempt to offset declines in income by inducing patients to use more services or a more complex bundle of services.

This issue has received a great deal of attention in the research literature, and space does not permit a review here.[10] The debate has been vigorous because the professional stakes to economists are high. At issue is the degree of applicability to physician services of classical models of economic behavior.

The issue of the quantity response to changes in fee levels is dealt with extensively in the policy context. Since 1984, the Congress has either frozen fees or restrained updates substantially. Each time, those in the federal government with responsibility for cost estimation must make their best judgment as to the effects of reductions in real prices on the utilization of services. The judgment on the part of both the Medicare actuary and the Congressional Budget Office (CBO) has been to assume a substantial offset from increases in quantity.

Recently, the work of CBO has been shared with the research community (Christensen, 1989). The policy assumptions have been based on an extension of previous analysis of the data base developed by Rice and McCall (1982) on the experiment in Colorado during the 1970s. The Medicare carrier for Colorado revised charge screen boundaries from nine localities to a single statewide unit. This led to changes in Medicare-allowed charges for each geographic area, with large increases for rural areas and a decline for Denver. Based on analysis of these data, the CBO assumes that induced changes in volume offset 56 percent of outlay reductions from reductions in Medicare charge screens and 38 percent of outlay increases from increases in charge screens.[11] The range of uncertainty in the projection is enormous, but one is probably better off with a careful point estimate of the behavioral response than assuming that there is none.

Assignment and Balance Billing

Concern about the determinants of balance billing is perhaps unique to the Medicare program. Private payors often deliberately set their payment schedules high enough so that most physicians are paid their billed charges. Medicaid, in contrast, prohibits balance billing.

Medicare has linked assignment and balance billing. Physicians seeking to be paid directly by the Medicare program must agree not to bill the patient for the difference between their charge and the amount that is approved by Medicare. Medicare has sought to encourage assignment by creation of the participating physician program, in which physicians who agree to accept assignment for all claims during the year receive fees that are 5 percent higher, face no limitations on increases in charges billed (but are still subject to screens for amounts allowed for payment), and are listed in a directory. Since 1984, nonparticipating physicians have faced restrictions on the amounts that can be charged for services.

For most of the history of Medicare, the assignment rate (percentage of claims or charges that are assigned) has been in the mid-50s. Since assignment is required for those beneficiaries who are also eligible for Medicaid, the assignment rate for other beneficiaries is somewhat lower. However, beginning in 1984 with the enactment of the participating physician program and restrictions on charges by nonparticipating physicians, the assignment rate has risen sharply, and now exceeds 80 percent (PPRC, 1989).

Much research has been conducted on the determinants of assignment and, more recently, participation. Descriptive work shows that assignment rates vary dramatically from one state to another (highest in the Northeast, lowest in the North Central states and the South) and vary by specialty (surgeons tend to have higher rates, and anesthesiologists—but not other hospital-based physicians—have particularly low rates) (PPRC, 1988). Regression analyses have found the expected positive relationship between payment levels and assignment (Paringer, 1980; Mitchell and Cromwell, 1982; Rice and McCall, 1983; Rice, 1984). Results on the socioeconomic status of patients have been mixed (Mitchell and Cromwell, 1982; Rodgers and Mussacchio, 1983; Rice and McCall, 1983). A recent survey of beneficiaries conducted for PPRC showed that once region is held constant, the probability of assignment does not vary with income (Nelson et al., 1989).

Although regression analysis has help researchers to understand assignment, it does not leave policymakers with a great deal of comfort concerning their ability to predict the effects of policy changes. Much of the regional variation remains unexplained. Also, the recent sharp increase in the assignment rate came during a period in which Medicare payment levels have fallen sharply compared to billed charges. Clearly, changes such as the participating physician program and charge limits have overpowered changes in variables for which the marginal impact on assignment has been studied.

Rising Expenditures for Physicians' Services

Data on outlays have documented the rapid increases in spending for physicians' services. For example, from 1980 to 1988, Part B outlays increased at an average annual rate of 17 percent. Physician services, which now account for 72 percent of Part B outlays, have grown almost as rapidly.[12] Although general inflation and growth of the enrollee population are responsible for a portion of this increase, services per enrollee have been growing at about 7 percent per year. Data from private insurers are more difficult to obtain, but many insurers report similar trends. However, data limitations have severely restricted the ability of researchers to study expenditure increases in more detail.

Medicare bill summary files show the differential rates of growth for broad categories of services. Between 1980 and 1987, the proportion of Medicare physician services classified as "medical" declined from 42 percent to 34 percent. The proportion classified as surgical was essentially unchanged, but diagnostic services increased from 15 percent to 21 percent (PPRC, 1988).

Two recent studies funded by the Department of Health and Human Services have increased our knowledge of the types of services that contribute disproportionately to rising expenditures. Because of limitations in the data that HCFA obtains from its carriers, the two research teams had to obtain and clean Medicare claims data from a number of carriers.

Mitchell, Wedig, and Cromwell (1989) examined Medicare spending on physicians' services from 1983 to 1986. Spending increased 29.5 percent over the period, with almost 75 percent attributable to increased services per beneficiary and changes in service mix. Spending for three types of services increased most rapidly: surgery, radiology, and specialized diagnostic tests.[13] Surgery services per beneficiary increased 35 percent during the period, with diagnostic surgical procedures such as colonoscopy and cardiac catheterization the most rapidly increasing subcategory. Radiology procedures increased at a rate similar to surgery, but nonsurgical diagnostic tests increased 67 percent. The latter include cardiac stress tests, pulmonary function tests, Holter monitoring, and echocardiography. In contrast to these procedures, visits were virtually unchanged.

Although the title of the study, "The Medicare Physician Fee Freeze," suggests that these increases in volume might have been induced by the 1984–1986 fee freeze, the data cover too limited a period to underpin solid conclusions. For example, the period coincided with the introduction of hospital prospective payment. In addition, much or all of the volume increase might have been a continuation of earlier trends. Finally, the increases in the volume of specific services appear to be several orders of magnitude larger than previous research results on induced demand would suggest as a likely result of the freeze.

McMenamin, West, and Marcus (1988) studied different carriers for the 1983–1985 period, using somewhat different techniques. Increases in claims for outpatient surgery accounted for 40 percent of the increase in total outlays. Both increased volume of surgery and a more expensive mix of services contributed to increased claims. Substitution for inpatient surgery accounted for only 8 percent of the increase in outpatient surgery.

Another factor was an increased number of claimants. While enrollment grew 4 percent, 11 percent more beneficiaries filed claims. The authors attribute 20 percent of the growth of services to increased claimants, but some contend that increased use of electronic billing by physicians during this period may have resulted in more beneficiaries' having claims (Greenberg, 1988).

The work of Schieber and Poullier (1989) on international comparisons of spending has been very influential in general discussions of cost containment. Many have been amazed by the magnitude of the difference in the proportion of gross national product spent on health services between the United States and other industrialized countries. In 1987, 11.2 percent of GNP was devoted to health care in the United States, compared to 9.0 percent in second-ranked Sweden and 8.6 percent in third-ranked Canada and France. The lack of universal coverage in the United States makes the differences in percentage of GNP even more stunning.

A historical series developed by these authors shows that this gap is a phenomenon of the 1980s. Before 1980, most Western countries were experiencing increases in the proportion of resources devoted to health care. But many countries were able to stabilize the proportion, while it continued to grow in the United States. This gap has been particularly worrisome to the business community and to labor because of its implications concerning the competitiveness of the U.S. economy.

Policy Directions

The many shortcomings in physician payment methods discussed in the first section make it unlikely that any single policy for reform would prove to be adequate. For example, policies to reduce distortions in relative payments are unlikely to solve the problem of rising expenditures as well. Thus, in its recent recommendations to Congress, the

PPRC emphasized use of a combination of policy tools (PPRC, 1989). It found that a combination of policies would not only have more potential to resolve the multiple problems but also could attract a broader spectrum of political support. The PPRC recommended a package of four policies to reform physician payment. These include a fee schedule based on resource costs, limits on balance billing, expenditure targets, and effectiveness research and practice guidelines. Each of the policies is directed at a partial reform of fee-for-service payment.

But broad-scale solutions need not be limited to fee for service. Broader payment units, such as physician DRGs and payments for episodes of care, have received attention and are being discussed. Alternative delivery systems such as HMOs are likely to play an important role over time. Policy toward alternative delivery systems is discussed by Harold Luft and Ellen Morrison in Chapter 8. To a large extent, such policy is not a physician payment issue, since HMOs and newer delivery systems are paid not as physicians but as entities responsible for organizing the delivery of comprehensive care. One issue concerning HMOs that is discussed here (as predominantly a physician payment issue) concerns whether Medicare should restrict the types of contracts between HMOs that serve Medicare beneficiaries and physicians. Recent legislation has imposed some restrictions on the magnitude of incentives to physicians to contain costs.

Medicare Fee Schedule

The PPRC developed a proposal for a Medicare Fee Schedule to replace payment according to the "customary, prevailing, and reasonable" (CPR) mechanism (PPRC, 1989). The fee schedule was developed in response to the evidence described earlier concerning distortions in relative payments for different services, for different specialties, and across different geographic areas. Much of the research that was instrumental in pointing out the distortions in the current pattern of payment was also used in the development of the proposed fee schedule. Also relevant was research on the design of and the experience with fee schedules in Canada, France, and West Germany (Rodwin, Grable, and Thiel, 1990). The legislation enacted in November 1989 followed the Commission's fee schedule proposal very closely.

A fee schedule consists of a relative value scale, which sets the value of each type of service relative to others, a conversion factor, which transforms the relative values into dollar payments, and various multipliers, which adjust the conversion factor by geographic area, specialty, or other considerations. In addition, a fee schedule requires clear and uniform standards for coding services. A policy mechanism to update the conversion factor and relative values is also required.

Relative Value Scale. If a relative value scale is to be based on costs, estimates must be developed for the two major types of costs—the time and effort of the physician and the nonphysician inputs that the physician often purchases. In response to a mandate from Congress to develop a relative value scale, HCFA commissioned William Hsiao to develop such a scale. Hsiao subcontracted a portion of the study to the AMA. The first phase of the study, which covered 17 specialties, was completed in September 1988 (Hsiao et al., 1988b).

Through a psychometric technique known as magnitude estimation, the Hsiao study developed estimates of the time and effort of physicians. For each specialty, approximately 25 vignettes were prepared describing the patient and, for services other than visits, what the physician did. Physicians were surveyed and asked to give the time involved and to rate the "work" involved relative to a reference vignette. The ratings for each specialty were then combined into a single scale through identification of services that are the same or equivalent in two or more specialties. The vignettes were then linked with Current Procedure Terminology (CPT), the coding system used by Medicare and most private insurers. A specialty training adjustment altered the relative values of procedures performed by specialists whose training differs in length from that of a reference specialty.

For nonphysician inputs, the Hsiao study used data from existing surveys on the ratio of practice costs to total revenues by specialty. A factor for each specialty was used to estimate practice costs for each service. The relative value scale based on services included in the physician survey was then extrapolated on the basis of charge data. Families of procedures were defined, and relative values within each family were based on relative charges.

The September 1988 report of the Hsiao study has been subjected to intensive review. Both the PPRC and HCFA asked in-house staff and outside experts to review the report. Various interest groups hired numerous consultants. Although the review by HCFA (Health Care Financing Administration, 1989) was not submitted to Congress until October 1989, well after each of the committees with jurisdiction over

Medicare had voted for a fee schedule based on resource costs, the reviews by the PPRC and many interest groups were discussed extensively at Commission hearings in November 1988 and February 1989. Compared to the review that most research receives (two or three journal referees), the degree of review was extraordinary.

This review process has been highly productive. The many constructive comments have led to modifications in the methodology for the next phase of the study by Hsiao and revisions by the PPRC of some aspects of the study. For example, many stated that the measurement of pre- and post-service work was not accurate enough. In addition, many specialty societies raised problems that were specific to services in their specialty.

The PPRC made a number of important changes in the relative value scale that were reflected in the data that it submitted to Congress for inclusion in the legislation.[14] It adjusted the relative values for all surgical services upward on the basis of a survey of Medicare carriers that it had conducted in connection with another project (Lasker et al., 1989). The survey indicated that the definition of a global service used in the Hsiao study was significantly narrower than in current practice. The Commission made a policy decision to omit the adjustment for specialty training both to avoid the use of specialty differentials in payment and because of a concern that much of the adjustment would reflect double counting—that the additional skill derived from specialty training is already reflected in the physician ratings of "work." Congress agreed with these changes and specified that the fee schedule not include specialty differentials.

The most important changes made by the PPRC came in the area of practice costs. Implicit in the formula used by Hsiao was an extreme assumption concerning how practice costs would change in response to a change in the valuation of the physician work. Thus, if the valuation of the physician work for a procedure was 40 percent less than under the current system, the Hsiao formula implied that practice costs should also be 40 percent lower than at present.

The PPRC revised the formula by which practice costs are incorporated into the relative value scale. It substituted an additive relationship, so that practice costs estimated for a service are unchanged when the valuation of the physician work is changed. This reduced the magnitude of change in relative values substantially. On the basis of additional editing of the physician survey data on practice costs, the PPRC also revised the practice cost factors used in the relative value calculations. The PPRC also separated out malpractice premium costs. This not only served to raise the visibility of these costs of the tort system but permitted the retention of specialty differentials for a component of costs that vary dramatically by specialty in conjunction with the elimination of specialty differentials for the other components of the relative value scale. The legislation reflects both the additive formula and the separation of malpractice premium costs.

Geographic Multipliers. Research by the Urban Institute (UI) and the Center for Health Economics Research (CHER), which was funded by HCFA under a mandate from Congress, was instrumental in the development of the geographic multipliers. Zuckerman, Welch, and Pope (1987, 1989) developed a Laspeyres index of costs of practice. The weights for the index were drawn from the AMA's periodic survey of physicians, and the price proxies were drawn from a variety of different sources. The preliminary (1987) version was used by the Commission to simulate its fee schedule proposal under alternative geographic policies (PPRC, 1989, chap. 9). The final version was used to provide data to the Congress on payment rates for the budget reduction provisions that revise prevailing charge screens in the direction of the fee schedule.[15]

The principle followed by the Commission throughout its development of the fee schedule was that relative payments should be based on relative costs. In applying the principle, the Commission had to decide whether the index should reflect only variations in practice costs, so that under the fee schedule physicians would derive the same net income from providing any given service in different locations, or whether the index should also include a component to be applied to the physician input. The UI/CHER index includes a component for the physician input, which is based on earnings of professionals other than physicians in each geographic area.

The Commission recommended that the geographic multiplier reflect variations in practice costs only. The recommendation was based in large part on testimony from physician and beneficiary organizations concerning what they regarded as "fair." It was also influenced by concern that the current payment system was limiting access to care in rural areas through lower payment rates than in urban areas. Although the Commission did not endorse the calls for uniform payment made by some organizations because of the UI/CHER data showing significant differences in practice costs, it did feel that a uniform physician input component would over time increase access to care in rural areas.

The Commission is concerned, however, that some of the additional costs of practice in remote rural areas are not reflected in the UI/CHER index. For example, some have suggested that the practices of one or two physicians in isolated rural areas have higher costs per service provided because of an inability to take advantage of economies of scale. If the community does not have a hospital, the physician often needs to provide laboratory and X-ray equipment, which will be underutilized. Maintenance of equipment is always more expensive in rural areas because of technicians' travel costs. Registered nurses must often be recruited from afar at salaries that can be higher than those in some urban areas. The Commission plans to consider whether a separate rural adjustment is called for.

The legislation passed by Congress reflects the reasoning described above, but the degree of change has been moderated. The index of professional earnings does enter the formula for geographic adjustment, but it is given only one-quarter of the weight that physician net income constitutes in the average medical practice. The legislation also specifies a 10 percent bonus in fees for services delivered in Health Manpower Shortage Areas, both rural and urban.

The Commission constructed models to simulate the impact of its fee schedule proposal on physicians and beneficiaries (PPRC, 1989, chap. 9; Colby and Juba, in press). Two models were required because of the interest in distributional impacts on both physicians and beneficiaries. Thus two files from the "BMAD" data system were used—a file including all Medicare claims for a sample of physicians and one including all claims for a sample of beneficiaries. The files were "aged" to reflect the likely impact of policy decisions from previous years that had gone into effect after the period for which the claims were filed.

The Commission decided not to incorporate behavioral assumptions concerning changes in utilization and assignment in response to the fee schedule. With the high degree of uncertainty concerning the magnitude of any response and the lack of consensus on the part of the research community, the Commission feared that the assumptions made would be so controversial as to obscure the important information that a model with static assumptions could yield. Subsequent modeling by CBO, which focused on the development of a "budget neutral" conversion factor, did incorporate an assumption concerning changes in utilization based on the Rice and McCall data on Colorado, but there were no significant qualitative changes in the results on distributional patterns (Christensen and Harrison, 1989).

Assignment and Balance Billing

As part of its fee schedule proposal, the Commission called for a uniform percentage limit on balance billing. Its simulation models and survey of beneficiaries played a role in this decision. The simulation model suggested that limits on balance billing would decrease balance billing in the aggregate, a result that surprised many. Additional analysis showed that the reduction in balance billing came principally from those unassigned claims for which the billed charge exceeded by a substantial proportion the allowed charge (both the previous allowed charge and the allowed charge under the fee schedule). This finding led some members of the Commission to drop their insistence on mandatory assignment, since a limit on balance billing has the potential to increase financial protection of beneficiaries by a substantial margin.

One of the principal reasons for surveying beneficiaries was to investigate the degree of protection that low-income beneficiaries have against balance billing. Many physicians had indicated to the Commission that they took patients' incomes into account when deciding whether to charge more than Medicare allows. As discussed earlier, analysis of the survey results did not find a relationship between beneficiary income and the probability that claims would be assigned. These results led some Commission members to be more willing to place limits on balance billing.

Some responded to the survey results by calling for mandatory assignment for low-income beneficiaries. Indeed, a number of specialty societies proposed this to the Commission, in some cases with income cutoffs that would mandate assignment for a majority of beneficiaries. The majority, however, were opposed to an income cutoff. Some found it philosophically inconsistent with a program that is not means-tested. Some were concerned that beneficiaries entitled to mandatory assignment would have reduced access to care because they would be less attractive to physicians. Research on patterns of physician services in the Medicaid program might have been relevant here, although Medicare fee levels have been much higher than those in Medicaid.

The Commission did not recommend a particular percentage amount to which balance bills would be limited; it simply endorsed the principle and provided simulations of a wide range of limits. In the legislation, Congress adopted the principle and chose a percentage amount toward the low end of the range. Beginning with a limit of 125 percent of the fee schedule amount for nonparticipating physicians (who receive 5 percent less than participating physicians), charges are ultimately limited to 115 percent of this amount.

Expenditure Targets and Practice Guidelines

The Commission's proposal for expenditure targets stemmed from an extensive review of cost containment options under Medicare. Whereas many on the Commission thought that HMOs and other alternative delivery systems would play a more significant role in the Medicare program over time, all agreed that the potential for HMOs to make a substantial contribution to cost containment in the short run was limited.

Increased patient cost sharing can restrain costs, but the option appeared not to be politically feasible, and many members were concerned about its potential to reduce access. On a number of occasions the executive branch has proposed increases in Medicare cost sharing, but Congress has never come close to legislating an increase. Congress has been more willing to increase premiums paid by beneficiaries than to increase cost sharing because of concern about placing the burden disproportionately on those who are sick. For the large proportion of beneficiaries with supplemental insurance, increased patient cost sharing is equivalent to a premium increase.

The Commission paid close attention to the research by Brook, Chassin, and others at the RAND Corporation on appropriateness of care and to research by Wennberg and others on small area variation. It decided that the major opportunity to contain costs in Medicare was to provide physicians with more and better information on the effectiveness of alternative treatments. This perception led to a number of proposals by the Commission, including expenditure targets. The Commission recommended federal support for the development of practice guidelines. The federal government should fund efforts by private entities such as medical societies, academic medical centers, and other research institutions to develop guidelines or parameters. These would be disseminated to practicing physicians and made available to organizations such as carriers and peer review organizations that perform utilization review.

Expenditure targets are designed to stimulate collective efforts on the part of the medical community to contain costs. The stimulus is a formula by which annual updates in fees depend on a comparison between the rate of growth of expenditures and a target rate of increase. Thus, if a target of an 11 percent increase is established and expenditures increase by 12 percent, the subsequent update in fees would be inflation less one percentage point.

Although such a formula would not change the incentive facing individual physicians—they would remain on a pure fee-for-service basis—it would provide more of a collective incentive for physicians to control costs. Tools that physicians could use would include development and dissemination of practice guidelines, additional participation in and support of peer review processes, and more support for other policies with the potential to contain costs.

Expenditure targets certainly do not reflect a "competitive approach" to cost containment. Instead, they attempt to coax physicians to work together as professionals to determine what are efficient forms of practice. Nevertheless, expenditure targets are compatible with competitive approaches. They are a tool for the traditional fee-for-service system to use in competing with organized systems. Of course, organized systems would benefit as well from increased knowledge concerning what is efficient practice.

Congress adopted a form of expenditure targets which they called "Medicare Volume Performance Standards." The major change from the concept proposed by the Commission is that the decisions on targets and fee updates are to be made by Congress after advice and deliberation rather than by HCFA on the basis of formulas. However, formulas are in place in case Congress does not act in any given year. Thus, the formulas are likely to play an important role in the decisions made by the Congress. Congress also set up a new entity in HHS, called the Agency for Health Care Policy and Research, to lead efforts to expand research on effectiveness of care and to support the developments of practice guidelines.

Broader Payment Units

Although fee for service leads to payments corresponding closely to what physicians do, the incentives to do more lead to higher costs. The Commission and others have examined payment units that are broader than fee for service, but not as broad as capitation.

Payment for physician services provided to hospital inpatients could be made on a per-case basis. At the time of enactment of hospital prospective payment, legislation called for a study of the feasibility and desirability of paying for physician services on the basis of diagnosis related groups (DRGs). This policy process was the reverse of the usual one in the sense that a major policy option was introduced prior to any analysis by health services researchers. Another problem was that different versions of the physician DRG proposal had very different implications, but the legislative mandate provided little guidance. For example, if the DRG payment is made to the admitting physician, the implications for incentives and relationships among physicians are very different from the situation where payment is made to a hospital medical staff that could then divide the revenue among physicians on the basis of fee for service.

As part of the effort to respond to the congressional mandate, HCFA commissioned a study by Janet Mitchell and colleagues that proved to be influential (1984). The research documented the wide variation of resources expended per patient and the limited ability of DRG classification to explain this variation for patients other than those admitted for surgery. The implication was that payment to individual physicians on a DRG basis would expose them to a large amount of risk and that factors outside the control of the physician might overwhelm the results of attempts to practice more efficiently. Analysis also pointed out the incompatibility of paying physicians on a per-case basis and the Medicare policy of voluntary assignment (Ginsburg, Newhouse, et al., 1986). If physicians not accepting assignment were to continue to bill patients on a fee-for-service basis, then the incentives of a broader payment unit would fall on patients rather than physicians.

In 1987, before the mandated study was completed, the Reagan administration proposed payment for inpatient services by radiologists, anesthesiologists, and pathologists (RAPs) on the basis of DRGs. The proposal, which appeared in the budget for fiscal year 1988, was never developed because the Department of Health and Human Services did not share the enthusiasm of the Office of Management and Budget for the concept. Organized medicine resisted strongly, seeing a broad threat to fee-for-service payment. The PPRC examined the issue and recommended against RAP DRGs. The Commission noted that RAPs have limited control over the rate of utilization of their services and that the real problem was the level of their fees and the exposure of patients to balance bills from physicians that they did not choose. The PPRC decided that these problems were best handled by a fee schedule that would include limitations on balance billing.

More recently, Welch (1989) has revived the physician DRG idea by emphasizing the medical staff version, which avoids most of the problems pointed out in the earlier work. Rather than making a DRG-based payment to an attending physician or a medical staff entity, carriers would continue to pay physicians on a fee-for-service basis but would adjust payments up or down based on their calculations of how all inpatient billings at a particular hospital compare to a DRG-based formula. In this form, DRG-based payment would resemble an expenditure target in that incentives of individual physicians would not be affected appreciably, but the entire medical staff of a hospital would now have an incentive to contain costs. Peer pressure, peer review, and restriction of medical staff privileges would be the tools used to respond to these incentives.

The limitation of DRG-based payment is that it deals with neither the hospital admission decision nor outpatient care. It could be combined with the expenditure target, however. Nested within the overall expenditure target could be a subtarget for growth in expenditures per admission for services delivered at a particular hospital. DRGs would be used only to adjust for changes in case mix over time.

We suspect that the concept underlying physician DRGs will resurface in policies that are more acceptable to physicians. If expenditure targets are applied rigorously, physicians will be looking for ways to contain costs in the context of fee for service. The concept of basing payment on the performance of a hospital medical staff may find use as a method to bring the incentives of expenditure targets that affect very broad segments of the physician community to smaller, more workable segments.

Physician Payment in Private Health Plans

We noted earlier that the Medicare policy of risk contracting with HMOs was not a physician payment policy, but rather a policy of delegating the responsibility to contain costs to private entities that compete both with traditional Medicare and with each other to serve Medicare beneficiaries. Within HMOs, methods of physician payment could range from salary to capitation to fee for service.

Policymakers have often displayed a schizophrenic attitude toward the issue of physician incentives. On the one hand, physicians need incentives to contain costs, but on the other hand, if the incentives are strong, there is fear that patient access to care and its quality will suffer.

In 1986 reports emerged that a California hospital was offering incentive payments to physicians to discharge Medicare patients early. The Congress reacted by prohibiting the offering of such incentives (OBRA86). But when some observers pointed out that HMO physicians often have incentives to contain costs, a provision was added prohibiting HMOs from using financial incentives. Congress did not intend that such an extreme limitation would actually go into effect; it set an effective date of 1990 and called for a report from HHS.

A number of studies were conducted to prepare for congressional consideration of this issue of financial incentives (ICF, 1988; Gold and Reaves, 1987; Hillman, 1987). But the research had an air of "looking where the lights are." While the key issue was the relationship between various incentive arrangements and access and quality, researchers reported that no serious prior attempts to measure the relationship had been made. Given the limitations in both time and resources, the researchers concentrated their efforts on exploring the frequency with which different incentive arrangements were used by HMOs. This provided useful information and called attention to the fact that certain financial incentives were sufficiently common that policymakers should recognize that prohibiting them would risk serious disruption.

OBRA89 did not resolve the issue (implementation of restrictions was deferred for another year), but the Ways and Means Committee, the committee that had raised the issue initially, suggested only limited restrictions on the use of financial incentives. The absence of research suggesting that patients would suffer and the data showing that some restrictions would be disruptive argue against broad-scale restrictions. This tendency is compounded by the relatively small role that Medicare risk contracts play in HMOs. The result of Medicare's prohibition of many arrangements that HMOs feel are important to their ability to contain costs could be that fewer HMOs will be available to Medicare beneficiaries.

Conclusion

Health services research has played a significant role in physician payment policy, both in helping to identify the problem and in providing the measurements needed for the solution. As we mentioned at the outset, research that measured things proved more important than research that tested hypotheses. Research on resource-based relative values, on geographic variation in payments relative to indexes of practice costs, and on patterns of increasing volume of services played particularly significant roles. So did simulations of the impacts of various payment reforms. Less important was research on how physicians respond to differences in fees. The lack of consensus concerning the relationship in this area prevented this research from being influential.

In physician payment, as in other policy areas, research did not determine the policy outcome. Traditional political forces and the values of policymakers played important roles. But research did serve two important functions: it informed policymakers about the consequences of alternatives, and it provided the essential information upon which to build the specifics of the policy that was adopted.

5

Financing Health Care for the Poor

Karen Davis and Diane Rowland

Unlike most industrialized nations, the United States does not have a national health insurance plan financing health care services for the entire population. The federal government's role in assuring access to health services for poor people, however, has expanded significantly since the mid-1960s. In 1965 the Medicaid program was enacted to provide public insurance coverage for selected groups of poor people—welfare recipients and the medically needy.

Medicaid was quite controversial in the early years. Criticism centered on rapidly rising expenditures, inefficiencies of operation, and instances of fraud and abuse by beneficiaries and health care providers. From this shaky start, however, Medicaid has come to be an accepted and established program. It is viewed as an essential complement to a market-oriented private health care industry in which access is critically dependent upon insurance coverage and ability to pay. Without major intervention by government, millions of poor people would go without needed health care or suffer severe financial hardship in obtaining care.

The acceptance and growth of governmental responsibility for assuring access to health care for the poor are linked in part to the contribution of health services research. This research has documented the extent and nature of health problems among the poor, barriers preventing access to the health care system and the implications for utilization of health services and health outcomes, and the effectiveness and efficiency of governmental health programs designed to improve access.

The national health policy process has also changed over time, providing an expanded forum for health services researchers. Congress and the executive branch have established units charged with developing and analyzing policy options. Special commissions and task forces established by public and private organizations have investigated the problems facing the poor and the effectiveness of alternative policy solutions. Advocacy groups have played an increasingly important role in promoting legislation expanding Medicaid coverage for the poor. These entities draw on data and research compiled by the health services research community in designing and articulating the case for policy initiatives.

Even in more recent times when pressures to restrict governmental health spending have been severe, programs for the poor have been relatively protected. This reflects in large part the documentation by health services research of the importance of assisting the poor in obtaining needed health care services, how well current programs are targeted on the poor, and the success of these programs in improving access to health care and health outcomes of the poor in an efficient manner.

In this chapter we document the contribution of health services research to policy regarding financing health care for the poor, especially Medicaid policy. We begin with a review of major Medicaid policy issues over the period from 1965 to 1990 and then review the findings of health services research with regard to the poor and their health care needs, the impact of governmental health programs on access to health services and health outcomes, and the program's overall effectiveness and efficiency. We conclude with our views on future policy directions for improving access to health care for the poor, and a discussion of research questions requiring further investigation.

Major Medicaid Policy Issues: 1965–1990

The Legislation

Medicaid was enacted in 1965 as Title XIX of the Social Security Act under P.L. 74–271, the Social Security Amendments of 1965. This legislation, signed into law by President Lyndon B. Johnson on July 30, 1965, included the Medicare program for the elderly. Medicaid was less extensively debated than Medicare; the former was viewed as an extension of the earlier Kerr-Mills legislation that provided assistance to states to pay health care providers for care of the poor (Stevens and Stevens, 1974). These so-called medical vendor payments began in 1950 for people on welfare and were expanded by the 1960 Kerr-Mills Act to "medically needy" aged. Medically needy aged were defined as persons aged 65 and over whose incomes exceeded the level that would have qualified them for cash assistance but who needed help paying for medical services.

Medicaid is a joint federal-state program under which the states provide medical benefits to low-income individuals who meet categorical criteria for eligibility as well as income and assets requirements. The federal government matches state payments according to a formula that varies inversely with the per capita income of the state. The federal government establishes minimum standards with regard to benefits and eligibility, but administration of the program, with fairly wide discretion, is left to the states.

Medicaid eligibility primarily follows the categorical criteria for welfare assistance: one-parent families with children, the elderly, and the disabled. States are required to extend Medicaid coverage to all recipients of cash assistance under Aid to Families with Dependent Children (AFDC), and to most elderly and disabled people who receive cash assistance from the Supplemental Security Income (SSI) program. States have the option of covering under AFDC, and therefore Medicaid, two-parent families in which both parents are unemployed. They also have the option of covering under Medicaid all children up to age 18 in families meeting state income standards (so-called "Ribicoff children" after Senator Abraham Ribicoff [D–Conn.], who offered this amendment). States have the option of covering medically needy families whose incomes net of medical expenses are within 133 percent of the income standard for AFDC and who meet the categorical requirements for welfare.

Variation among states in terms of Medicaid eligibility is greatest for poor children and families. Many poor families are not covered because state income standards for AFDC and Medicaid eligibility are well below the poverty level. One-third of the states have income standards below half the federal poverty level, and 85 percent have income standards below 75 percent of the poverty guideline (Congressional Research Service, 1988b). Many states do not extend coverage to two-parent families or to medically needy individuals who are impoverished by large medical expenses (CRS, 1988b). Federal legislative changes in recent years may lead to greater uniformity among states by extending Medicaid eligibility to additional groups—pregnant women, young children, elderly and disabled low-income people—and by tying eligibility income levels to the federal poverty level.

Medicaid coverage of the aged, blind, and disabled is more consistent nationally than coverage of poor children because the Supplemental Security Income cash assistance program has uniform national eligibility criteria, leaving states with less discretion. SSI income eligibility levels are set at 76 percent of poverty for single beneficiaries and 90 percent of poverty for married couples (Commonwealth Commission, 1987). Fourteen states do not extend Medicaid coverage to all SSI beneficiaries (CRS, 1988b). States have the option of supplementing federal SSI payments and may extend Medicaid to those SSI beneficiaries receiving only supplementary payments. Aged, blind, and disabled Medicaid beneficiaries are also generally eligible for care under Medicare and primarily use Medicaid to supplement acute care services financed by Medicare and to pay for long-term care.

Services covered by Medicaid also vary among states. All states cover hospital and physician services, but states often impose limits on the number of hospital days or physician visits covered during the year. The extent of coverage of other services also varies widely (CRS, 1988b). Payment levels and utilization controls on hospital and physician care also vary among states, making the scope of Medicaid benefits far from uniform. As a result, Medicaid neither covers all the poor nor provides those who are covered with comprehensive benefits.

Medicaid: 1965–1990

Medicaid's original goal was to encourage the states to provide comprehensive medical care coverage to the nation's poor (Davis and Schoen, 1978). From enactment in 1965 to 1971, expenditures grew rapidly from $1.6 billion to $6.3 billion, as states initiated their programs and expanded coverage (HCFA, 1986).

Amendments in 1967 expanded Medicaid coverage of preventive services for children and instituted the Early and Periodic Screening Diagnosis and Treatment (EPSDT) program (see Table 5–1 for more information on legislative changes in Medicaid over the period from 1965 to 1990). The 1972 Amendments to the Social Security Act provided the first major changes in Medicaid coverage. In response to some states' concern about the growing cost of the program, the goal of comprehensive coverage of the poor by Medicaid was eliminated. States were permitted to assess patients on welfare a charge for optional services and to assess medically needy patients a charge for both basic and optional services. The legislation also established Professional Standards Review Organizations (PSROs) to review the quality and necessity of care rendered to Medicaid and Medicare patients and instituted penalties for fraud and abuse.

At the same time, coverage of the aged, blind, and disabled was expanded as most states elected to provide Medicaid coverage to beneficiaries of the Supplemental Security Income (SSI) program, the new federal cash assistance for the aged, blind, and disabled. In addition, intermediate care facilities for the mentally retarded were added as a benefit. As a result, Medicaid spending increased at an annual rate of 25 percent from 1971 to 1975 (U.S. Department of Health and Human Services, HCFA, 1986).

By 1976, the Medicaid program had 22.9 million beneficiaries and expenditures of $14.1 billion (U.S. Department of Health and Human Services, HCFA, 1986). The years from 1976 to 1980 saw two major trends in Medicaid: a decline in program eligibility and a rapid increase in spending due to inflation. The decline in eligibility was partially a result of state failure to index income eligibility standards to inflation. By 1980, the number of people eligible for Medicaid had dropped to 21.6 million, but spending had increased to $23.3 billion. Rising prices and increased intensity of medical services accounted for almost all of the increase in Medicaid spending during this period—despite state efforts to institute cost containment measures.

In 1981, in response to both rapidly escalating program costs and a proposal by the Reagan administration to cap federal Medicaid expenditures, Medicaid entered a period of fiscal retrenchment (Rowland, Lyons, and Edwards, 1988). Medicaid is an open-ended entitlement program under which states pay for medical care services on behalf of eligible beneficiaries; the federal government matches state spending with no upper limit on what the federal government will match. The Reagan administration proposal would have ended the entitlement nature of Medicaid by placing an upper limit or "cap" on what the federal government would spend in any given year on Medicaid. State expenditures would only have been matched up to the federal maximum; once that fixed amount was reached, the states would be faced with the choice of cutting their Medicaid spending to stay within the federal limits or paying for the additional spending solely with state funds. If implemented, this cap would have resulted in an estimated cut of $9 billion in federal Medicaid spending from 1981 to 1985 (Iglehart, 1985).

Table 5-1. A brief legislative history of Medicaid

Year	Legislation	Provisions
1965	Social Security Amendments of 1965 (PL 89–97)	Established Medicare and Medicaid.
1967	Social Security Amendments of 1967 (PL 90–248)	Required coverage for children of Early and Periodic Screening, Diagnosis, and Treatment Services (EPSDT).
1972	Social Security Amendments of 1972 (PL 92–603)	Repeal of comprehensive coverage goal; instituted optional patient cost-sharing; limited federal participation for capital expenditures not approved by health planning agencies; improved federal matching for Medicaid management information systems; established penalties for fraud and abuse; established PSROs.
1981	Omnibus Budget Reconciliation Act of 1981 (OBRA 81) (PL 97–35)	Provided for reductions in federal Medicaid funding over the FY 1982–1984 period; modified hospital reimbursement requirements; permitted competitive bidding for laboratory services and medical devices; authorized agreements with prepaid entities other than federally qualified HMOs; modified requirements for medically needy programs; authorized "freedom-of-choice" waivers which can restrict providers from whom beneficiaries may receive services; authorized waivers for provision of home and community-based services to individuals who would otherwise require institutionalization.
1982	Tax Equity and Fiscal Responsibility Act of 1982 (TEFRA) (PL 97–248)	Facilitated coverage of home care for certain disabled children; modified groups of persons on whom copayments could be imposed by states; provided for replacement of PSROs with a new utilization and quality control peer review organization (PRO) program.
1984	Deficit Reduction Act of 1984 (DEFRA) (PL 98–369)	Legislation which began yearly expansions to coverage of certain groups of pregnant women and young children.

Table 5-1 (continued)

Year	Legislation	Provisions
1985	Consolidated Omnibus Budget Reconciliation Act of 1985 (COBRA) (PL 99–272)	Required states to provide coverage to pregnant women in two-parent families that meet AFDC standards even where the principal breadwinner was employed; required 60 days postpartum coverage of eligible pregnant women; allows optional coverage of hospice services.
1986	Omnibus Budget Reconciliation Act of 1986 (OBRA 86) (PL 99–509)	Provided optional coverage of pregnant women and infants up to age 1, and on an incremental basis, children up to age 5 with family incomes below a state-established level (between AFDC level and 100 percent of federal poverty line); provided optional coverage of either buy-in or full benefits to poor elderly and disabled people; mandated coverage of eligible homeless people; allowed presumptive eligibility for pregnant women.
1987	Omnibus Budget Reconciliation Act of 1987 (OBRA 87) (PL 100–203)	Permitted acceleration of coverage of poor pregnant women and children up to age 5; established option to cover pregnant women and infants up to 185 percent of poverty; required coverage of children up to age 7 who meet AFDC eligibility; established a separate home and community-based waiver for elderly; revised nursing home quality requirements.
1988	Medicare Catastrophic Coverage Act of 1988	Mandated coverage of pregnant women and infants with incomes below 100 percent of poverty; mandated buy-in coverage of Medicare beneficiaries with incomes below 100 percent of poverty.
1988	Family Support Act of 1988	Required states to extend Medicaid coverage for 12 months to families who lose cash assistance because of earnings; required states to extend Medicaid coverage to two-parent families where the principal breadwinner is unemployed.

Table 5-1 (continued)

Year	Legislation	Provisions
1989	Omnibus Budget Reconciliation Act of 1989 (OBRA 89)	Mandated state coverage of pregnant women and children up to age 6 with incomes up to 133 percent of poverty; specified that payment for obstetrical and pediatric services be sufficient to ensure access to providers; established standards for EPSDT services and for follow-up treatment.

Sources: Congressional Research Service, May 1986, Summary of Enacted Health Legislation 1959–1985, Report no. 86–113 EPW; Congressional Research Service, July 24, 1984, Medicaid Legislative History, Program Description, and Major Issues, Report no. 84–140 EPW; Committee on Ways and Means, March 1988, Background Material and Data on Programs within the Jurisdiction of the Committee on Ways and Means, 1988 edition (Washington, D.C.: U.S. Government Printing Office); Committee on Ways and Means, 1989, Background Material and Data on Programs within the Jurisdiction of the Committee on Ways and Means, 1989 edition (Washington, D.C.: U.S. Government Printing Office).

Congress did not enact the Medicaid cap proposal. Strong opposition from the states as well as from advocates of the poor and health care providers saved the entitlement nature of Medicaid. The states were concerned that a ceiling on federal spending would result in pressure for additional spending of state dollars to compensate for federal reductions. Advocates were concerned that a spending ceiling would limit the scope of program coverage and lead to an erosion in benefits and eligibility. Both groups argued that the Reagan administration's proposed cap represented an abandonment of the federal government's commitment to help finance medical care for the poor. Their arguments, coupled with growing recognition of the importance of Medicaid financing for the poor, ultimately persuaded Congress to retain the existing structure of Medicaid.

However, the drive to cut federal spending meant that although the structure of Medicaid was preserved, it was not protected from deep spending cuts. The Omnibus Budget Reconciliation Act (OBRA) of 1981 imposed a temporary reduction in the federal share of Medicaid spending in each state of up to 3 percent in 1982. In 1983, the reduction level increased to 4 percent and in 1984 to 4.5 percent. States were able to offset some of the reductions by meeting quantitative targets for cost containment or having an all-payor rate-setting program. It is estimated that these reductions cut federal Medicaid spending by more than $4 billion from 1980 through 1984 (House Committee on Energy and Commerce, 1986). OBRA also reduced Medicaid eligibility indirectly by restricting AFDC coverage for the working poor. It further eliminated AFDC coverage for young people of ages 19 and 20 living at home. These provisions had the effect of removing almost one million Medicaid beneficiaries from coverage (Swartz, 1988; Rowland, Lyons, and Edwards, 1988).

Along with reduced federal aid, the OBRA legislation gave states greater flexibility over the scope and design of their Medicaid programs in order to provide additional options to reduce program spending. Much of this new authority concerned state discretion over provider payment and ability to restrict use of services by beneficiaries. Specifically, the OBRA legislation gave states new authority over hospital payment under Medicaid and allowed states to experiment with alternative delivery systems as a means of restructuring care to reduce expenditures. Before 1981, states had been required to pay hospitals using the Medicare principles of hospital payment. States were allowed to apply for permission to use alternative payment systems, but the process was cumbersome and few states implemented alternative systems. In addition, states gained additional authority to experiment with alternatives to fee-for-service payment for physicians involving case management, capitated payment, and limitations on freedom of choice of physicians or other health care providers. With the new authority, states could design prepaid enrollment systems for the poor without being constrained by the requirements associated with federally qualified HMOs.

After OBRA81, Medicaid continued to be a target for restructuring and deep cuts in each of the Reagan budgets. However, after 1981 the Congress protected the program from major legislative cutbacks and did not extend the temporary reductions in federal matching share after they expired in 1984. Thus, by 1984, federal program financing had been restored to its former matching rate.

Despite the economic recession in 1981 and the high levels of unemployment as well as the increased number of people living in poverty, the states did not permit the number of people covered by Medicaid to increase. One study found that although poverty among children increased 35 percent between 1979 and 1983, the number of children on Medicaid increased by only 4 percent (Swartz, 1988). Similarly, although poverty among women of ages 18 to 40 increased 60 percent, the number of young women on Medicaid increased by only 20 percent.

Overall from 1980 to 1985, Medicaid eligibility increased only modestly from 21.6 to 21.7 million beneficiaries, but expenditures grew from $23.3 billion in 1980 to $37.5 billion in 1985 (U.S. Department of Health and Human Services, HCFA, 1986). The annual rate of increase in Medicaid expenditures during this period was 8 percent. Price increases accounted for a 10 percent annual rate of increase, but expenditures were moderated by a 2 percent decrease in Medicaid utilization—reflecting increased state efforts to contain costs through limits on benefits and restricted access to health care for Medicaid beneficiaries (Muse, 1987).

Beginning in 1983, congressional attitudes toward Medicaid began to shift. Democrats gained seats in the Congress in the 1982 elections and began to mount more effective opposition to Reagan administration proposals. A growing consensus developed that cuts in programs for the poor had gone too far and that the "safety net" of programs assisting the poor needed to be protected. The deep recession of 1981–1982 and increased unemployment and poverty intensified this concern—as well as disturbing new data showing that access to health care and the health of the poor were beginning to deteriorate (American Academy of Pediatrics, 1982).

Beginning in 1984 Congress responded to heightened concern about infant mortality and poor child health by amending Medicaid annually to expand coverage of poor pregnant women and children. These expansions in Medicaid coverage increased the number of Medicaid beneficiaries from 21.7 million in 1985 to 24.2 million in 1988. Medicaid program costs were estimated to increase to $55.1 billion for 1988 (U.S. Congress, House Ways and Means, 1989).

The expansion of Medicaid eligibility to poor pregnant women, children, and the elderly and disabled in the 1980s is the most important of the Medicaid changes in its 25-year history. The initial impetus for this expanded coverage began during the Carter administration with the proposal in February 1977 of a Child Health Assurance Plan (CHAP), to expand Medicaid to poor pregnant women and children (U.S. Department of Health, Education, and Welfare, 1977). This plan was developed in the early days of the Carter administration as part of its revision of the Ford Fiscal Year 1978 Budget. The proposal was an outgrowth of earlier work by Karen Davis (Davis, 1973 and 1976) documenting gaps in care for poor children. Secretary Joseph A. Califano, Jr., a long-time advocate of Medicare and Medicaid, embraced the proposal as a way to put the stamp of the Carter administration on a revised budget that would reflect a concern with improving access to health care for the poor—rather than the Ford budget's preoccupation with cutting federal budgetary outlays.

The CHAP proposal was seriously considered by the Congress and was expanded during congressional consideration to include a minimum eligibility standard based on the federal poverty level, coverage of pregnant women and children up to age 18, expanded benefits for mental health and dental care, and minimum standards on payment of pediatric services (U.S. Congress Committee on Interstate and Foreign Commerce, 1979). The Carter administration expanded its 1979 bill to include a minimum income standard tied to the federal poverty level and other provisions developed during legislative consideration in 1977–1978 (Davis, 1979). This legislation was eventually stalled, however, over a controversial amendment in the House of Representatives to ban funding for abortions.

In 1983 the American Public Health Association (APHA) urged Congress to expand Medicaid by establishing a minimum income eligibility level for pregnant women and children linked to the poverty level and to mandate coverage of all pregnant women and children meeting state AFDC income standards or the minimum income eligibility level (Davis, 1983). Henry Waxman (D–Cal.), chairman of the Subcommittee on Health and the Environment, agreed to put forward a bill, following the earlier Carter CHAP proposal but focused primarily upon Medicaid eligibility expansions. The bill laid out a blueprint for year-by-year incremental additions to expand Medicaid eligibility. With the support of numerous interest groups concerned with the health of children, particularly the Children's Defense Fund and the American Academy of Pediatrics, Medicaid legislation was enacted in 1984 to expand coverage to additional groups of poor pregnant women, children, and elderly and disabled people.

The Deficit Reduction Act of 1984 (DEFRA) required states to cover eligible pregnant women from the time of pregnancy verification and to cover pregnant women in families with an unemployed head and children born after September 30, 1983, up to age 5 in families with incomes below the AFDC income and asset standards. This legislation was followed by the Consolidated Budget Reconciliation Act of 1985 (COBRA), which expanded the requirement that all pregnant women in families meeting the AFDC income and asset standards be covered from the time of pregnancy verification through 60 days postpartum regardless of the employment or welfare status of the family.

In the Omnibus Reconciliation Act of 1986 (OBRA86), Congress made federal Medicaid matching funds available if states, at their option, expanded coverage to pregnant women and children up to age 5 and to elderly and disabled individuals with incomes up to the federal poverty level. This was the first important legislative action to link eligibility explicitly to the federal poverty level, and it represented the first important step away from the welfare eligibility nature of Medicaid.

In 1987, Congress included provisions in the Omnibus Reconciliation Act (OBRA87) that permitted states to increase coverage for pregnant women and infants up to 185 percent of the poverty level. It also raised the age of coverage of children in requiring states to extend Medicaid coverage to all children meeting AFDC income standards under age 7 (with the option for states to cover under age 8) and also gave states the option of covering all children below the poverty level up to age 8.

The Medicare Catastrophic Coverage Act of 1988 further expanded Medicaid by requiring state Medicaid programs to pay the Medicare premium, deductibles, and coinsurance for all Medicare elderly and disabled beneficiaries with incomes below the poverty line. The states were also required to cover all pregnant women and children under age one below the poverty line on a phased-in basis. Although this law was subsequently repealed in 1989, the Medicaid provisions were left intact.

In 1989 the Omnibus Reconciliation Act mandated state coverage of pregnant women and children up to age 6 with family incomes up to 133 percent of the federal poverty level, effective April 1, 1990. In addition, it specified that payment for obstetrical and pediatric services must be sufficient to enlist enough providers so that covered services will be as accessible to Medicaid beneficiaries as to the general population, and it established standards on Early Periodic Screening, Diagnosis, and Treatment (EPSDT) services for children and follow-up treatment of conditions detected in children undergoing screening. These provisions regarding payment and comprehensiveness of preventive care services followed the provisions developed in consideration of the Carter Child Health Assurance bills in the late 1970s.

Thus, in an incremental fashion, the states have been encouraged or required to add additional needy individuals to Medicaid coverage. The pattern is clearly to raise the age of coverage of children over time so that poor children born after September 30, 1983, remain eligible for

Medicaid as they grow older. Medicaid eligibility has also been extended to many near-poor pregnant women and young children. In addition, Congress has balanced expanded coverage for poor pregnant women and young children with expanded coverage for poor elderly and disabled persons.

Other Medicaid changes improved coverage of certain groups of disabled individuals. The Tax Equity and Fiscal Responsibility Act of 1982 (TEFRA) allowed states to extend Medicaid coverage to certain disabled children under age 18 who were living at home and would be eligible for SSI if they were institutionalized. OBRA86 required states to continue Medicaid coverage for disabled persons with severe impairments who lost their eligibility for cash assistance because of earnings from work. While not explicitly expanding coverage to the homeless, OBRA86 clarified the fact that an individual without a permanent or fixed address who met other requirements for eligibility could not be excluded from coverage.

Contribution of Health Services Research to Medicaid Policy Issues

Acceptance of Medicaid

One of the first contributions of health services research to Medicaid policy was the literature documenting the effectiveness and efficiency of the program. Perceptions of the program in its early years were clouded by expenditures that rose far more rapidly than had initially been projected, reports of abuse of the program by some beneficiaries and health care providers, and a general feeling that the program was excessively expensive (Davis, 1973, 1976; Freund, 1984; Holahan, 1978; Mitchell and Cromwell, 1980; Reinhardt, 1985; Spiegel, 1979).

Although it was certainly true that the cost of Medicaid exceeded initial expectations, careful analysis of the program's expenditures revealed the fact that the initial growth in Medicaid expenditures was largely attributable to growth in number of beneficiaries as those eligible enrolled in the program, as well as to increases in general medical care inflation. Medicaid expenditures per person did not exceed comparable costs of health care for the general population (Blendon and Moloney, 1982; Davis and Schoen, 1978; Rogers, Blendon, and Moloney, 1982). This helped make the point that Medicaid was costly because health care was costly, and not because of any flaws specific to the program (Moloney, 1982). Moreover, early research documented the overall impact of the program in improving access to health care for those it covered, particularly access to ambulatory physician services and to preventive care (Aday and Andersen, 1984; Aday, Andersen, and Fleming, 1980; Blendon and Moloney, 1982; Congressional Budget Office, 1981; Davis, 1976; Davis and Reynolds, 1976; Davis and Schoen, 1978; Rabin and Schach, 1975; Rogers and Blendon, 1977; Rogers, Blendon, and Moloney, 1982).

Criticism of the program then began to shift to its failure to cover all of the poor in need of health care. The failure of states to index income eligibility levels to inflation came in for particular criticism (Rowland and Gaus, 1982). This criticism gained force when more sophisticated studies began to document the adverse health consequences of the lack of health insurance coverage for the poor (Braveman et al., 1989; Lurie et al., 1984).

Medicaid Expansion to Poor Pregnant Women and Children

The Medicaid policy changes in the 1980s that expanded coverage to additional groups of poor pregnant women and children were a direct result of a significant body of health services research. One of the most important contributions of this research was simply documenting the fact that large numbers of poor children were not covered by Medicaid. The research showed that children are more likely to be uninsured than adults, and that Medicaid reaches only about half of all children in poverty (Burwell and Rymer, 1987; Butler, Winter, et al., 1985; Congressional Budget Office, 1979; Congressional Research Service, 1988a, 1988b; Davis, 1975; Davis and Rowland, 1983; Davis and Schoen, 1978; Kasper, 1986a, 1986b; Rosenbach, 1985; Schoen, 1984; Short, Cantor, and Monheit, 1988; Swartz, 1988; Walden, Wilensky, and Kasper, 1985).

Research also documented the fact that the absence of health insurance coverage led to lower utilization of physician services and preventive care (Davis and Schoen, 1978; Davis and Rowland, 1983; Freeman et al., 1987; Gortmaker, 1981; Howell, 1988; Kasper, 1986a, 1986b; Kleinman, Gold, and Makuc, 1981; Newacheck, 1988; Orr and Miller, 1981; President's Commission on Ethics, 1983; Rowland and Lyons, 1989a; Wilensky and Berk, 1982). For example, low-income children without Medicaid coverage were more likely to go without physician care (32.6 percent) than those with Medicaid coverage (24.8 percent) (Rosenbach, 1985). Low-income children without either private health insurance or Medicaid were the least likely to receive physician care (36.3 percent).

Perhaps the most significant research contributing to a major policy change in coverage was literature documenting the importance of prenatal care for reducing infant mortality (Institute of Medicine, 1985). The report on preventing low birth weight in infants by the Institute of Medicine was a particularly important contribution to the policy debate. This report, which synthesized research from a number of studies, demonstrated that investment in prenatal care would save three dollars for every one dollar spent by reducing the costs associated with low-birth-weight infants. Prenatal care was important in counseling pregnant women regarding smoking and nutrition during pregnancy, as well as in detecting medical conditions such as hypertension and anemia that lead to premature births if not treated early in pregnancy (Griffith and Cislowski, 1986). Other studies documented gaps in health insurance coverage for maternity care and inadequacies in prenatal care (Alan Guttmacher Institute, 1987; U.S. General Accounting Office, 1987; Rosenbaum and Hughes, 1988). This research made a compelling case for the expansion of coverage of pregnant women under Medicaid to ensure adequate financial access to prenatal care and delivery.

The impact of the IOM report was further amplified by the release of a number of reports by public agencies and private organizations that called for action to improve health insurance coverage for pregnant women and young children. One of the most influential was a report of the Southern Governors' Association on infant mortality (SGA, 1985), as well as reports by the House Ways and Means Committee (U.S. Congress Committee on Ways and Means, 1985), the House Select Committee on Children (U.S. Congress Select Committee on Children, 1985), and the Children's Defense Fund (CDF, 1985).

The expansion of Medicaid to young children was also precipitated by research on the importance of preventive health care in childhood— including the areas of immunization, vision, hearing, nutrition, development, and dental screening (Axnick, Shavell, and Witte, 1969; Berwick and Komaroff, 1982; Butler, Winter, et al., 1985; Office of Technology Assessment, 1988; Rosenbaum and Johnson, 1986). Research on the effectiveness of medical interventions for children served to underscore the importance of ensuring access to health care for children (Starfield, 1985a, 1985b). This research also appealed to the rationale that investment in the health of children would pay dividends to the nation in the form of increased economic productivity as well as reduced future health care outlays.

Other research provided estimates of the cost of expanding Medicaid coverage (Congressional Research Service, 1988a; Thorpe, Siegel, and Dailey, 1989; Torres and Kenney, 1989). These studies helped policy officials understand the fiscal implications of expanded Medicaid coverage and the cost trade-offs of expanded coverage of different groups of low-income persons.

Medicaid has also been expanded in recent years to certain groups of disabled children. Again, health services research has made a major contribution by estimating the number of children with varying levels of disability, assessing their need for different types of health and social services, describing current utilization and cost of acute health care services received by children with chronic conditions, depicting financial burdens on families, and highlighting the inadequacy of Medicaid and private health insurance to meet the needs of this vulnerable population (Butler, Budetti, et al., 1985; Butler, Rosenbaum, and Palfrey, 1987; Gortmaker and Sappenfield, 1984; Iryes, 1981; Newacheck, 1987; Newacheck and McManus, 1988; Office of Technology Assessment, 1987; Perrin, 1985; Rowland, 1989). Studies pointing out the marked variation across states in Medicaid services for disabled children led to greater policy support for federal standards applicable to all states (Fox and Yoshpe, 1987; Rymer and Adler, 1987).

Medicaid Expansion to Poor Medicare Beneficiaries

The states were permitted to expand Medicaid benefits to all poor elderly and disabled persons with incomes below the federal poverty level in OBRA86. In part this policy change was based on the desire to alleviate the financial hardship of the poor elderly and to assure that states improved Medicaid coverage simultaneously for poor children and poor elderly people. In part it was based on research demonstrating that only a small fraction of the elderly poor were covered by Medicaid, and that as a consequence many poor and near-poor elderly faced serious barriers to the receipt of necessary health care or incurred excessive financial burdens in obtaining acute health care services (Commonwealth

Fund Commission, 1987; Davis, 1986; Davis and Rowland, 1986, 1990; Rowland and Lyons, 1989b). Research documented that the burden of illness is a serious problem for low-income elderly people. They are more likely than higher-income elderly people to be in fair or poor health, since chronic illness is much more common among poor elderly people. Those with chronic conditions often require medications or supplies that are not included in Medicare benefits (Commonwealth Fund Commission, 1987).

Medicare provides basic health insurance protection for hospital and physician services for nearly all elderly people. However, for many of the elderly, Medicare coverage is an essential but inadequate protection against burdensome medical bills. First, Medicare requires beneficiaries to pay a premium ($398 per year in 1989) for coverage under the physician services component of Medicare (Part B). Second, Medicare requires substantial cost sharing for covered services, including a hospital deductible ($560 per year in 1989), a physician deductible ($75 per year), and 20 percent coinsurance on all physician charges allowed by Medicare, plus any excess charges for those physicians who do not accept Medicare assignment. In addition, Medicare does not cover many acute care services such as prescription drugs, dental care, eyeglasses, hearing aids, and other services. Medicare covers only very limited long-term care services, including limited stays in skilled nursing homes and home health services for elderly people recovering from an acute health problem. As a result, Medicare picks up less than half of all medical expenses of the elderly (U.S. Congress Committee on Ways and Means, 1989).

Gaps in Medicare benefits have led many elderly to purchase private health insurance, or MediGap policies, to supplement Medicare. About 72 percent of all elderly persons purchase private health insurance or have it provided by former employers as a retirement benefit (Commonwealth Fund Commission, 1987). However, only 42 percent of the poor elderly and 65 percent of the near-poor elderly have private supplementary policies, and they are much more likely to purchase these policies themselves rather than having them provided by former employers than are higher-income elderly. As a result, they can incur substantial financial burdens in meeting premium payments.

Medicaid is an important supplement to Medicare for many poor and near-poor elderly people. About 3.2 million aged persons qualify for Medicaid benefits (Congressional Research Service, 1988b). For these individuals, Medicaid pays the Medicare premiums and cost-sharing requirements. In many states, elderly Medicaid beneficiaries also receive coverage for prescription drugs, dental care, and nursing home services. For the few elderly poor who are not covered by Medicare (for example, immigrants without sufficient work history to qualify for Social Security and Medicare), Medicaid provides basic health care coverage.

Studies have shown, however, that the impression that Medicaid supplements Medicare for all poor elderly people is false. Only 29 percent of poor elderly people and 8 percent of the near-poor elderly have Medicaid coverage (Commonwealth Fund Commission, 1987). Qualifying for Medicaid is linked to eligibility for SSI and shares all the problems and complexities of that system. Medicaid eligibility, moreover, is determined in part by state rules, and states vary widely in their coverage of the poor and near-poor elderly. As a result, Medicaid coverage of the aged poor and near-poor varies widely by state despite the uniform standards of the SSI program. Eleven states cover not only virtually all of the aged poor but also some near-poor, while 39 states do not even cover all of the aged poor (Davis, 1986). All but 14 states provide Medicaid coverage to all SSI beneficiaries (Congressional Research Service, 1988b).

Research has also documented that the absence of coverage supplemental to Medicare results in reduced access to health care services. Low-income elderly people who have no Medicaid or MediGap insurance to supplement Medicare use less medical care than those with more comprehensive coverage. Even adjusting for differences in health status, those relying only on Medicare to pay their bills receive less medical care. For example, poor elderly people in fair or poor health without Medicaid see physicians 25 percent less frequently than similar poor elderly people with Medicaid (Commonwealth Fund Commission, 1987).

Studies have also shown that for poor and near-poor elderly people, out-of-pocket costs are a substantial burden. In 1986, such estimated spending was more than 10 percent of income for poor and near-poor elderly people. Medicaid coverage substantially alters the financial burden of medical expenses for this group. Poor elderly people without Medicaid coverage spend more than twice as much for out-of-pocket expenses, twice as much for prescription drugs, and 50 percent more for physician services than poor elderly people with Medicaid (Commonwealth Fund Commission, 1987).

For many near-poor elderly people, medical expenses can reduce meager incomes to levels that, in effect, shift them into poverty. In 1987, 12 percent of elderly Americans had incomes below the federal poverty threshold. However, the impact of out-of-pocket spending for medical care is not included in the official poverty calculations. When medical expenses are considered and deducted from available income, 17 percent of elderly Americans are living on incomes below the poverty threshold (Commonwealth Fund Commission, 1987). Many near-poor elderly people are, in fact, the hidden poor. One-third of this group are reduced to poverty by their out-of-pocket payments for medical care (Commonwealth Fund Commission, 1987). To a large extent these payments are for insurance premiums to ensure protection against unexpected or large medical expenses. Medicare premiums and payments to purchase private MediGap coverage account for 40 percent of out-of-pocket spending by the medically impoverished. However, without the Medicare Part B or MediGap coverage, the out-of-pocket spending for direct medical services would be even greater. Finally, near-poor elderly people who are impoverished by their medical out-of-pocket spending are more likely to be in poor or fair health than nonimpoverished near-poor elderly people, with their medical care spending accounting for, on average, more than 20 percent of income (Commonwealth Fund Commission, 1987).

This research was instrumental in convincing the Congress to take firmer steps to expand Medicaid coverage to poor elderly people. By March 1988, only the District of Columbia, Florida, and New Jersey had elected to provide Medicaid coverage for poor aged and disabled persons permitted under the OBRA86 legislation (Congressional Research Service, 1988b). Florida provided coverage for persons below 90 percent of poverty, while the District of Columbia and New Jersey provided coverage up to 100 percent of poverty.

In 1988, therefore, Congress required states to "buy-in," through the Medicaid program, Medicare coverage for all beneficiaries with incomes below the poverty level. Specifically, states are required to pay Medicare premiums, deductibles, and coinsurance for elderly and disabled enrollees whose incomes are at or below the poverty level and whose assets are at or below twice the resources standard used in the SSI program. This provision was included in the Medicare Catastrophic Health Care Coverage Act and was to be phased in over time. By January 1989 the states were required to cover persons with incomes at or below 85 percent of poverty; by January 1, 1990, 90 percent of poverty; by January 1, 1991, 95 percent of poverty; and by January 1, 1992, states are required to cover all persons with incomes at or below 100 percent of poverty (Congressional Research Service, 1988b). A somewhat slower phase-in schedule applies to Section 209b states. Under this provision the states are only required to pick up Medicare premiums and cost sharing; they are not required to provide full Medicaid benefits including supplemental services such as prescription drugs, dental care, eyeglasses, and hearing aids.

This provision, which was not repealed by action of the Congress in November 1989, is an important expansion of Medicaid to poor elderly persons. However, it fails to provide complete Medicaid benefits to this group, and it does not address the impoverishment that medical expenses can inflict on the near-poor.

Medicaid Cost Containment and Managed Care

Fiscal Pressures on States. The major policy issue facing the Medicaid program since its inception is how to curb its rapid rate of increase in expenditures. Research documented that the growth in Medicaid expenditures in the early years was largely attributable to expansion of enrollment. Inflation in the health care sector for all patients helped assuage policy concerns that the program was inefficient, wasteful, or exceptionally subject to abuse. However, the unanticipated financial drain represented by the program has led to ongoing attempts—particularly at the state government level—to institute cost saving measures. Health services research has been particularly important in assessing the effectiveness of these measures.

Throughout the 1970s the states attempted to cut Medicaid outlays by imposing restrictions on benefits, not indexing income eligibility levels to inflation, holding down provider payment rates, especially for physicians, and experimenting with HMOs and cost sharing to reduce Medicaid beneficiary utilization of services (Blendon and Moloney, 1982). Attempts to impose cost sharing on welfare patients on an experimental basis were opposed and eventually defeated on the grounds that they represented experimentation with human subjects without their informed consent (*Crane vs. Matthews,* 42 USCA 1315). Extensive experimentation with placing Medicaid beneficiaries in HMOs in California in the early 1970s was particularly controversial. Scandals and instances in which Medicaid patients were denied essential care eventually led to reduced reliance on this approach to curtail costs.

The pressure to cut Medicaid spending became especially strong in 1981 when the Reagan administration took office with a public mandate to decrease taxes and cut federal nondefense domestic spending (Blendon and Moloney, 1982). In response to reduced federal support for Medicaid and other domestic programs as well as their own economic and budgetary problems, many states cut back or altered their Medicaid programs and also achieved saving by instituting changes in provider payment levels and methods and by instituting managed care features in their Medicaid programs (Rowland, Lyons, and Edwards, 1988).

The Medicaid programs in the various states have undergone significant changes in response to the federal financing cutbacks as well as to state fiscal problems (Bovbjerg and Holahan, 1982; Feder and Holahan, 1985; Holahan and Cohen, 1986). With the enactment of the Omnibus Budget Reconciliation Act of 1981, states had to accept a temporary reduction in federal financial support as the price for greater flexibility over program design. Many responded to the federal reductions by enacting cuts in their programs instead of making up the difference with state revenues.

Benefit and Eligibility Cutbacks. Restrictions on eligibility and benefits are, on the surface, a direct and easily designed method to reduce state expenditures under Medicaid. Limits on income eligibility standards, coverage of optional groups, and amount of covered services are familiar strategies to states seeking to constrain costs. Most states turned to these familiar techniques when fiscal pressures and federal cutbacks made reduced spending a top priority in 1981. Many also turned to new ways to pay for hospital care and alternative delivery systems to supplement the saving that could be achieved from direct cuts in eligibility and benefits (Bachman, Altman, and Beatrice, 1988; Bachman, Beatrice, and Altman, 1987).

For poor children and their families, Medicaid provides for most acute medical care as well as long-term care services. The states have substantial freedom to determine the range and level of benefits but are required to cover inpatient and outpatient hospital services, physician services, laboratory and X-ray services, family planning, screening and diagnostic services for children, and home health and nursing home care in skilled nursing facilities for adults (Congressional Research Service, 1988b). States can elect to provide other services including prescription drugs, dental care, and nursing home care in intermediate care facilities.

States can restrict the use of required and optional benefits by limiting the numbers of physician visits or days of hospital care, or by imposing utilization controls or nominal copayments. Prior to the OBRA81 legislation, restrictions on benefits were the major way in which states tried to limit Medicaid utilization and costs. During the 1980–1985 period, states continued to utilize benefit restrictions to restrain costs, but now coupled these restrictions with payment limits on providers and new delivery mechanisms (Davis, Anderson, Rowland, and Steinberg, 1990).

For hospital care, states can employ two types of benefit limitations: a limit on the number of days of hospital care covered per admission or per year, and a requirement for prior authorization for specific procedures or elective surgery. Prior authorization is a more popular approach, with 22 states now imposing such limits as compared to 12 states in 1980. From 1980 to 1986, the number of states imposing some limit on the range of services that can be provided and the locational setting increased from 14 to 43 states. In 1986, only 4 states (Maine, Massachusetts, North Dakota and South Dakota) were without any inpatient hospital utilization controls (U.S. Department of Health and Human Services, HCFA, 1987).

Limitations on physician services and hospital days are also common state cost-containment strategies. Limits on covered days of service mean that when hospitals treat Medicaid patients, the full cost of care may not be recovered if the patient's care requirements exceed the limits of Medicaid coverage. The excess would become uncompensated care and counted as bad debt or charity care.

Hospital Payment Limits. The most direct way to reduce Medicaid spending for hospital care is to limit the amount hospitals are paid for care to Medicaid beneficiaries. However, from the enactment of Medicaid in 1965 until the Omnibus Budget Reconciliation Act of 1981, state Medicaid programs had only limited control over hospital payments. States were required to use the Medicare principles of reimbursement on the basis of reasonable costs as the method to determine payments to hospitals for services to Medicaid beneficiaries.

The close link between Medicare and Medicaid policy for hospital payment resulted in Medicaid hospital payment levels that were comparable to those of Medicare and private insurers. As a result, hospitals did not face the kinds of reductions in payment levels under Medicaid that physicians had encountered since the early seventies, when states attempted to contain Medicaid costs by freezing physician payment levels or setting the levels well below private rates.

With the passage of OBRA in 1981, Congress removed the requirement that a waiver was needed to decouple Medicaid hospital payment from Medicare reasonable cost principles. States were given more flexibility to develop and implement new Medicaid hospital payment methods as long as those payments were reasonable and adequate to meet the costs of efficiently and economically operated facilities. The payment levels were to take into account the circumstances of hospitals that served a disproportionate number of low-income patients and were to be sufficient to ensure that Medicaid patients would have reasonable access to services of adequate quality (Bovbjerg and Holahan, 1982).

These conditions were intended to protect hospitals, especially public hospitals, serving large numbers of the poor by requiring states to give special consideration to such facilities in their payment methodologies. This provision meant that states could set payment rates that were independent of the costs of any particular hospital and that were not related to increases in the costs of goods and services purchased by the hospitals. Prior to OBRA81, the Health Care Financing Administration would not have approved such alternate plans. In addition to modifying the conditions for approval, OBRA81 also streamlined the HCFA approval process for alternative plans to make state changes faster and easier to implement.

Implementation of the 1981 OBRA hospital payment provisions by the states was accelerated by the changes in Medicare hospital payment enacted in 1982 and 1983. In 1982 TEFRA set a ceiling on Medicare hospital payment levels, and in 1983 Congress enacted the Medicare prospective payment system using DRGs to replace payment on a cost basis. The Medicare hospital payment changes meant that many states could no longer rely on Medicare payment methodology to avoid revisions to their own Medicaid hospital payment systems. With the implementation of prospective payment for hospitals under Medicare, most states moved to develop their own payment methodology for Medicaid. All the new plans were directed solely at Medicaid hospital payments and did not tie Medicaid to all-payor reforms as most of the earlier alternative systems had done, and as many health policy analysts recommended (Cohen, 1982; Vladeck, 1982). By 1986, only 16 states continued to use the Medicare principles of reasonable cost reimbursement as their Medicaid payment policy (U.S. Department of Health and Human Services, HCFA, 1987). Twenty-four states developed new plans between 1980 and 1986. Both California and Michigan, with alternative Medicaid plans approved prior to 1981, implemented new payment methodologies in January 1982 under the new OBRA authority (Bovbjerg and Holahan, 1982).

In general, the new payment plans implemented after the OBRA81 legislation appear to have slowed the growth of hospital expenditures in the short time since their implementation. One study shows that average annual growth in hospital expenditures in states with new payment methods dropped from 15.7 percent from 1979 to 1981 to 8.5 percent from 1981 to 1983 (Cromwell and Hurdle, 1984). The states that implemented new systems did not restrain cost increases quite as well as the states that changed their hospital payment systems prior to OBRA81 legislation, but they did hold cost increases lower than the states that continued to use Medicare methods of reimbursement.

Medicaid hospital policy changes appear to have been effective in reducing the growth in expenditures per beneficiary from 3.8 percent from 1978 to 1981 to less than one (0.9) percent from 1981 to 1984 (Holahan, 1987). When aged, blind, and disabled beneficiaries who are covered by both Medicare and Medicaid are excluded, real growth in hospital spending per beneficiary fell to zero percent during this period.

However, differences appear to exist in the relative effectiveness of reimbursement methods. All-payor rate-setting has achieved lower rates of growth in total hospital expenditures, lower levels of cost per day and cost per admission, and a reduction in labor intensity over other methods (Cromwell and Kanak, 1982; Kidder and Sullivan, 1982; Zuckerman and Holahan, 1988). States that use all-payor rate-setting are able to force down hospital prices for all payors, so growth in total expenditures may decline further than in states relying solely on Medicaid hospital payment systems. The states with payment systems that only apply to Medicaid may be more successful in containing Medicaid outlays than in curtailing the rate of growth in hospital expenditures overall. Over the longer term, hospitals' willingness to provide quality care to Medicaid beneficiaries may be markedly reduced in those states that restrict Medicaid hospital payments but do not effectively control the growth in total hospital costs.

In sum, the states have embarked on new and often untested

approaches to hospital payment reform ranging from minor modifications in cost reimbursement to prospective payment on the basis of case mix. Given the recent nature of many of these changes, very little is known about the impact. However, the decoupling of the Medicaid payment levels from those of Medicare has the potential for creating differentials between the rates Medicaid pays for care of the poor and the payment rates for those who are on Medicare or are privately insured. If Medicaid rates drop significantly below the market rate for hospital care, these payment methods could have deleterious effects on access to hospital services by the poor and may cause serious financial problems for the providers who care for a high volume of poor patients.

Managed Care. As the states have looked for new ways to restrain costs, restructuring the provision of care in a more cost-effective manner has emerged as a potential solution to the difficult choices confronting most states (Spitz, 1982). The Medicaid population's use of hospital emergency rooms for routine care and relatively high inpatient hospital admission rates and lengths of stay have led some states to explore various forms of managed care. In a managed-care situation, the Medicaid beneficiary no longer has full freedom of choice of provider. Instead, a medical care provider or organization arranges and coordinates all care.

Providing Medicaid beneficiaries with a physician or other provider who can provide continuity and coordination of care is viewed as a way of both improving quality of care and constraining costs. Health maintenance organizations (HMOs) and other prepaid care systems as well as "case management" systems that link the Medicaid enrollee with a specific provider or set of providers are models of managed care. It is argued that, if effective, these systems of care could help to stretch limited state dollars for care of the poor.

Before 1981, individual Medicaid beneficiaries were assured freedom of choice in the selection of (qualified) providers. As part of the increased flexibility given to the states in OBRA81, Congress authorized the states to experiment with alternative methods of organizing and delivering care that included limiting care to a specified set of providers. OBRA81 permitted states to apply to the Health Care Financing Administration for "freedom of choice" waivers. With such a waiver, the state was permitted to limit the number and types of providers that a Medicaid beneficiary could select for care and to "lock-in" the beneficiary to a single provider entity for a given period of time. This change permitted states to use case management and prepaid care systems for their Medicaid population.

The 1981 legislative changes also broadened the definition of an HMO as a Medicaid provider and relaxed the requirements on states for contracting with HMOs for care of Medicaid patients. Prior to 1981, states were only permitted to enroll Medicaid beneficiaries in prepaid plans that had no more than 50 percent of their enrollees on Medicare or Medicaid and that were federally qualified HMOs or federally funded community health centers. Under the OBRA81 legislation, states were allowed to establish their own qualification standards for Medicaid HMOs, and these HMOs were permitted to have up to 75 percent Medicare and Medicaid enrollment (Neuschler, 1985).

Medicaid programs have begun to use their authority to waive freedom of choice to test various approaches to case management, capitation, and primary care networks. Managed care has been implemented for a limited population of 1.5 million in 29 states and the District of Columbia (Anderson and Fox, 1987). Managed care encompasses a wide variety of approaches, including not only HMO enrollment of Medicaid beneficiaries but risk-sharing arrangements with other types of organizations such as health insuring organizations (HIOs), and primary care physician gatekeeper or medical case management approaches as well. OBRA85 required HIOs to meet all of the federal requirements for HMOS because of congressional concern with abuses and poor quality of care. As a result, only the five states that had HIOs in 1985 will be able to continue to operate (Anderson and Fox, 1987).

Twenty-one state Medicaid programs had contracts with HMOs in the fall of 1986 (Spitz, 1987). Seventy percent of Medicaid HMO enrollment in 1986 was in six metropolitan areas: Los Angeles, Phoenix, Madison, Milwaukee, Detroit, and Chicago (Spitz, 1987). Wisconsin has mounted a major effort to enroll its AFDC-Medicaid population in HMOs, but only preliminary evidence on effectiveness and access implications is available (Rowland and Lyons, 1987).

Medical case management in which a primary care physician designated by the beneficiary must approve utilization of specialty or hospital services is also growing. As of December 1986, 19 states had enrolled 655,138 Medicaid beneficiaries in case-management programs (Spitz, 1987). The largest was in Kentucky, with more than 200,000 Medicaid patients. The responsibilities of physicians and patients in case-management systems have not been well defined. To date, any saving would appear to be the result of reduced access to care or the selection of relatively healthier patients (Spitz, 1987). Development of medical protocols and specification of expectations for gatekeeper physicians will be required before performance can begin to meet the rhetoric and promise of this approach (Spitz, 1987).

One study analyzed managed care contracts and interviewed Medicaid, managed care plan, and local public health officials in 30 states in the summer of 1987 (Rosenbaum et al., 1988). The study included HMOs, other prepaid plan arrangements, and primary care case management approaches. The study found that managed care plans suffered from many of the problems intrinsic to Medicaid generally—such as high turnover in eligibility, absence of adequate benefits, and shortage of qualified providers. In addition, however, managed care plans often introduced difficulties caused by delays in enrollment and disenrollment and mass dislocation of beneficiaries from known and trusted community providers. Also, managed care plans have not addressed the requirements for appropriate maternity care, which are of major importance to the younger Medicaid population (Rosenbaum et al., 1988).

In 1982 Arizona implemented a managed care system for the state's poor population called the Arizona Health Care Cost Containment System (AHCCCS). The Arizona AHCCCS project has been implemented on a demonstration basis as an alternative to a full-scale Medicaid program and, as such, is unique among the states. The system combines prepaid capitation, competitive bidding for provider contracts, strict eligibility determinations, nominal copayments, and freedom of choice restrictions into a single system. However, major changes since its inception make it difficult to draw conclusions about its impact on access and costs (Bachman, Beatrice, and Altman, 1987; Christianson, 1984; Vogel, 1984).

Managed care approaches offer promise if care can be delivered to the Medicaid population more cost effectively without compromising quality or access to care. Experiences to date have been mixed. A few demonstrations have failed, either in the initial stages because of political opposition or in later stages because of financial or administrative difficulties. It is too early to know how effective the demonstrations have been in assuring access to quality health care for Medicaid beneficiaries at costs lower than the prevailing fee-for-service system (Anderson and Fox, 1987; Bachman, Beatrice, and Altman, 1987; Freund and Hurley, 1987; Freund and Neuschler, 1986; Spitz, 1987). But, despite the obvious merits of capitated plans with coordinated services, putting providers at risk for care to the poor requires cautious implementation and monitoring to avoid underutilization of services, poor treatment, and denial of emergency services (Iglehart, 1983; Neuschler, 1985; Rowland and Lyons, 1987).

These studies, by pinpointing administrative difficulties that have kept cost-containment initiatives from living up to their original promise, should be helpful to federal and state policy officials in improving and redirecting cost-containment efforts.

Summary

Health programs for the poor have been subjected to more extensive scrutiny than those covering more politically powerful middle-class groups, such as employer health insurance coverage and Medicare. This reflects in large part the lack of political clout of the poor and their advocates, and also in part the tension between liberals and conservatives regarding the responsibility of the public sector to assure adequate health care for the poor.

As a result, health services research has had a particularly significant impact on shaping policy changes and public attitudes toward Medicaid. It is health services research that is largely responsible for the gradual political acceptance of Medicaid as an essential and effective program that ensures access to needed health care services for millions of impoverished Americans. Research has also played an important role in the expansion of Medicaid to poor pregnant women, young children, the elderly, and disabled people. This research has depicted the barriers to access to health care services caused by gaps in insurance coverage, and the gains in terms of improved health from expanded access. Health services research has also addressed the legitimate concerns of policy officials that steps should be taken to lower costs where possible, at the same time minimizing any adverse effect on beneficiaries. Limits on benefits, provider payments, and managed care approaches have all been extensively studied by the research community, providing guidance to federal and state policy officials with information on both the effectiveness and the possible adverse consequences of alternative cost-containment strategies.

Research and Data Limitations

Despite this progress, health services research on programs designed to improve health care for the poor has been hampered by inadequate data systems, the low funding priority given to research on Medicaid and other health care programs for the poor, and the lack of methodological development that would permit sophisticated analyses evaluating the health impact of programs improving access to health care. Since Medicaid is a federal-state program, each state is responsible for collecting and reporting a minimum data set on Medicaid beneficiaries and expenditures. These reports typically generate counts of Medicaid beneficiaries and expenditures by type of service and basis of eligibility. This information, while useful, is inadequate to evaluate the effectiveness of the program. Little is known about the health status of beneficiaries. Although limited information on utilization of health care services by Medicaid beneficiaries is collected, this is not linked to other beneficiary characteristics such as income, presence of any supplementary types of insurance coverage, race/ethnicity, geographic location, health needs, or health care provider characteristics. The data collected vary in their reliability and may reflect differences among states in definitions and data collection procedures.

Research would be greatly facilitated by an ongoing sample survey of low-income individuals—including both those covered by Medicaid and those excluded from coverage. This would permit analyses of the impact of Medicaid coverage on utilization of health care services, holding constant for health status and other factors affecting use. Such a survey would provide a much better basis not only for assessing the differential contribution of Medicaid to access to health care services but also for pinpointing disparities among Medicaid beneficiaries for example, rural versus urban residents. It would be invaluable in improving estimates of the impact of expanding Medicaid to additional groups of low-income individuals and assessing both the costs and benefits of such expansions.

One major gap in knowledge has been the extent to which eligible persons participate in Medicaid, and the barriers that impede eligible nonparticipants from taking advantage of Medicaid benefits. More research is also needed on new directions for the program, that is, how Medicaid might be restructured to improve the delivery of health care services to the poor.

A fundamental problem is the lack of adequate measures of effectiveness with which to assess the benefits of Medicaid coverage. Most research that has tried to evaluate the health benefits of improved access to health care has focused on a limited number of measures, such as infant mortality. Yet most policy choices, such as raising the income eligibility level for infants to, say, 200 percent of poverty versus expanding coverage of children aged 7 to 12 up to 100 percent of the poverty level, require a more sophisticated approach to measurement of health outcomes. To date, the methodological development that would be required to assess the importance of improved access to health care for older children as well as adults has been particularly deficient.

Throughout the 1980s the Health Care Financing Administration has devoted an extremely small percentage of its budget to research on Medicaid policy issues, mainly because such analysis has been viewed as primarily a responsibility of the states. Yet the states have faced budgetary pressures that have made it difficult for them to support health services research—nor is it particularly efficient for each state to fund research on Medicaid issues independently.

Future Policy Issues and Directions

Whether by design or default, Medicaid has become the major health policy vehicle for assuring access to health care for the poor. Medicaid expenditures far outweigh governmental support of health care delivery programs for the poor, including federal outlays for primary care centers and state and local government support of public hospitals and clinics. Although a case could be made that an ideal health system would encompass a single health financing plan that would provide the same benefits, payment rates, utilization, and quality controls to all Americans regardless of income, family composition, age, welfare status, or place of employment, health policy in the United States has thus far evolved in a more incremental fashion, building on existing programs rather than on sweeping radical change.

Medicaid seems likely, therefore, to continue for some time to be the primary way in which low-income persons obtain health insurance coverage. As policy options for expanding and improving Medicaid continue to be considered, a much expanded research effort on Medicaid and the health problems of low-income individuals needs to be mounted.

One issue that seems likely to dominate the national agenda for the rest of this century is the expansion of Medicaid eligibility to additional groups of low-income individuals. To date, Congress has mandated coverage of pregnant women and children under age 6 up to 133 percent of the federal poverty level, and coverage of Medicare premiums and cost sharing for elderly and disabled beneficiaries up to 100 percent of the federal poverty level. States have the option of covering pregnant women and infants up to 185 percent of the federal poverty level, and children up to age 8 under 100 percent of the federal poverty level, children up to age 18 under the state AFDC income standard, and of providing a full range of Medicaid benefits to all elderly and disabled persons with incomes below 100 percent of the federal poverty level.

One important area of research investigation would involve evaluation of the impact of the Medicaid eligibility expansions that have been enacted to date. How many people have been newly covered? Is the change in eligibility known to low-income people, and what are participation rates? Why do some eligible people not participate? Would non-Medicaid approaches to insurance coverage reach more individuals? How effective have outreach measures, if any, been? What has been the change in the receipt of health care services by these newly enrolled Medicaid beneficiaries? Have there been detectable changes in health outcomes for those newly covered, such as changes in infant mortality or low-birth-weight babies? What has been the change in financial burden on families who have been newly covered by Medicaid? What has been the impact of uncompensated care and financial distress on hospitals and other primary care providers serving the poor? How do states respond to expansion of federal mandates in coverage? Are the advantages of expanded eligibility offset by new limits on available services or substandard payment rates to providers? What are the administrative problems faced by states in implementing incremental changes in Medicaid eligibility?

Equally important is research to assist policy officials in setting priorities for future expansions of Medicaid eligibility. What are the costs and potential benefits of bringing in additional groups of low-income children or adults? What should guide decisions about raising income eligibility levels for young children versus expanding coverage to older children or to adults? What particular difficulties are posed by terminating coverage of low-income women 60 days after delivery of a baby? What would be the health and administrative advantages of covering poor women of childbearing years, regardless of pregnancy status? What health problems do low-income uninsured people have? Are there important segments of the low-income population not eligible for Medicaid coverage who face serious barriers to receipt of health care? What is the health consequence of this gap in coverage? Does primary care of chronic health problems for uninsured poor adults get neglected, with consequent adverse health impacts? What expansion of eligibility would have the greatest impact on improving health or reducing morbidity? How can comparisons between the health gains of one group be made with those of another?

Another research issue involves coverage of the near-poor and medically needy under Medicaid. How does the spend-down in Medicaid currently work? What would be the advantages and disadvantages of permitting near-poor individuals to purchase Medicaid coverage? What are the financial burdens faced by seriously ill near-poor Medicare beneficiaries? What would be the advantages and disadvantages of permitting near-poor Medicare beneficiaries to obtain Medicaid by contributing to the cost of coverage on a sliding scale? Should federal and state governments subsidize continuation of Medicaid coverage for those who would otherwise become ineligible?

One important issue that has not been addressed is the high rate of turnover in Medicaid enrollment. Recent studies have shown that a high fraction of Medicaid beneficiaries are covered for relatively brief periods of time (Short, Cantor, and Monheit, 1988). For example, only 44 percent of Medicaid beneficiaries at the beginning of a three-year period were still covered 32 months later. More than one-third were enrolled less than eight months. Changes in employment and earnings are major factors affecting Medicaid enrollment. The majority of newly covered Medicaid enrollees (56 percent) were uninsured before qualifying for Medicaid; the majority of individuals leaving Medicaid (55 percent) were subsequently uninsured. The Family Support Act of 1988 permits individuals to retain their Medicaid benefits for one year following their move from welfare to work. Has the new law reduced the number of people who become uninsured when they lose Medicaid coverage? What problems are created for continuity of primary health care, preventive care for children, and sound maternity care by the high turnover in Medicaid eligibles? What are the health and access problems of families undergoing constant changes in employment, residence, family structure, and health insurance coverage? What implications does high turnover in Medicaid eligibility have for states trying to institute managed care approaches? How could employer health plan coverage and Medicaid coverage be better coordinated to avoid gaps in health insurance coverage? What would be the cost and administrative implications of permitting employers to purchase Medicaid for employees?

Another important research area is more careful evaluation of the impact in terms of health, access, and quality of care of cost-containment measures instituted by the states. Have reduced hospital and physician payment rates reduced the availability of Medicaid participating providers? What are the consequences of having Medicaid payment rates fall well below those of other payors? Are there thresholds below which adverse consequences occur either to beneficiaries or to providers? What other barriers to provider participation—such as delays in payment and Medicaid provider relations—reduce availability of care? Would minimum standards on provider payment rates increase access to services? Would the use of emergency rooms be reduced by greater participation of primary care physicians? What would be the potential offsetting saving from reduced emergency room use or early use of preventive and primary care? What has been the impact on quality of care of managed care approaches? Should HMOs be required to have a mix of patients, including a minimum share of non-Medicaid and Medicare patients? Should HMOs be federally qualified, meeting quality and financial soundness criteria, to participate in Medicaid? Are there health care delivery systems that can deliver quality care at lower cost to Medicaid beneficiaries? What are their characteristics? Does designation of a primary care provider by Medicaid beneficiaries improve the continuity of care? Does it reduce costly doctor shopping or inappropriate use of specialty care?

Clearly, a much expanded research effort will be needed both to guide policy decisions that place greater reliance on Medicaid as a vehicle for assuring access to health care for the poor and to ensure that the Medicaid coverage actually succeeds in improving access to quality health care for beneficiaries.

6

Financing Health Care
for Elderly Americans

Diane Rowland

With the enactment of Medicare in 1965, universal government-spon-sored health insurance coverage was provided to almost all Americans age 65 and over. Today, health care policy for the nation's 31 million elderly people is virtually synonymous with Medicare policy. Issues of access, cost, and quality of care for the elderly population have inevitably become linked to evaluations of the effectiveness of Medicare. As a result, gaps in Medicare's protection, most notably lack of long-term care, preventive health measures, and prescription drug coverage, are the driving force shaping health policy for the elderly population.

The Medicaid program fills notable gaps in the scope of Medicare cov-erage. Medicaid helps to pay medical bills that are not fully covered by Medicare for nearly 3 million low-income elderly Americans and provides for assistance with nursing home bills for almost half of the 1.3 million elderly people now in nursing homes (Commonwealth Fund Commis-sion, 1987; Rivlin and Wiener, 1988). Medicaid is today the primary source of financing for long-term home care and the major force shaping public policy. The scope of assistance available from Medicaid to the low-income population and its role in financing long-term care are critical elements in assessing health care for the elderly population.

Legislative changes and policy debates related to Medicare and Med-icaid over the 25 years since enactment provide the policy framework for an examination of the interaction between health services research and health care policy for the elderly population (Table 6–1). Although direct links are often difficult to establish, research directed at evaluating the impact of the Medicare program and designing approaches to rem-edy coverage gaps or access differentials has helped shape the policy

Table 6-1. Health legislation and the elderly: 1965–1989

Year	Legislation	Provisions
1965	Social Security Amendments of 1965 (PL 89–97)	Established Medicare and Medicaid
1967	Social Security Amendments of 1967 (PL 90–248)	Expanded hospital coverage and durable medical equipment under Medicare
1970	Public Health Service Amendment of 1970 (PL 95–515)	Authorized grants and contracts for research on provision of home health services
1972	Social Security Amendments of 1972 (PL 92–603)	Added disabled and ESRD for Medicare Increased premiums and deductibles Established Medicaid ICFs Medicare ECF converted to SNFs
1975	Special Health Revenue Sharing Act of 1975 (PL 94–63)	Demonstration grants for home health services agencies Set up committee to look at mental health needs of elderly
1977	Rural Health Clinics Act (PL 95–210)	Medicare coverage of rural health clinics
1980	Social Security Disability Amendment of 1980 (PL 96–265)	Voluntary certification of Medicare Supplementary Health Insurance Policies
1980	Omnibus Budget Reconciliation Act of 1980 (PL 96–499)	Medicare Home Health (unlimited visits, no cost-sharing, dropped prior hospitalization requirement) Medicare "swing-bed" option
1980	Pneumococcal Vaccine Coverage (PL 96–611)	Medicare coverage for pneumoccocal vaccines
1981	Omnibus Budget Reconciliation Act of 1981 (PL 97–35)	Medicaid Home- and Community-Based Waivers (§2176)
1982	Tax Equity and Fiscal Responsibility Act of 1982 (PL 97–248)	Medicare Hospice Benefit
1986	Comprehensive Omnibus Budget Reconciliation Act of 1985 (PL 99–274)	Medicare Prevention Demonstration
1987	Omnibus Budget Reconciliation Act of 1986 (PL 99–509)	Medicaid option to poverty-level for full coverage or Buy-in

Table 6-1 (continued)

Year	Legislation	Provisions
1987	Omnibus Budget Reconciliation Act of 1987 (PL 100–203)	Nursing Home Reform; Medicaid LTC Waiver
1988	Medicare Catastrophic Coverage Act of 1988 (PL 100–360)	Expanded Medicare benefits, including drugs and respite care and cap on out-of-pocket spending Medicaid Buy-In and Spousal Impoverishment
1989	Omnibus Budget Reconciliation Act	Medicare mental health benefits; Pap smears
1989	Medicare Catastrophic Coverage Repeal	Repeals all of PL100–360 except Medicaid provisions

environment and contributed to changes in eligibility and the scope of coverage under the Medicare and Medicaid programs.

This chapter examines the role of health services research in the development of health policy for elderly Americans. I identify the major acute and long-term care policy issues, review the health services research base to address these issues, and assess the overall contribution of health services research to the major policy initiatives for the elderly since the enactment of Medicare and Medicaid.

The Policy Framework

The major health policy issues for elderly people emanate from analysis of the adequacy of Medicare in addressing the health financing needs of elderly Americans. The adequacy of acute care coverage and options for reform are assessed in terms of the impact of Medicare in improving access to care, alleviating financial burden, and remedying gaps in acute care coverage. Long-term care policy, on the other hand, is shaped by the absence of Medicare coverage. Assessment of the gaps in Medicare and analysis of options to improve or reform coverage, especially for long-term care services, provide the framework for analysis of the contribution of health services research to the health policy agenda for elderly Americans.

Policy Issues

Medicare was designed and enacted in 1965 to meet the acute health care needs of the elderly population. Fairly extensive coverage of short-term hospital care and limited coverage of post-acute skilled nursing facility and home health services were provided under the Hospital Insurance or Part A component of the program. Physician and other ambulatory services were covered under the voluntary Supplementary Medical Insurance or Part B component of the program.

The design and scope of the Medicare benefit package were modeled after private health insurance coverage for the under-65 population. Benefits are focused on acute episodes of illness, with required cost sharing and limits on the amount of covered benefits. The benefit package excludes prescription drugs, routine eye examinations, eyeglasses, hearing aids, dental care, dentures, and most preventive care as well as long-term care services that are not related to acute care needs.

Critical concerns with the scope of Medicare coverage have arisen with regard to remaining gaps in acute care coverage, the extent of financial burden associated with care, and the notable lack of coverage for long-term care assistance. Long-term care reform has become a particularly prominent policy issue as the aging of the population focuses new attention on gaps in financing both community-based long-term care and nursing home care.

Most long-term care services are financed directly by the elderly or their families, often at substantial cost. Medicare pays for only limited home health and skilled nursing services related to acute illness. The means-tested Medicaid program is the primary source of public financing for long-term care. It pays for nursing home services and some home and community-based care, but only for those poor enough to qualify for services. Private long-term care insurance has not been generally available, and there is little experience with the policies currently being marketed.

The policy issues in long-term care relate to the need for this type of care, the organization and delivery of services, and the appropriate mix of public and private financing for such care. Much attention has been given to developing home and community-based alternatives to institutional nursing home care. Concerns over the quality of care in nursing homes and the heavy financial burden on those who need institutional care have been central to the evaluation of Medicaid coverage of long-term care. The examination of gaps in both public and private financing of long-term care services has stimulated efforts to reform financing and improve coordination of care.

Thus, the two major policy priorities emerging since the enactment of Medicare are filling the remaining gaps in the adequacy of acute care coverage under Medicare and addressing the lack of public or private insurance coverage for long-term care. The role of health services research is to help improve understanding of the scope of these problems and to propose and test alternative approaches to address these gaps. In undertaking this task, health services research is substantially strengthened by the availability of program experience and data collection and demonstration efforts that have facilitated analysis.

Analytical Framework

Evaluation of the effectiveness of Medicare has been aided by the development of a strong programmatic data base to supplement survey data and the use of pilot demonstration projects to assess specific benefit changes. Research on health and long-term care coverage of the elderly population thus has had a strong base that provided a framework for research and analysis.

With the enactment of Medicare, there was a major expansion of data on the elderly population. To meet the administrative requirements of the Medicare program, a research base was built to use claims data for analyzing the elderly population's use of hospital and medical services and their expenditures under Medicare (West, 1971; Lave et al., 1983; U.S. DHHS HCFA Reports, 1982–1989). When coupled with national health surveys of the population, these data sets provided an unprecedented capacity to examine health care utilization by the general elderly population as well as by specific subgroups.

National surveys of health care utilization and expenditures of the general population, including the over-65 population, permit analysis of differences in health status and use of care between the elderly and the non-elderly populations and provide the ability to analyze utilization by the elderly population of services not covered by Medicare. The annual Health Interview Surveys (HIS) by the National Center for Health Statistics permit both cross-sectional and trend analysis. The 1984 Supplement on Aging and the 1986 longitudinal follow-up to the Supplement on Aging of the Health Interview Survey are particularly useful because they permit both cross-sectional and longitudinal analysis and provide data on both acute and long-term care services for the elderly population living in the community.

Special one-time surveys, such as the 1977 National Medical Care Expenditure Survey (NMCES) by the National Center for Health Services Research and the 1980 National Medical Care Utilization and Expenditure Survey (NMCUES) by the National Center for Health Statistics and the Health Care Financing Administration, provide more detailed national estimates, utilization and expenditure information, and a rich analytical base for special studies. Merging the household interview results with Medicare claims files provides in-depth utilization data on aged individuals.

Special efforts have been undertaken to develop a data base for the analysis of long-term care issues and options. The 1982 and 1984 National Long Term Care (NLTC) Surveys and the 1985 National Nursing Home Survey (NNHS) provide information on the population in need of long-term care services. The NLTC surveys provide detailed information on the health and functional limitations of older people living in the community and include a companion survey of informal caregivers who provide unpaid assistance to the frail elderly. The 1985 NNHS is a nationwide sample survey of the nursing home industry and patient population. It is a follow-up to the 1973 and 1977 nursing home surveys and thus permits some analysis of changes in the characteristics of the nursing home population over time.

Results from the 1987 National Medical Expenditure Survey (NMES) are just becoming available to the research community. This household interview survey of the entire population will update the 1977 NMCES and 1980 NMCUES surveys and provide an in-depth profile of the characteristics of health care insurance, utilization patterns, and expenditures of both the elderly and non-elderly populations in 1987. The new survey has already been used to provide estimates of the potential utilization and cost of the prescription drug benefit under the Medicare Catastrophic Coverage Act (U.S. Congress CBO, 1989). It also provides additional opportunities for analysis because the sample included both the community-based and institutional elderly population.

These data bases form the research base for analysis of the impact of Medicare on health status and the use of medical care services by the elderly population (U.S. DHHS HCFA, 1982–1989 and 1982–1987). Findings from these national data bases have often been augmented by results from demonstration projects designed to test the effects of specific changes in Medicare benefits. The demonstration efforts provide valuable insights into the number of potential beneficiaries and the level of induced demand to be anticipated in changes in Medicare coverage and benefits (U.S. DHHS HCFA Demonstration Summaries, 1977– 1989).

Linking Health Services Research to Acute Care Policy

The principal objective of the Medicare program was to ensure equitable access to health care services for the nation's elderly population and lighten the burden of medical expenses. Lack of health insurance after retirement and differentials in access to care among the elderly population by income, race, and residence were the major problems that Medicare was designed to address.

Health services research evaluated the impact of Medicare on increasing access to care, alleviating the financial burden, and remedying gaps in acute care coverage. This evaluation provided an assessment of the program's effectiveness in providing mainstream medical care to the nation's elderly and helped to identify areas requiring additional policy action. Research evidence on gaps in access to care and scope of benefits combined with studies assessing the extent of financial burden incurred by Medicare beneficiaries provided the policy framework for proposals to provide improved acute care coverage under Medicare.

Access to Care

The chief goal of the Medicare program was to remedy the failure of the private market to provide adequate health insurance for elderly people. When Medicare was enacted, only 38 percent of the aged who were no longer working had insurance (Greenfield, 1968). As individuals retired, they lost their employer group health insurance coverage. Insurance companies were reluctant to write individual comprehensive policies for the elderly for fear that they would insure an excessive number of poor risks. Available policies often limited coverage, exempted preexisiting conditions, and in general offered inadequate protection (Merriam, 1964).

Medicare has clearly been highly successful in providing health insurance protection for the elderly population. With its passage, universal

access to insurance was assured for the 95 percent of the elderly population who were recipients of Social Security or Railroad Retirement
benefits. Thus the extensiveness of insurance coverage among the
elderly population was removed as a policy issue. The focus shifted to
evaluating the impact of Medicare on access to care and on the health
and economic well-being of the elderly population and to identifying
remaining inequities and gaps in coverage (U.S. Congress Committee
on Finance, 1970; U.S. Congress Committee on Ways and Means,
1975).

Medicare program data were used to examine medical care and to
document expenditures under Medicare by type of service (Scharff,
1967; West, 1971; Gornick, 1976; Gornick et al., 1985). Both cross-
sectional and trend analyses of patterns of utilization and expenditures
within the elderly population were conducted. The findings of these
studies helped to document Medicare's role in increasing access to medical care and removing differentials in use within the elderly population.
By combining Medicare claims data with household interview data,
researchers have also been able to identify the remaining gaps in Medicare coverage (Schlenger, Wadman, and Corder, 1983; Cafferata, 1984;
Schlenger and Corder, 1984; Kovar, 1986).

Research studies have shown a remarkable increase in access to care
for the nation's elderly population (Davis, 1973; Peel and Scharff, 1973;
Davis, 1975; Gornick, 1976; Davis and Shoen, 1978; Aday, Anderson,
and Fleming, 1980; Ruther and Dobson, 1981; Long and Settle, 1982;
Long and Settle, 1984; Gornick et al., 1985). In 1958, 32 percent of the
elderly did not see a physician, but by 1976 this was reduced to 21
percent (Aday, Anderson, and Fleming, 1980). Medicare also resulted
in a substantial increase in use of hospital services, with the population
over age 65 using more hospital services than the non-elderly population
(Lubitz and Deacon, 1982). Utilization of health care services by the
elderly increased in the post-Medicare era to levels equal to or above
those of the non-elderly population.

The major debate about access to care centered on whether
subgroups of the elderly experienced differentials in access despite the
overall increase enjoyed by the general elderly population. In essence,
was Medicare financing sufficient to overcome barriers to care, or did
specific subgroups such as the poor elderly or rural residents require
additional interventions to achieve equitable access?

Davis examined the distribution of Medicare benefits among elderly persons on the basis of income, race, and geographic location and investigated the importance of cost sharing, reimbursement, and nondiscrimination policy on differentials (Davis, 1975). Using data from 1968 and 1969, she concluded that even though the same set of benefits was available to all persons regardless of income, race, or geographic location, wide differences existed in the use of services. The lowest utilizers of medical services were the population groups with the poorest health—the poor, minorities, and residents of the South. However, use of medical services by the poor with supplementary coverage from Medicaid was substantially higher than that of the poor without such assistance (Davis and Reynolds, 1976).

Later work by Ruther and Dobson (1981) examined use of services by race from 1967 to 1976 and found a noteworthy decrease in the racial disparities found by Davis in the early days of program implementation. By examining utilization patterns pre-Medicare (1963–1966) and under a mature program (1977), Long and Settle documented the accomplishments of Medicare in removing the most severe inequities in access to health care that had led to Medicare's enactment (Long and Settle, 1984). By 1977, substantial income-related and racial barriers to equal access had, with minor exceptions, disappeared. However, persistent differentials in access to hospital services for southern blacks in contrast to southern whites and between urban and rural elderly beneficiaries continued.

Concerns over the differential in access to care in urban and rural areas led to legislation to expand care options in rural areas (Ecosometrics, 1981; Coward and Cutler, 1989). In 1977 Congress enacted the Rural Health Clinics Act (PL 95–210), which authorized direct Medicare payment for medical care provided by nurse practitioners and physician assistants in rural health clinics. Research documented the need for additional personnel in rural areas and the cost-effectiveness and quality of care provided by nurse practitioners and physician assistants.

Demonstrations were also initiated to evaluate the effectiveness of converting unused acute care capacity in small rural hospitals to provide services to long-term care patients (Wiener, 1987; Shaughnessy et al., 1988). As a result of the positive findings from the swing-bed experiment, Congress added the swing-bed option to Medicare coverage in the 1980 Omnibus Budget Reconciliation Act (PL 94–499).

In sum, health services research has helped to show that Medicare has been successful in expanding access to care and eliminating differentials in care among subgroups of the elderly population. By documenting Medicare's role in the elimination of barriers by income and race, these studies became important measures of the overall effectiveness of Medicare in achieving, to a great extent, its original objectives. By showing the remaining problems that faced residents of rural areas, health services research helped in the development and evaluation of strategies to expand access to care in these areas. By providing baseline information to compare with current patterns of utilization, health services research continues to provide a mechanism for monitoring progress and identifing access problems.

The Financial Burden of Medical Care

The second major objective of the Medicare program was to reduce the financial burden faced by elderly people. As noted, at the time of enactment of Medicare, less than half of the elderly population had private health insurance coverage. Spending for medical care consumed a major portion of the income available to the elderly population and constituted a major financial burden (Merriam, 1964; Greenfield, 1968).

Assessment of changes in the financial burden of payments for medical care with enactment of Medicare became another contribution of health services research to the overall evaluation of Medicare's effectiveness. Early studies showed that Medicare substantially eased the out-of-pocket spending burdens of the elderly, but noted that Medicare's cost-sharing requirements could be an onerous burden to the poor (Davis, 1973; Davis and Schoen, 1978; Link, Long, and Settle, 1980; Long, Settle, and Link, 1982). The need for additional coverage to help fill in for Medicare's cost sharing and deductibles became evident soon after enactment of the program. For the poor elderly population, Medicaid provided this coverage by paying the Medicare premium, deductibles, and cost sharing as well as providing supplementary benefits under Medicaid such as prescription drug coverage. For those able to afford coverage, a private health insurance market developed that offered "MediGap" policies to supplement Medicare coverage.

The major policy issues related to supplementary coverage have focused on the adequacy of the private insurance coverage and the need to improve Medicaid coverage for the low-income population. Almost three-quarters (72 percent) of all elderly people have Medigap plans, 8 percent receive assistance through the Medicaid program, and the remaining 20 percent rely solely on Medicare (U.S. Congress CBO, 1986). The likelihood of having private supplementary coverage is lower for the very old and minorities and for the less well off among the low-income population than for other elderly people (Long and Settle, 1982).

Early reports of abuse in the marketing of private plans led to a GAO investigation, culminating in the enactment of standards and a voluntary certification program for private supplementary plans enacted as part of the Social Security Disability Amendments of 1980 (PL 96–265) (DeNovo and Shearer, 1978; U.S. Congress House Select Committee on Aging, 1978). These amendments have come to be known as the Baucus Amendments after the chief sponsor of the legislation.

As part of the Baucus legislation, Congress required the Department of Health and Human Services to evaluate the effectiveness of the new standards on the private supplementary insurance market by surveying consumers and state regulators. The study undertaken by the Stanford Research Institute (SRI) reviewed the scope of coverage in individual policies, evaluated the effectiveness of state regulatory efforts, and assessed consumer awareness of extent of coverage (McCall, Rice, and Hall, 1983; Rice and McCall, 1985; McCall, Rice, and Sangl, 1986). Other work drawing on the 1980 NMCUES data analyzed coverage and provided a model to predict possible effects of the Baucus regulatory approach (Cafferata, 1984a, 1984b, 1985a).

The adequacy of these plans continues to be a major policy issue (Consumers Union, 1984; U.S. GAO, 1986a; Consumers Union, 1989). Health services research has analyzed the scope of supplementary insurance coverage and the characteristics of those most likely to be covered (Long and Settle, 1982; McCall, Rice, and Hall, 1983; Cafferata, 1984; Corder and Garfinkel, 1985). It has contributed to the private coverage debate by documenting the extent of consumer knowledge about private Medigap insurance, assessing the scope of coverage available from private plans, and lending analytic support to the efforts at regulation (Cafferata, 1984a, 1984b, 1985a; Rice and McCall, 1985; McCall, Rice, and Sangl, 1986; Garfinkel, Bonita, and McLeroy, 1987; McCall, Rice, and Hall, 1987).

For the low-income population, health services research has helped to document the importance of Medicaid coverage and the variations in availability of Medicaid assistance by state (McMillan et al., 1983; McMillan and Gornick, 1984; Davis and Rowland, 1986; Davis, 1986).

Medicaid coverage fills the major gaps in Medicare for the poor by covering Medicare premium and cost-sharing requirements and providing supplementary benefits, including both prescription drugs and long-term care services. The poor with Medicaid coverage spend substantially less out of pocket than those without Medicaid, yet only a third of the poor elderly have Medicaid coverage (Commonwealth Fund Commission, 1987). Medicaid eligibility levels in most states are set below the poverty level, and many states fail to provide full coverage to their elderly poor population.

In response to the evidence on the inadequacy of Medicaid coverage of the poor elderly population, Congress moved to expand the availability of Medicaid assistance. As part of the Omnibus Budget Reconciliation Act of 1986 (PL 99–509), Congress provided states with the option of extending full Medicaid coverage or partial assistance with Medicare premiums and cost-sharing to elderly and disabled people with incomes up to the poverty level. The partial assistance option is known as Medicare buy-in. Later, as part of the 1988 Catastrophic Coverage Act (PL100–360), Congress required the states to buy-in all elderly and disabled Medicare beneficiaries with incomes below the poverty level. Despite the subsequent repeal of the catastrophic law, the Medicaid buy-in provisions remain in force.

As Medicare premiums and cost sharing have continued to increase, the adequacy of Medicare's protection against financial burdens for medical care has emerged as a policy concern (U.S. Congress Special Committee on Aging, 1984). In 1989, the House Select Committee on Aging reported that the elderly were spending more of their incomes on out-of-pocket health care costs in 1987 and 1988 than they had a decade earlier or, more notably, in 1966 at the time of Medicare's implementation (U.S. Congress Select Committee on Aging, 1989).

Analysis of the elderly's out-of-pocket health expenses before and after Medicare's enactment showed a corrosive trend in the protection against out-of-pocket liability (Rosenblum, 1985). Out-of-pocket expenses for physician services and drugs remained prominent components of overall out-of-pocket spending. These trends lent support to efforts to reduce the financial burdens from Medicare's cost-sharing requirements. However, studies based on the 1980 NMCUES showed that for the elderly with catastrophic health expenses, defined as expenses exceeding $2000 in a year, 80 percent of the catastrophic burden was due to spending for nursing home care (Rice and Gabel, 1986). This research showed that alleviation of the financial burden could best be addressed by extending coverage for long-term care services.

Scope of Medicare Benefits

With few exceptions, the Medicare benefit package remained unchanged from enactment in 1965 until the expansions legislated under the Medicare Catastrophic Coverage Act of 1988 (Blumenthal et al., 1988; Lave, 1988). Essentially, the covered benefits were physician and hospital care with some limited extended home health care and skilled nursing facility benefits associated with an acute episode of illness. During the 1970s, legislation was passed to liberalize the home health benefit and adopt a hospice benefit for the terminally ill (Schlesinger and Wetle, 1988; Lave, 1988).

When enacted in 1988, the Medicare Catastrophic Coverage Act represented the most extensive benefit expansion in Medicare coverage since the inception of the program. Although now repealed, the provisions of the catastrophic act restructured the cost-sharing obligations and expanded the scope of acute care benefits under Medicare to include mammography examinations, prescription drug coverage, respite care, and unlimited hospital care.

One of the major contributions of health services research to the debate over expanding the scope of Medicare benefits has been the documentation of the number of people who use specific benefits and the financial barriers they face as a result of gaps in Medicare coverage. The 1977 National Medical Care Expenditure Survey and the 1980 National Medical Care Utilization and Expenditure Survey were important sources of information on the impact of socioeconomic factors and insurance adequacy on the use of uncovered Medicare benefits. The new 1987 National Medical Expenditure Survey provided previously unavailable information on prescription drug use and expenditures.

A significant amount of research related to the scope of Medicare benefits has been undertaken to determine whether it is feasible and cost-effective to extend Medicare coverage by adding specific benefits. In some cases, this research has been specifically requested by Congress in response to pressure from organized groups advocating specific benefit changes, such as the coverage of orthopedic shoes and foot care to assist elderly diabetics (Lave, 1988).

In the aftermath of the Catastrophic Coverage Act, expansion of the Medicare benefit package remains an unresolved policy issue in health coverage of the elderly population. There is a growing consensus that the current system does not provide adequate coverage, but much remains to be learned about the impact of benefit changes on consumer and provider behavior and on health outcomes (Pauly and Kissick, 1988).

The research evidence in support of expanding the scope of Medicare coverage is extensive for some benefits and limited for others. Changes in scope of coverage are generally constrained by the cost of expansion and are enacted on an incremental basis. Coverage of home health care, hospice care, preventive health services, mental health care, and prescription drugs have been the major areas of legislative action with regard to the scope of the Medicare benefit package.

Home Health Benefits. Home health care has been the major area of legislative activity with regard to Medicare benefits. Home health services under Medicare have been tightly controlled and tied to the acute-care nature of Medicare benefits. In the struggle to provide some measure of long-term care assistance under Medicare, the home health benefit has been seen as a policy wedge that could eventually be broadened to offer long-term home care (Dunlop, 1980). The studies of the home care benefit thus focused on who qualified for existing benefits, how services were utilized, and the cost of such care (Hedrick and Inui, 1986).

Research helped to document the impact of the conditions that users of the Medicare home health benefit had to meet prior to becoming eligible for reimbursable home health services under Medicare. Drawing on the results of community-based long-term care demonstrations as well as the program experience under Medicare, these studies assessed the cost-effectiveness of home care services, provided profiles of the users of home health services, and documented the gaps in care for many disabled elderly people (U.S. General Accounting Office, 1974; Lavor and Callender, 1976; U.S. General Accounting Office, 1977; Ricker-Smith and Trager, 1978). These studies provided the foundation for legislative efforts to liberalize the home health benefit throughout the late 1970s (U.S. Department of HEW, 1976).

The 1980 Omnibus Reconciliation Act (PL 96–499) drew on this research base to change the requirements for Medicare home health services in order to facilitate use of the benefit. It removed the 100-visit limit on home health services and provided for an unlimited number of home health visits under either Part A or Part B. It eliminated all cost sharing for home health services and dropped the requirement of a prior hospitalization as a condition for Part A services. However, the provisions requiring the need for skilled services, the provision of services on an intermittent basis only, and the homebound requirement were retained and served to continue to limit eligibility for such assistance.

Studies of the use of home care services continue to focus on the evaluation of potential changes in scope of benefit, including redefining the homebound and skilled care requirements for services and permitting care to be delivered on a daily basis (U.S. General Accounting Office, 1982, 1986b; Leader, 1986; Ruther and Helbing, 1988; Kane, 1988). Changes in the intermittent care requirement that prohibits daily home health visits on an extended basis have been attempted several times and were incorporated in the Medicare Catastrophic Coverage Act. However, this provision was subsequently repealed along with the other provisions of the act.

Hospice Care. Research on Medicare expenditures in the last year of life stimulated discussion of the possible need for alternatives to the high-technology hospital-based care offered to the terminally ill under Medicare. Using Medicare program data, researchers showed that a small proportion of Medicare beneficiaires consumed a large proportion of Medicare expenditures and that many of the highest utilizers were beneficiaries in their last years of life (Piro and Lutins, 1973; Lubitz and Prihoda, 1984; McCall, 1984; Riley et al., 1987; Scitovsky, 1988).

The hospice movement grew out of the quest for more humane and cost-effective ways of caring for the terminally ill. In the late 1970s, research on care for the terminally ill focused on the advantages and disadvantages of recognizing hospice care as a reimbursable service under Medicare. An Ohio study found that terminally ill cancer patients in hospice care used 50 percent less hospital care and ten times more home care than patients in traditional treatment and had lower overall expenditures (Brooks and Smyth-Staruch, 1984).

In 1980 the National Hospice Study, sponsored by the Robert Wood Johnson Foundation, was undertaken to determine the cost-effectiveness of hospice care and assess the feasibility of offering hospice services as an alternative to traditional technology-oriented care (Kane, 1988). Employing a quasi-experimental design, the study set out to compare the cost of hospital-based and home-based hospice care with traditional care in 40 sites. Twenty-six sites had Medicare benefit waivers from the Health Care Financing Administration to investigate the cost-effectiveness of offering hospice care as a Medicare benefit (U.S. DHHS HCFA, 1987a). These demonstrations laid the groundwork for enactment of the Medicare hospice benefit in the 1982 Tax Equity and Fiscal Responsibility Act (PL 97–248). Although Congress moved to enact the benefit before the demonstrations had been completed, the experience from the demonstration implementation helped to facilitate making hospice care available to terminally ill Medicare beneficiaries by demonstrating that the benefit was feasible (Mor and Birnbaum, 1983; Mor, Greer, and Kastenbaum, 1988).

Research has shown that home-based hospice care is less expensive than hospital-based care and that recipients of hospice care have a higher level of satisfaction than their counterparts receiving traditional care (Birnbaum and Kidder, 1984; Greer et al., 1986). The evaluation of the hospice demonstration has provided valuable insights into the administration of the hospice benefit under Medicare as well as guidance in program modifications and refinements (Dunlop, 1983; Kane et al., 1984; Davis, 1988; Bulkin and Lukashok, 1988; Mor, Greer, and Kastenbaum, 1988). A modest improvement in the hospice benefit was included in the Medicare Catastrophic Coverage Act of 1988, but this has now been repealed.

Preventive Health Services. Medicare coverage specifically excludes preventive health services, including routine physical examinations, most immunizations, screening examinations, and health education and counseling services. The lack of preventive care coverage under Medicare has been criticized as an example of penny-wise and pound-foolish policy that warrants further examination (Breslow and Somers, 1977; Somers, 1978; White House Conference on Aging, 1981; Somers, 1984; Kane, Kane, and Arnold, 1985; Russell, 1986; Rovin and Boniface, 1988).

Congress has shown increased interest in expanding the scope of Medicare to provide preventive services coverage, but only if the provision of those services can be shown to be cost-effective. In 1980, the Congress added coverage of pneumococcal vaccinations to the Medicare benefit package based on evidence that using the vaccine among the elderly population would reduce disability and save lives (PL 96–611). In the 1985 Consolidated Omnibus Budget Reconciliation Act, Congress sought to provide a more systematic evaluation of the effectiveness of a broad range of preventive services (PL 99–274). Demonstration projects to test the cost-effectiveness of offering Medicare coverage for health screening, health risk appraisals, immunization, and health counseling were initiated.

One of the problems in assessing the appropriateness of expanding Medicare coverage to include preventive health services is that much of the research evaluating preventive health services has been conducted on the non-elderly population and may not be generalizable to the elderly population (Kane, Kane, and Arnold, 1985). At the request of Congress, the Office of Technology Assessment reviewed the cost-effectiveness of a wide range of preventive health services for the elderly, including screening for cholesterol level, glaucoma, cervical cancer, colorectal cancer, and breast cancer (U.S. Congress OTA, 1989).

As part of the now-repealed portion of the Medicare Catastrophic Coverage Act of 1988, Congress had added routine mammography screening as a benefit for all Medicare beneficiaries. The research evidence supporting the benefit helped to get the provision included in the original legislation and will undoubtedly play a role in efforts to restore the benefit in the wake of the repeal of the broad bill. The 1989 Omnibus Budget Reconciliation Act did add coverage for routine Pap smears to the Medicare benefit package, effective July 1, 1990.

Mental Health Benefits. One of the most notable gaps in Medicare coverage of acute care problems is the very limited coverage for mental health benefits. Lifetime coverage under Medicare is limited to 190 days of inpatient care in a psychiatric facility. There is also a limit of $250 per year for outpatient services, subject to a 50 percent copayment. The limited coverage under Medicare leaves many elderly people with mental health problems uncovered unless they can qualify for services from Medicaid or the Veteran's Administration (Cohen and Hastings, 1989).

Several recent studies have found that Medicare beneficiaries are not receiving adequate mental health benefits (Schlesinger and Wetle, 1988). Elderly people with mental health problems are more likely to go without care than individuals in other age groups and use fewer mental health services (Leaf et al., 1985; Shapiro et al., 1985). These studies point to the need to address the adequacy of Medicare's mental health benefit.

Improved mental health coverage under Medicare is a long-standing issue on the policy agenda (Scallet, 1983; EBRI, 1985). Limited improvements in the benefit to permit coverage for reimbursement to be extended to services of clinical psychologists and social workers and to eliminate the annual dollar cap were enacted as part of the 1989 Omnibus Budget Reconciliation Act.

Prescription Drug Coverage. The lack of prescription drug coverage under Medicare was noted from the time of enactment but remained a notable gap in coverage (Greenfield, 1968; Avorn, 1983; U.S. Congress CBO, 1983; Lave, 1988; Rowland, Lyons, and Davis, 1989). Outpatient prescription drug coverage was finally added as a limited benefit subject to a substantial deductible in the Catastrophic Coverage Act of 1988. With congressional consideration of the benefit, numerous studies were undertaken to estimate the impact and help shape the deliberations (Lingle, Kirk, and Kelly, 1987; U.S. General Accounting Office, 1987; U.S. Congress OTA, 1987a; Waldo, 1987). The extent of out-of-pocket spending by the elderly population and the lack of prescription drug coverage under most private insurance supplementary plans were well documented (Rice and Gabel, 1986).

One of the most controversial aspects of the debate over the inclusion of prescription drugs developed over the cost estimates for the new benefit. The estimates prepared by the Congressional Budget Office were substantially lower than those of the admininstration as a result of differing assumptions on cost and use of services (U.S. Congress CBO, 1989). In part, the estimates were made more difficult because they had to be based on extrapolations of data from the late 1970s and early 1980s. When the 1987 NMES data become available with essential utilization and cost data, the CBO was able to develop new estimates with a greater degree of reliability. By the time new estimates were available, catastrophic coverage had been repealed.

Options for Reform

Interest in restructuring the Medicare program to address gaps in benefits and lack of financial protection for individuals with high levels of medical care utilization has led to the development of proposals for comprehensive reform. Concern over the long-range fiscal solvency of the Medicare trust funds has further stimulated efforts at reform by offering the prospect of both streamlining coverage and containing costs. Major reform options were set forth and debated at a 1983 conference sponsored by the Congressional Budget Office and the House Committee on Ways and Means (U.S. Congress Special Committee on Aging, 1984).

Health services research has played a major role in this debate by documenting the increasing financial burden faced by Medicare beneficiaries and developing proposals to improve protection for the general elderly population (U.S. Congress CBO, 1983; Hsiao, 1984; Ginzberg, 1984; Davis and Rowland, 1986; Harvard Medicare Project, 1986; Blumenthal et al., 1986; U.S. Congress CBO, 1986; Rice and Gabel, 1986; Feder, Moon, and Scanlon, 1987). These studies showed that the low-income elderly and those without supplementary coverage were particularly at risk for high medical costs, but that inadequate catastrophic and long-term care coverage were problems for all elderly people (U.S. Congress Energy and Commerce Committee, 1986a).

Concern over the lack of catastrophic coverage under Medicare has been a recurring policy issue. President Ford called for a limited form of "catastrophic insurance" protection combined with increases in Medicare coinsurance and deductible in the FY 1977 Budget (U.S. Congress CBO, 1976). The lack of adequate catastrophic protection under Medicare was repeatedly raised in discussions of the adequacy of Medicare coverage (U.S. Congress CBO, 1977, 1983). The need to expand protection for high-end catastrophic medical costs became a particularly high priority of the Reagan administration with the appointment of Dr. Otis Bowen as Secretary of the Department of Health and Human Services. Drawing on the analysis of the Social Security Advisory Council, which he chaired in 1982, Bowen sought to reform Medicare coverage by limiting out-of-pocket payments for cost sharing and expanding coverage of hospital care (Advisory Council on Social Security, 1983; Bowen and Burke, 1985; U.S. DHHS, 1986a). The administration's initiative relied on earlier research findings and proposals as well as additional research on the distributional effects of catastrophic expenses, using the national surveys and Medicare data bases at Department of Health and Human Services (U.S. DHHS, 1986b). The administration's proposal became the basis for congressional consideration of Medicare expansion.

In enacting catastrophic coverage, one of the critical policy issues faced by the Congress was to determine the extent of the financial burden faced by elderly Medicare beneficiaries and to analyze options for reform in terms of the numbers and types of Medicare beneficiaries who would benefit and the potential cost of expanded coverage. Health services research was a critical component in assessing the need for catastrophic protection, analyzing options for reform, and estimating the cost of various reform options (U.S. Congress CBO, 1983; Gornick et al., 1983; Christensen, Long, and Rodgers, 1987; U.S. Congress Committee on Ways and Means, 1987; Feder, Moon, and Scanlon, 1987; Christensen and Kasten, 1988).

When signed into law on July 2, 1988, the Medicare Catastrophic Coverage Act (PL 100–360) addressed the major financial burdens stemming from Medicare's cost-sharing requirements. Expenditures by Medicare beneficiaries for hospital care were limited to a single hospital deductible per year, and an overall cap was placed on out-of-pocket spending for Part B services. With the repeal of catastrophic coverage these benefits were eliminated, and beneficiaries are still liable for payment of a hospital deductible with each separate admission and have no limit on Part B cost sharing. However, the expansion of Medicaid buy-in assistance to the elderly with incomes below the federal poverty level was retained.

Linking Health Services Research and Long-Term Care Policy

The major gap in comprehensive health care coverage of the elderly population is the lack of coverage for long-term care services. Unlike acute care services, financing for long-term care remains largely unaddressed by the Medicare program or private insurance programs (Doty, Liu, and Wiener, 1985; Rivlin and Wiener, 1988). The burden of procuring and paying for long-term care services falls heavily on those who require these services. More than half of the $33 billion spent on nursing home care for the elderly population in 1987 was paid directly by impaired elderly people and their families (Waldo et al., 1989).

The Medicaid program has emerged, almost by default, as the major public source of financing for nursing home services, but Medicaid is a means-tested program that requires virtual impoverishment to establish eligibility for coverage. Many nursing home residents are forced to turn to Medicaid for assistance as they struggle to pay bills that are often in excess of $28,000 per year. However, for disabled elderly people seeking care in the community, Medicaid offers only limited assistance, creating a bias toward institutional care.

Long-term care is a more undefined and unresolved policy area than acute care services for the elderly. In acute care, the universal protection offered by Medicare provides a policy framework that can be used to examine the adequacy of coverage and needed modifications. In long-term care, the universal policy framework is absent and much of the debate centers around the identification of public and private strategies to reform long-term care financing.

Policy issues in long-term care thus have both a short-term and a long-range perspective. In the short term, policy initiatives have focused on expanding the availabilty of home and community-based services as an alternative to institutional care for those who are disabled but prefer to remain in the community. For those who are institutionalized, the major policy issues concern the quality of care in nursing homes and the economic burden faced by those who need care in these facilities. Initiatives in these areas have been targeted primarily at the Medicaid program because it is the current source of almost all public financing for long-term care.

The long-range policy perspective in long-term care goes beyond the framework of Medicaid coverage and policy to examine alternative public and private approaches to finance both home care and nursing home services for a growing elderly population. Critical issues in developing future financing policy for long-term care include defining the population eligible to receive long-term care services, designing and organizing a delivery system for community-based as well as institutional long-term care services, determining the extent of public versus private sector responsibility for long-term care, and finding the public and private resources to finance such care. Helping to provide answers to these questions remains one of the major challenges facing the health services research community.

Despite increasing policy interest in the answers to these questions, health services research has been hampered by the limitations of the data bases and by the program experience available to apply to this analytical task. Detailed information on the disabled elderly population living in the community has only recently become available as a result of the 1982 National Long-Term Care (NLTC) survey and the 1984 Supplement on Aging (SOA). The 1982 NLTC survey of the disabled Medicare population also included a special survey of their caregivers, providing new insights into the dynamics and burden of caregiving. Data on the nursing home population has also been limited, with the 1985 follow-up to the 1977 National Nursing Home Survey just beginning to be available for use.

As a result, long-term care policy has largely been shaped by data bases that were not specifically designed to address long-term care issues, and by the results of important but limited demonstration projects that attempted to evaluate the effect of various home care options. Analysis of the community-based long-term care demonstrations undertaken in the 1970s and 1980s played a valuable role in improving our understanding of the unmet needs of the physically and cognitively impaired elderly population and permitted some analysis of the impact and cost of alternative approaches to delivering long-term care. However, the lack of national data and program experience to evaluate the need for and use of long-term care services has left policymakers with many unanswered questions that impede broad-scale reform efforts.

Home and Community-Based Services

As long-term care emerged on the policy agenda, it quickly became clear that an alternative to nursing home placement for disabled individuals was a high policy priority. The provision of services in the home or community that could reduce the need for institutionalization became an objective of public policy, but there was much uncertainty about who needed home and community-based care and the cost-effectiveness of providing services.

The policy debate over improving Medicare or Medicaid coverage of long-term care services in the community has largely been driven by questions related to benefit design, the organization and delivery of services, and the cost implications of improved coverage. In essence, this debate has centered on the potential size of the long-term care population, on whether expanding noninstitutional coverage would supplement or supplant informal caregiving, and on the cost-effectiveness of in-home and community-based services as an alternative to nursing home care.

The Home Care Population. Determining the size and characteristics of the population in need of home and community-based services provides the foundation for examination of policy options for home care reform. Yet in the late 1970s, as policymakers and analysts began to develop proposals for home care coverage, critical information on how many elderly people needed home care services and the nature of their needs was lacking (U.S. Congress CBO, 1976; U.S. DHHS HCFA, 1981; Palmer and Vogel, 1981). The need for better information led to the undertaking of the 1982 National Long-term Care survey to provide better data on the disabled population and stimulated additional demonstration efforts to provide program experience.

In addition to survey design and demonstration evaluation

health services research has contributed to the definition of the home care population by helping establish methods to define disability levels within the population and then using these measures in national data sets to estimate the size and characteristics of the disabled population. With these estimates of the size and composition of the noninstitutional long-term care population, researchers could then estimate the number of people served and the potential cost of various options to expand public financing of home care services through Medicare or Medicaid.

Initially, the home care population was defined in general terms reflecting lost capacity for self-care and potential need for a broad range of personal care services (Nagi, 1976; U.S. DHHS HCFA, 1981; Institute of Medicine, 1977). The lack of specificity in the definition of those needing care made assessments of the extent of impairment in the population difficult. Health services research has helped to advance the home care policy debate by providing a mechanism for identifying and categorizing the potential home care population.

Researchers and policymakers are increasingly defining the population in need of long-term care services in the community on the basis of functional impairment as measured by limitations in Activities of Daily Living (ADL) and Instrumental Activities of Daily Living (IADL). The ADL scale, originally developed by Sidney Katz, measures functional impairment by examining degree of difficulty in eating, bathing, using the toilet, dressing, and transferring from a bed or chair (Katz et al., 1963). IADLs were developed to assess the level of cognitive as well as physical disability, and include home care mangement activities such as using the telephone, shopping, housekeeping, doing laundry, taking medications, and managing finances (Lawton and Brody, 1969). The functional approach to assessing disability has gained acceptance over more medically oriented approaches because disability measures, such as the ADL scale, have been found to be strong predictors of institutionalization and reflect the types of deficits that long-term care services are intended to fill (Katz et al., 1970; Spector et al., 1987; Liu and Cornelius, 1989).

National estimates of the size of the community-based long-term care population have been developed using the 1982 and 1984 National Long Term Care surveys and the Supplement on Aging to the 1984 National Health Interview Survey. With this information researchers have estimated the number of elderly people suffering from one or more limitations in ADLs at about six million people (Weissert, 1985; Macken,

1986; Rivlin and Wiener, 1988; Rowland, 1988). More recent research has focused on defining and further examining the characteristics of the community-based long-term care population by evaluating the number, type, and severity of ADL limitations (Rowland et al., 1988; Wiener and Hanley, 1989).

Research has also pointed out the importance of addressing the needs of the cognitively impaired population, including those with Alzheimer's disease. Estimates of the extent of cognitive impairment in the elderly population can be derived by using the Short Portable Mental Status Questionnaire (SPMSQ) in the 1982 and 1984 National Long Term Care Survey (Pfeiffer, 1975; Kasper, 1990). Many of those individuals who have Alzheimer's disease and related dementias also require assistance to remain in the community, but do not have ADL limitations (U.S. Congress OTA, 1987b; Commonwealth Fund Commission, 1989). Although extending long-term care coverage to the cognitively impaired is a policy priority, additional research is required to establish a mechanism for establishing eligibility for a long-term care benefit on this basis (Rowland, 1989).

One of the most important contributions of research to the policy debate has been to demonstrate the tremendous toll of caregiving on the families of the disabled elderly. Research has highlighted the importance of informal sources of support and documented the burden of caregiving by showing that most long-term care is provided on an unpaid basis by family and friends, with more than half of the care provided by wives and daughters (U.S. General Accounting Office, 1977; U.S. DHHS HCFA, 1981; Doty, 1986; Stone, Cafferata, and Sangl, 1987; Commonwealth Fund Commission, 1989).

Research related to the large emotional, financial, and physical strain of caregiving helped to lay the foundation for the provision of a limited respite care benefit under Medicare. Using the informal caregivers supplement to the 1982 National Long Term Care Survey, researchers showed that many of the caregivers are elderly themselves and most are of modest financial means, with nearly one in ten caregivers having to quit employment because of caregiving responsibilities (Stone, Cafferata, and Sangl, 1987). The respite benefit included as part of the Medicare Catastrophic Coverage Act (PL 100–360), but now repealed, was intended to provide a modicum of relief to these caregivers.

Although informal care predominates, 30 percent of the severely disabled elderly living at home use formal paid long-term care services to supplement assistance from family and friends (Commonwealth Fund Commission, 1989). Formal care includes that provided by home health workers, homemaker and personal care workers, adult day care, and respite services. The most severely disabled are those most likely to use paid home care. As a result, people with the highest level of ADL dependencies and those who live alone have higher out-of-pocket expenses than other impaired persons (Liu, Manton, and Liu, 1985; Feder, 1989; Liu and Cornelius, 1989).

In sum, health services research has advanced our understanding of the disabled population living in the community by estimating the size of this population; profiling their characteristics in terms of age, sex, race, income, and living arrangement; and analyzing their sources of both informal and formal support. By using ADLs as a measure of liability, health services research helped to establish a common framework that could be applied to this analysis. By profiling the population in need of long-term care and their caregivers, health services research has helped policymakers understand who stands to benefit from home care reform.

Evaluating Alternative Approaches to Community Care. Concern about inappropriate nursing home placement and rising long-term care costs led to a series of government-financed demonstrations to study whether substituting care at home for care in a nursing home could reduce costs and improve quality of life for the disabled elderly population. During the last 15 years, demonstrations sponsored by the Health Care Financing Administration tested the impact of expanded Medicare and Medicaid coverage of community-based services. The evaluations of these demonstration efforts can be used to assess the effectiveness of alternative approaches to delivering home-based services (Hamm, Kickham, and Cutler, 1982; Vertrees, Mantor, and Adler, 1989).

Demonstration projects on home- and community-based services evolved in three phases. In the first phase, individual projects at selected sites were initiated to test the concept of a single entry point for long-term care delivery and the effectiveness of a case manager as a gate-keeper for community-based care. In this approach, the case manager provides an in-depth assessment of the services required by an individual to remain in the community and then arranges for the delivery of appropriate care (Applebaum, Seidl, and Austin, 1980; Eggert, Bow-lyow, and Nichols, 1980; Skellie, Mobley, and Coan, 1982; Weiss and Monarch, 1983; Hughes, Cordray, and Spiker, 1984; Yordi and Waldman, 1985; Haskins et al., 1985; Zimmer, Groth-Juncker, and McCusker, 1985; Gaumer et al., 1986). Others tested the impact and cost of providing specific benefit expansions, such as homemaker and adult day health services (Weissert et al., 1980).

These early demonstrations operated under different research protocols, making comparability of results difficult. The need for a well-designed multi-site study using a common procedure led the Department of Health and Human Services to undertake the National Long-term Channeling Demonstration in 1980. This 10-site project used a common protocol to test the effect of case management alone and with service expansion. A major evaluation of the project was included as part of the original design (Kemper et al., 1986).

A review of the experience of 16 community-care demonstrations showed that expanding public financing for home care was likely to increase public costs, but that the expanded services made people feel better off and did not serve to reduce family caregiving (Kemper, Applebaum, and Harrigan, 1987). Most of these studies have shown slight reductions in nursing home use, although in many cases the results are not statistically significant and the research designs are not rigorous. The strongest evidence was found in South Carolina's Community Long-Term Care project, which used a randomized research design and concluded that significantly fewer people entered nursing homes among those receiving the expanded community services than among the control group (Nocks et al., 1986).

One of the critical concerns underlying the implementation of the demonstration projects was whether the provision of paid care was a substitution for unpaid care, but this issue was not extensively studied in most demonstration projects. Information from the Channeling Demonstration project indicates that in most cases, formal paid services are used to supplement rather than to replace informal care (Christianson, 1986). On the issue of cost-effectiveness, comparisons of the public cost of services for people eligible for expanded home and community-based services with the cost for those who are not indicate that expansion of home care services increases costs overall (Stassen and Holahan, 1980; Haskins et al., 1985; Kemper et al., 1987).

The mixed results from the community care demonstrations led others to propose alternative models for long-term care delivery. One such model, the Social/HMO or S/HMO, pools financing for acute care and community-based long-term care services. Modeled on the HMO for acute care, the S/HMO integrates community-based long-term care into a prepaid, managed HMO model. Backed by funding from 20 private foundations and congressionally required participation by the Health Care Financing Administration, the S/HMO was implemented on a demonstration basis at four sites in 1985. Early results are promising, but the final evaluation will not be available until the demonstration is completed in 1992 (Greenberg et al., 1985; Greenberg et al., 1988; Leutz et al., 1988).

Although the community-based care demonstrations, including the channeling project, were ongoing and seemingly producing mixed results with regard to the cost-effectiveness of offering home care as an alternative to nursing home care, Congress moved in 1981 to expand Medicaid coverage of home care (U.S. Congress Energy and Commerce Committee, 1981). Concerns about the institutional bias in Medicaid and growing interest in community care led to the enactment of community care legislation as part of the 1981 Omnibus Budget Reconciliation Act (PL 97–35). Under this provision, known as the 2176 waiver, states can apply for waivers to provide services that are not ordinarily available to Medicaid beneficiaries, such as homemaker, personal care, and rehabilitation services, respite care, and case management. The Secretary of the Department of Health and Human Services is authorized to grant waivers to allow states, on a budget-neutral basis, to use federal Medicaid funds to purchase long-term care services for Medicaid individuals who are at risk of nursing home placement (U.S. Congress Energy and Commerce Committee, 1986b). As of 1988, 37 states were offering home and community-based services to approximately 59,000 elderly Medicaid beneficiaries under the 2176 waivers (Neuschler, 1988).

The size and scope of the state waiver programs have been severely limited by state fiscal concerns and by the federal requirement that they not increase increase Medicaid long-term care expenditures above levels that would have been incurred had the waivers not been granted. Demonstrations have shown that it is difficult to control expenditures by limiting services to those who would have been institutionalized without services, because many people satisfy nursing home eligibility requirements but would not enter a nursing home even if home care services were not provided (Lave, 1985; Kemper et al., 1987; Rivlin and Wiener, 1988; Feder, 1989). As a result, Congress recently enacted new waiver authority (Section 1915d) that eliminates the constraint on the number of people served if the states accept a cap on federal funds for nursing home and waivered services (U.S. Energy and Commerce Committee, 1988).

Improving Nursing Home Care

The primary focus of policy reform efforts throughout the 1970s and 1980s has been on the cost and quality of nursing home care. Issues with regard to the cost of care arise largely because of the limited sources of financing for long-term institutional care services (Cafferata, 1985b). The notable lack of long-term care coverage for nursing home services under Medicare has been a major focus of research. Studies have assessed the limited scope of the Medicare skilled nursing facility benefit and variations in its administration across the country (Loesser et al., 1981; Smits et al., 1982; Vladeck, 1987). Research related to the distribution of health care expenditures shows that nursing home services constitute a major out-of-pocket burden and that only limited assistance is available from Medicaid (Waldo et al., 1989). Yet, despite the substantial cost of nursing home care, concerns have grown over the quality of care provided in these homes and have stimulated efforts to strengthen the regulation of quality standards as well as provide assistance with the financial burdens associated with nursing home care.

The Nursing Home Population. A major policy issue with regard to nursing home services concerns who uses nursing home care and who is at risk of nursing home placement. The 1985 National Nursing Home Survey provides the most recent information on the institutionalized elderly population and updates information collected in the 1973 and 1977 National Nursing Home surveys. These data bases provide information on the number of elderly people who are institutionalized and their sociodemographic characteristics. Less information is available on payment sources, length of nursing home stays, and transitions between nursing homes and the community (Sirrocco and Koch, 1977; Van Nostrand et al., 1979; Hing, 1981). This lack of data has hindered policy development addressing the financing of nursing home care and the integration of acute and long-term care services. Recent research has focused on describing the characteristics of nursing home residents and discharges, examining the factors that predict nursing home admission, analyzing trends in nursing home utilization, and developing policy options (Fox and Clauser, 1980; Scanlon, 1980; Harrington, 1985).

The percentage of the elderly population living in nursing homes has been relatively stable over the last ten years, with approximately 5 percent of the elderly population in nursing homes on any given day in 1985 (Hing, 1981, and 1987). Among the 1.3 million institutionalized elderly, almost half (45 percent) are age 85 or older, and three-quarters are female. The risk of being admitted to a nursing home rises dramatically with age, from 1 percent for those age 65 to 74 to 22 percent for those age 85 and over. Racial differences have been found in the use of nursing homes by the elderly population, with lower utilization levels by minorities (Institute of Medicine, 1981; Hing, 1987).

Research examining the factors that contribute to nursing home placement has highlighted functional decline and lack of support within the community. Studies have shown that dependence in ADLs or cognitive impairment may be an important reason for entering a nursing home (Kane, Mathias, and Sampson, 1983; Cohen, Tell, and Wallack, 1986; Liu and Cornelius, 1988). In 1985, more than 90 percent of elderly nursing home residents were ADL-impaired and almost two-thirds were reported to be disoriented or have memory difficulties (Hing, 1987).

The composition of nursing home patients has become more functionally dependent over time. Elderly nursing home patients in 1985 were older and more likely to experience limitations in ADL than those in 1977 (Hing, 1987). This may in part reflect the impact of the Medicare Prospective Payment system (PPS) incentives that encourage earlier discharge of hospital patients (Meiners and Coffey, 1985).

Research has also focused on the importance of lack of support within the community in predicting institutionalization. Elderly persons living without spouses may be unable to obtain the personal assistance needed to remain in the community. Eighty-four percent of those who were institutionalized were without spouses compared to 56 percent of the functionally impaired living in the community (Macken, 1986).

Quality of Nursing Home Care. Throughout the 1970s and 1980s, the issue of quality of care in nursing home facilities remained on the forefront of the health policy agenda. The nursing home scandals in New York resulted in the Moreland Act Commission on Nursing Homes and the Residential Facilities investigation and helped highlight the issue nationally in the mid-1970s. The need for improvement in both nursing home quality and enforcement of standards became a policy concern at both the federal and state level (Vladeck, 1980; Caldwell and Kapp, 1981; Smith, 1981).

Protection of patients' rights and improvements in nursing home certification requirements under Medicaid and Medicare have been the subject of both litigation and advocacy. Controversial regulations on nursing home quality and certification standards promulgated by the Department of Health and Human Services were tabled pending a congressionally authorized study of nursing home quality by the Institute of Medicine of the National Academy of Sciences. The report of the Institute of Medicine provided a blueprint for reform (IOM, 1986).

In the Omnibus Reconciliation Act of 1987 (PL 100–203), Congress enacted a complete overhaul of the Medicare and Medicaid programs' approach to ensuring the quality of care for nursing home residents. The requirements that nursing home facilities must meet in order to receive Medicaid and Medicare payment were substantially revised as a result of the recommendations in the Institute of Medicine's report.

Financial Burdens of Nursing Home Care. The public and private cost of nursing home care is substantial. Research has helped to delineate the role of public versus private financing for nursing home care and has helped to improve our understanding of the financial burdens associated with such care. The cost of nursing home care and the impact of this cost on the disabled elderly and their families remain the overwhelming policy issues in long-term care (Rivlin and Wiener, 1988). Because of the lack of private insurance coverage for nursing home care and the means-tested nature of Medicaid benefits, more than half of all nursing home expenditures are direct out-of-pocket payments by the elderly and their families.

The way in which Medicaid serves as a long-term care program has been the most active policy area in the nursing home debate in recent years. In the 1970s, anecdotal reports of transfer of assets to obtain Medicaid eligibility were investigated and led to legislation implementing a prohibition on shifting assets to relatives or friends in order to meet Medicaid eligibility criteria. Some called for greater family responsibility for the cost of nursing home care. As part of the examination of relatives' contribution to the care of their disabled family member, researchers showed that little cost saving would be gained by shifting a greater burden of the cost of nursing home care to families because 20 percent of nursing home residents had no living relatives and most were unmarried, divorced, or widowed (Callahan et al., 1980). The study did, however, point out that spouses of nursing home residents already bore a heavy burden for care of their spouses, and as a result many were left to live an impoverished existence in the community.

Growing concern over the required impoverishment of a spouse of a nursing home resident in order to qualify for Medicaid benefits led to enactment of changes in Medicaid eligibility standards for nursing home coverage as part of the Medicare Catastrophic Coverage Act of 1988 (PL 100–360). This provision requires states to protect the income and assets of the community spouse up to certain minimum levels, with an increase to 150 percent of the poverty level by 1992. Although the general Medicare provisions of the catastrophic coverage act have now been repealed, these Medicaid changes remain in force.

Concern over the impoverishment requirement embodied in Medicaid eligibility for nursing home assistance, however, goes beyond the concern for protecting assets and income for the community spouse. Spending down one's income and assets to become eligible for Medicaid coverage is the only means of securing assistance to pay nursing home bills for most Americans because of the general lack of private insurance (U.S. GAO, 1979). Only very limited information is available about the spend-down process. The NNHS does not collect information on when Medicaid becomes the primary payor for care. As a result, little information is available about who is spending down and the dynamics of the process.

A General Accounting Office report which reviewed case studies and conducted other analyses estimated that between one-quarter and two-thirds of Medicaid nursing home patients initially entered as private paying patients and subsequently became eligible for Medicaid, and that this conversion was more likely to occur among patients with longer stays (U.S. GAO, 1983). Analysis of the 1985 NNHS indicates that 40 percent of elderly patients have Medicaid as their primary source of payment when they enter the nursing home. Among the 60 percent who rely on other sources, one-fifth convert to Medicaid at some point during their stay (Sekscenski, 1987).

Researchers at the Urban Institute have taken a different approach and constructed a microsimulation model that estimates the length of time required before elderly persons spend their income and assets down to the federal poverty line. According to this model, it is estimated that 70 percent of elderly persons living alone have their incomes reduced to the poverty level after 13 weeks in a nursing home and 90

percent are impoverished within one year (U.S. Congre
Committee on Aging, 1987).

The potential of private long-term care insurance to
erishment to obtain Medicaid assistance has been exam
prototype policies and estimating the number of people
tially benefit (Meiners and Trapnell, 1983; Meiners, :
concerns over the affordability of private insurance limit the saving for
Medicaid that is likely to accrue from greater private insurance coverage
(Rivlin and Wiener, 1988).

In sum, research has helped to delineate the role of public versus
private financing for nursing home care and to improve our understanding of the financial burdens associated with such care. By furthering
understanding of the extent to which long-term care is a burden for many
families, research has helped to provide a basis for future policy action
to reform financing.

Options for Reform

The long-range policy agenda for long-term care is to develop and evaluate comprehensive reform strategies to improve the financing and
delivery of long-term care services. The development of major proposals will be aided by the growing body of research on both home care and
nursing home care. Analysis of reform options will be possible as the
major national data bases provide a previously unavailable capacity to
develop policy simulation models incorporating measures of disability.

Future reform efforts will also be strengthened by health services
research that has helped to lay out the options for reform. Broad
approaches for long-term care financing reform were presented and contrasted in a 1977 options paper prepared by the Congressional Budget
Office (U.S. Congress CBO, 1977). Subsequent work during the late
1970s and early 1980s provided insights into the advantages and disadvantages of alternative strategies for long-term care reform (Callahan
and Wallack, 1981; Meltzer, Farrow, and Richmond, 1981).

A major effort to develop an analytical framework to examine the
major options for reforming the way long-term care is financed was
undertaken by the Brookings Institution during the 1980s (Rivlin and
Wiener, 1988). A policy simulation model was developed to project the
population of disabled elderly over the next three decades and to estimate their financial resources and likely use of long-term care. This

model was used to explore the future potential for private-sector long-term care alternatives and their impact on the need for a public role. Numerous private and public options were analyzed. The researchers concluded that private alternatives should be encouraged, but that a public insurance long-term benefit under Medicare should be enacted to replace the means-tested Medicaid program.

Despite budgetary concerns that have restricted willingness to consider major expansions in public financing, proposals for long-term care reform have continued to be developed and advanced. Approaches have ranged from comprehensive social insurance coverage of both nursing home and community-based services to targeted proposals limited to home care under Medicare (Rivlin and Wiener, 1988; Commonwealth Fund Commission, 1989). Other approaches call for the integration of both acute and long-term care financing under Medicare (Somers, 1982; Davis and Rowland, 1986; Harvard Medicare Project, 1986; Somers, 1987).

Prospects for the Future

From enactment in 1965 until the Catastrophic Coverage Act of 1988, the scope of Medicare benefits remained essentially unchanged. During the 1970s and early 1980s, the major policy issues related to Medicare involved provider payment policy revisions, most notably implementation of a new hospital payment system and revisions of physician payment (U.S. Congress Senate Committee on Finance, 1970; Committee on Ways and Means, 1975). Long-term care and coverage of prescription drugs and preventive services remained outside the scope of the acute-care-focused Medicare program.

During the 1970s and 1980s, much attention was given to the gaps in Medicare coverage of acute care services resulting from cost-sharing requirements and uncovered services. Research was conducted to analyze the extent of financial burden and assess the impact of proposed reforms. This research helped to create the policy environment leading to the Medicare Catastrophic Coverage Act of 1988. During this same period, growing concern over the cost of long-term care services and the lack of public or private financing became a major policy issue. The push for long-term care expansions resulted in modest expansions of the home health benefit under Medicare in 1980 (PL 96–499). However, the major research and policy activity during this time has involved documentation of the need for improving long-term care financing and development of options for reform.

The short-lived Medicare Catastrophic Coverage Act of 1988 represented the most significant expansion in Medicare's scope and the first major restructuring of benefits since enactment. The introduction of a ceiling on out-of-pocket spending for cost sharing, the elimination of restrictions on days of covered hospital care, and the addition of benefits including outpatient prescription drug coverage, respite care, and mammography screening as a preventive service, closed gaps in Medicare's protection that had been noted since the program's inception.

Health services research helped to identify those vulnerable to catastrophic expenses under Medicare and offered alternative proposals to address these gaps. Research thus played a key role in the debate surrounding the benefits and cost associated with catastrophic coverage. Yet, ultimately, the politics of the issue and the resentment of many elderly people over the financing approach, which relied solely on Medicare beneficiaries to support the cost of expanded coverage, led to the successful move to repeal the new law.

An examination of the research base underlying the catastrophic coverage debate is nonetheless instructive because the policy issues that the Catastrophic Coverage Act addressed touch virtually every area of Medicare's coverage. Health services research helped to provide the underpinning for the expansion of benefits embodied in the Catastrophic Coverage Act. The extensive financial burdens faced by many elderly people were well documented by health services researchers, and this helped to lay the framework for expanded hospital benefits, limits on out-of-pocket spending, coverage of prescription drugs, and mandatory Medicaid buy-in assistance for the low-income elderly. Research on the efficacy of preventive health services, most notably mammograms for the detection of breast cancer, provided the foundation for the coverage of mammography under Medicare.

The repeal of the benefit expansions in the catastrophic legislation reopens the research agenda related to Medicare acute care coverage but also casts a long shadow over long-term care reform. However, the aging of the population will undoubtedly serve to keep long-term care reform high on the policy agenda throughout the 1990s. Research can help to provide the analytical underpinning for the consideration of both public and private initiatives. In the aftermath of the catastrophic legislation, more caution about expanded benefits and more concern about the accuracy of cost estimates and the sources of financing are likely to be high priorities of health services research in long-term care over the coming years.

· 7 ·

Controlled Experimentation
as Research Policy

Joseph P. Newhouse

The Health Insurance Experiment (sometimes referred to as the RAND Health Insurance Experiment), a controlled trial in health care financing, was probably the largest and one of the longest-running health services research projects ever undertaken. The field work spanned nearly a decade, and the analysis of the data that were collected is still continuing. In this chapter I first describe the policy and research context in which the project took place and then turn to the major findings of the Health Insurance Experiment. I next consider the implications of the results and conclude with thoughts on the role of a controlled experiment in formulating health care policy.

The Health Insurance Experiment (HIE) sought to improve federal and private policy toward the financing of medical care services. Policy decisions on health care financing take place along at least five dimensions: (1) what services should be covered; (2) how well they should be covered (how much cost sharing there should be); (3) how much and on what basis providers should be reimbursed; (4) how care should be financed (the mix of taxes and premiums); and (5) administrative issues. The HIE was directed primarily at the first two dimensions, especially the second, with some attention to the third and fifth. Before presenting the design and results of the HIE, I will describe the state of the debate over health care financing when it began, the policy milieu within which it evolved, and the knowledge base of health services research at the time.

The Health Care Financing Debate in the 1970s and 1980s

Planning for the HIE began in mid-1971. At that time the role of cost sharing was widely debated, usually in ideological terms. The left generally saw cost sharing as a barrier to obtaining necessary care; the right generally saw free care as leading to overuse and abuse. Neither side had much evidence, although anecdotes abounded.

The appropriate scope of services was also debated. The left saw comprehensive coverage as preferable; in particular, coverage of outpatient services might encourage patients to seek preventive care when well and, when sick, to seek care at a time when such care might be crucial. The right argued that outpatient care did not generally lead to large bills and that high administrative expense made insurance coverage an expensive way to pay for outpatient care. In addition, there was a fear that total costs would rise, not fall, if outpatient services were covered.

In Washington the Nixon administration faced choices with respect to what national health insurance plan, if any, it should propose and what it should do, if anything, to reform the Medicaid program, which was perceived in several quarters as unsatisfactory. By contrast, the Medicare program was viewed as generally successful. Some proposed that there should be income-related cost sharing (Feldstein, 1971a), but others, such as the Committee for National Health Insurance, saw this as an administrative nightmare and advocated free care for all.

A somewhat different theme was introduced into the debate by the Nixon administration's white paper of 1971, which advocated the spread of HMOs on the ground that they were more efficient. The white paper, however, could not answer two key questions because the answers were unknown: the degree to which the observed lower use of health care in HMOs was due to enrollment of better risks (favorable selection), or, if HMO medical care really was different and the lower use was not due to favorable selection, its effect on health status.

Shortly after the effort to design the HIE began, there was considerable activity in Congress to enact a national health insurance program. There were several proposed approaches, ranging from the Health Security Act sponsored by Senator Kennedy and Representative Corman, which covered most services with minimal or no cost sharing but restricted reimbursements, to the Nixon administration's Comprehensive Health Insurance Plan, which consisted of a mandate that employers provide insurance to their employees combined with a residual publicly supported plan for those not covered through their place of work, to a so-called catastrophic bill sponsored by Senators Long and Ribicoff. None of these proposals attracted enough support to be enacted into law. In 1975 a compromise bill, sponsored by Senator Kennedy and Representative Mills, failed on a close vote in the House Ways and Means Committee.

During the Carter administration there was lessened interest in national health insurance plans, although the Department of Health and Human Services constructed a cost estimation model for such a plan. During the Reagan administration there was no executive branch interest in national health insurance. Nonetheless, even if there was to be no single national health insurance plan, the generic issues of what services should be covered, how well they should be covered, and how providers should be reimbursed had to be addressed by all existing private and public plans. Hence, improving the knowledge base with respect to these issues was important, irrespective of whether there was new national health insurance legislation.

What Health Services Research Said about These Issues in the Early 1970s

At the time the HIE began in 1971, the research literature provided little guidance on how varying the amount of cost sharing affected use or health outcomes. Nor did it say much about the effect of covering or failing to cover specific services, such as physician outpatient services. Some rudimentary research was available comparing use among those with and without insurance, but if someone wanted to know what would happen, for example, if there were a per-charge visit in the Medicaid program, no certain answer could be provided, even as to its effect on use. One measure of how responsive use is to insurance is the price elasticity of demand, which is simply the percentage change in use relative to the percentage change in price. The price elasticity estimates in the literature at the time the HIE began differed by a factor of ten (Feldstein, 1971b; Davis and Russell, 1972; Phelps and Newhouse, 1972, 1974; Scitovsky and Snyder, 1972; Rosett and Huang, 1973).

There were good reasons why the literature was so inconclusive. To begin with, in some studies those who expected to make more use of medical services had probably obtained better insurance. If so, comparing use between those with different amounts of insurance would overstate the response to insurance. Indeed, this problem has plagued employer plans with multiple options, such as the Federal Employees Health Benefits Plan, in which average use across plans is driven to a large degree by the characteristics of the enrollees in each plan rather than the coverage provisions of the plan (Price, Mays, and Trapnell, 1983; Enthoven, 1989; Jones, 1989). For example, one cannot infer from the average use of federal employees enrolled in the Blue Cross High Option plan what use would be if everyone were enrolled in such a plan because the sickest employees are disproportionately represented in that plan.

There were other problems with the studies reported in the literature. Claims or other administrative data sets yielded no information on uncovered services or on the patterns of use of those who did not satisfy a deductible and therefore did not take the trouble to file a claim for any use they may have had below the deductible. Furthermore, although insurance policies differed almost endlessly in minor details, most provided full or nearly full coverage of hospital services. Although there was variation in the coverage of physician services, many other services, such as prescription drug and dental services, tended not to be covered at all. Thus, it was difficult to quantify the effect of variation in coverage of hospital services or drug and dental services. In the case of physician services, data from insurance files could not be obtained if the services were not covered, and household surveys were plagued by difficulty in obtaining details of the insurance policy from the household and by errors in the recall of usage and charges.

Problems became more acute if one was interested in particular subgroups, such as the poor. Because of the Medicaid program, there was disproportionate policy interest in the poor, but Medicaid data themselves did not offer much basis for analysis. There was mandatory coverage of a number of services and no cost sharing at the time of service. Thus, there was no basis for projecting the effects of varying the scope of the covered services that were mandated or estimating responses to modest cost sharing. In addition, the monthly changes in eligibility made it very difficult to draw inferences from Medicaid data, because people could defer visits until they were eligible and crowd in visits if they anticipated losing eligibility. Claims data on privately insured groups were also not very helpful, because they generally did not contain information to identify low-income persons.

Even when analysts could agree on how much utilization would change if a service were covered to a greater or lesser extent, there was no agreement on whether the resulting change in utilization was good or bad—that is, was it comprised of mostly "necessary" or mostly "unnecessary" services? In other words, there was no research on how health status changed if coverage or cost sharing changed. Nor could it be determined whether health status effects differed by income group.

As pointed out earlier, the Nixon administration's white paper emphasized health maintenance organizations (HMOs). The literature on HMOs (see Luft, 1978, 1981 for a summary) suggested that those enrolled in HMOs went to the hospital much less frequently but made approximately the same use of ambulatory care. Whether the reduction in hospital use was due to the fact that HMO enrollees were healthier or that HMOs practiced a different and less hospital-intensive style of medicine was not known. If the reduction in use was attributable to a less hospital-intensive style, no systematic study had been undertaken to determine whether such a style affected enrollees' health. The lack of answers to these questions did not prevent the Congress from embracing the HMO concept by passage of the 1973 Health Maintenance Organization Act; nonetheless, it was clear that fundamental questions remained.

Public Policy Experimentation and Objectives of the HIE

Although the randomized controlled trial had by 1970 become the standard for clinical research, the methodology had been little used in research directed at public policy. The first major public policy experiment was the New Jersey Negative Income Tax (NIT) Experiment, begun in 1968, to determine the effects on hours worked (labor supply) of individuals who were guaranteed a minimum income, with the minimum reduced by a specified percentage for each dollar earned. More specifically, the NIT Experiment sought to determine how hours worked varied as both the guarantee levels and income reductions varied.

Although the NIT Experiment produced equivocal results, it nonetheless served an important function by bringing to light several issues that had not been addressed in the debate over the negative income tax, such as the sensitivity of the cost of the plan to the length of the accounting period for income (Munnell, 1986). Moreover, it demonstrated the feasibility of policy experiments. As a result, a number of other policy experiments were launched, including additional income maintenance experiments as well as experiments in housing allowances and peak-load pricing of electricity and telephones. The Office of Economic Opportunity, which had sponsored the New Jersey Experiment, agreed to sponsor a similar experiment in health insurance.

Although the design of the Health Insurance Experiment began in mid-1971, enrollment in a pilot sample was not begun until late 1973 and the first regular sample families were not enrolled until late 1974. Enrollment was staggered over time and ended in early 1977. Because families participated for either three or five years (length of enrollment was randomized), the last families completed their participation in early 1982. All told, the experiment enrolled nearly 7,700 people in six sites; around 2,000 of the enrollees received their care through a staff model HMO.

The Health Insurance Experiment had several objectives:

1. To estimate how the use of various services responded to plans that varied cost sharing. In particular, what were the consequences of alternative levels of cost sharing for the total amount spent on medical care?
2. To estimate the consequences for health status, assuming that use varied with cost sharing. In the rhetoric of the policy debate, to what degree was additional care "necessary" if care was free at the point of use, and hence to what degree was free care desirable?
3. To determine if the answers to the first two questions varied by income group. In particular, should the poor be exempt from cost sharing? Was income-related cost sharing administratively feasible? The interest of the original sponsoring agency, the Office of Economic Opportunity, was in fact centered on the poor, and hence the original design of the experiment was limited to families with incomes under $12,000 per year. When the research operations of the Office of Economic Opportunity were abolished, however, the experiment was transferred to the Department of Health, Education, and Welfare. The design of the experiment was then broadened to include almost the entire range of income because of the interest at the time in a comprehensive national

plan. There remained, however, some oversampling of the poor in an attempt to estimate with greater precision the response of the poor to cost sharing. However, the elderly were omitted, because it was felt that Medicare was a successful program that did not need changing. (Indeed, at the time Senator Javits proposed making the entire population eligible for Medicare as a national health insurance program.)

4. To determine the effects of covering outpatient as well as inpatient services. This led to the inclusion of plans in the HIE that differentially covered outpatient services.
5. To estimate the reduction in use, if any, and the resulting health status effects in a well-established HMO. Was greater reliance on HMOs a desirable strategy?

The Design of the Experiment[1]

Between November 1974 and February 1977 the HIE enrolled families in six sites: Dayton, Ohio; Seattle, Washington; Fitchburg/Leominster, Massachusetts; Charleston, South Carolina; Franklin County, Massachusetts; and Georgetown County, South Carolina. The sites were selected to represent: (1) the four major census regions; (2) both northern and southern rural sites (Franklin and Georgetown counties); (3) the range of city sizes, which also acts as a surrogate for the complexity of the medical care delivery system because the concentration of specialists varies with city size; and (4) the range of waiting times to appointment and physicians per capita to test for the sensitivity of the results to the degree to which delivery systems were operating at capacity. Table 7-1 summarizes these characteristics of the six sites chosen.

Families participating in the experiment were assigned to one of fourteen different fee-for-service insurance plans, which varied the amount of cost sharing, or to a prepaid group practice, the Group Health Cooperative of Puget Sound, located in Seattle, Washington. In addition, some existing members of the prepaid group practice were enrolled as a comparison group for those randomly assigned to receive services at the prepaid group.

The fee-for-service insurance plans varied the coinsurance rate (the percentage of the bill paid by the patient) and the stop-loss provision, called the Maximum Dollar Expenditure in the HIE. The coinsurance

Table 7-1. Characteristics of HIE sites

Site	Census region	Population of urbanized area or county (1970)	Primary care physicians per 100,000 population (1972)[a]	Days spent waiting for an appointment with a primary care physician new patient[b] (1973, 1974)	Median family income (in dollars) (1969)	Percent over age 24 with less than 5 years education (1970)	Percent black (1970)	Number of enrollees
Seattle, WA	West	1,200,000	59	4.1	11,800	1.8	3	1,220[c]
Dayton, OH	North central	690,000	41	7.5	11,400	3.3	13	1,140
Charleston, SC	South	230,000	33	15.9	8,300	6.2	25	780
Fitchburg/Leominster, MA	Northeast	78,000	30	25.0	10,000	4.3	1	724
Franklin County, MA	Northeast	59,000	46	9.2	9,900	2.8	1	891
Georgetown County, SC	South	34,000	44	0	6,400	20.6	48	1,061
United States	—	—	46	7.1	9,600	5.5	11	—

a. Includes general practioners, family practitioners, internists, and pediatricians.
b. Physicians who do not use appointment systems and take patients on a first-come, first-served basis are valued as having zero wait time. All physicians sampled in Georgetown County at the time of the survey accepted patients on this basis. For other sites, the values are negligibly changed if only physicians using appointment systems are included.
c. An additional 1892 participants were enrolled in the Group Health Cooperative of Puget Sound.

Table 7-2. HIE enrollment sample, by site

Plan	Dayton	Seattle	Fitchburg	Franklin County	Charleston	Georgetown County	Total
Free	301	431	241	297	264	359	1,893
25 percent[a]	260	253	125	152	146	201	1,137
50 percent	191	0	56	58	26	52	383
95 percent	280	253	113	162	146	166	1,120
Individual deductible	105	285	188	220	196	282	1,276
Subtotal	1,137	1,222	723	889	778	1,060	5,809
Group Health Experimental		1,149					
Group Health Control		733					
Total	1,137	3,104	723	889	778	1,060	7,691

a. Includes those with 50 percent coinsurance for dental and mental health and 25 percent coinsurance for all other services.

rate was either 0, 25, 50, or 95 percent. For most families the Maximum Dollar Expenditure (MDE) was $1,000 per family per year, but it was reduced for low-income families. Specifically, the MDE was 5, 10, or 15 percent of income, or $1,000, whichever was less. Families were randomized among the 5, 10, and 15 percent figures. In one plan the MDE was $150 per person per year to a maximum of $450 per family. This provision was used only with 95 percent coinsurance; thus, this plan approximated a $150 per person deductible and is referred to below as the Individual Deductible plan.

Covered expenses included virtually all medical services. In general, the same coinsurance rate applied to all medical services, but there were two exceptions. In the Individual Deductible plan the cost sharing applied only to outpatient services; inpatient services were free. In some plans with 25 percent coinsurance for medical services, the coinsurance rate was 50 percent for dental and mental health services.

Table 7-2 gives the distribution of the 7,691 persons who participated in the HIE by plan and site. Approximately 70 percent participated for three years and the remainder participated for five years.

Main Findings of the Experiment

I begin with the findings from the fee-for-service part of the experiment and then turn to the HMO findings.

Effects on Use: Fee-for-Service

As shown in Table 7-3, individuals on the various plans differed substantially in their rate of use. The table shows variation by coinsurance; the MDE levels have been pooled because variation in the MDE percentage had only minor effects. The dollars spent per person per year were almost 50 percent higher if care was free at the point of use than in the least generous plan, the plan that required participants to pay 95 cents on the dollar up to the stop-loss figure. There were nearly two more face-to-face visits per person per year on the free care plan than on the 95 percent coinsurance plan, and the hospital admission rate was around 25 percent higher.

Because 70 percent of those admitted to the hospital exceeded their Maximum Dollar Expenditure, the effective cost sharing for those hos-

Table 7.3. Annual use of medical services per capita by type of plan, sample means

Plan	Outpatient Visits[a] (no.)	Outpatient Expenses[b] ($)	Inpatient Admissions (no.)	Inpatient Expenses[b] ($)	Total expenses[c] Unadjusted ($)	Total expenses[c] Adjusted ($)	Probability Any medical (%)	Probability Any inpatient (%)
Free	4.55 (0.168)	340 (10.9)	0.128 (0.0070)	409 (32.0)	749 (38.7)	750 (39)	86.8 (0.817)	10.3 (0.45)
Coinsurance rate								
25 percent	3.33 (0.190)	260 (14.70)	0.105 (0.0090)	373 (43.1)	634 (52.8)	617 (49)	78.8 (1.38)	8.4 (0.61)
50 percent	3.03 (0.221)	224 (16.8)	0.092 (0.0116)	450 (139)	674 (143.5)	573 (100)	77.2 (2.26)	7.2 (0.77)
95 percent	2.73 (0.177)	203 (12.0)	0.099 (0.0078)	315 (36.7)	518 (44.8)	504 (47)	67.7 (1.76)	7.9 (0.55)
Individual deductible	3.02 (0.171)	235 (11.9)	0.115 (0.0076)	373 (41.5)	608 (46.0)	630 (56)	72.3 (1.54)	9.6 (0.55)
Chi-square (df=4)	68.8	85.3	11.7	4.1	15.9	17	144.7	19.5
P value for chi-square (df=4)	< 0.0001	< 0.0001	0.02	n.s.	0.003	0.002	< 0.0001	< 0.0006

Note: Numbers in parentheses represent standard error, corrected for intertemporal/intrafamily correlation.

a. Visits are face-to-face contacts with MD, DO, or other health providers, excluding dentists and office psychotherapists as well as visits made for radiology, anesthesiology, or pathology services only.

b. Expressed in June 1984 dollars.

c. These figures are adjusted for the imbalance of plans across sites. The site-specific responses on each plan (simple means by site) are weighted by the fraction of the sample in each site and summed across sites. In the case of the 50 percent plan, which has no observations in Seattle, the weights are renormalized excluding Seattle.

pitalized on the 25, 50, and 95 percent coinsurance plans was not very different; for the typical person on those plans it cost $1,000 (the MDE) to go to the hospital. Hence, it is not surprising that admission rates were not much different among those three plans, nor that the admission rates were significantly lower on those plans than on the free care plan.

The cost per person admitted was not very different on any plan. Because most persons admitted to the hospital exceeded their stop-loss provision, the cost to most participants of an additional day, an additional procedure, or an additional test while hospitalized was zero, irrespective of the plan to which they were assigned.

The Individual Deductible plan had free inpatient care and costly outpatient care (95 percent coinsurance to a maximum of $150 per person). Comparison of the results on this plan with those of the free care plan allows one to determine whether more comprehensive coverage of outpatient care would save money. There were two reasons why this might be true. Because of the deductible, participants in the Individual Deductible plan did indeed visit the physician less, about six fewer visits per year for a family of four. As noted earlier, those arguing for more comprehensive care (for example, Roemer et al., 1975) feared that persons who had to pay for office visits would defer visiting the physician, thereby making it ultimately more costly to treat their malady. In addition, some argued that the asymmetric coverage of inpatient and outpatient services encouraged physicians to hospitalize patients for routine diagnostic procedures in order to minimize the cost to the patient. Such hospitalization, however, would raise the costs of medical care to society.

The results of the Individual Deductible plan disproved the notion that comprehensive coverage of outpatient services would save money. Although some patients manifestly did defer visiting the physician, this was not, on average, "penny-wise and pound-foolish"; total expenditures under the Individual Deductible plan were about 20 percent less than under the free care plan. Of course, the reduction in use may have been harmful to health; before turning to those results, I examine whether the response differed by subgroup, using a four-equation model described in Manning et al. (1987).

The pattern of reduced use by plan was found for each third of the income distribution (Table 7-4). Indeed, the percentage differences in expenditure between the two extreme plans, the free care plan and the 95 percent coinsurance plan, are largest for the highest third of the income distribution and smallest for the lowest third (this difference is not statistically significant at conventional levels). Although the response of the likelihood of *any* use to plan was greatest among the lowest third of the income distribution, the response of the likelihood of hospitalization was greatest among the highest third (results not shown), and the latter more than offsets the former in terms of total expenditure.

It should be remembered, however, that the responses shown in Table 7-4 are to the experimental insurance plans, and with the exception of the Individual Deductible plan, many of those in the lowest third of the income distribution had lower stop-loss values (because of the percentage-of-income feature of the Maximum Dollar Expenditure). For example, a poor family with $5,000 of income and a 10 percent of income limit on the Maximum Dollar Expenditure faced only a $500 maximum out-of-pocket expense, whereas a family with a $20,000 income, approximately the median family income in 1979, faced a $1,000 out-of-pocket limit. Thus, it would cost the poor family half of what the middle-class family would pay to go to the hospital. By contrast, if a member of the poor family were not admitted to the hospital, the chances were good that the family would not exceed its Maximum Dollar Expenditure, so both it and the middle-class family would probably face an expenditure of 95 cents on the dollar for outpatient care.

Table 7-4. Predicted annual use of medical services by plan and by income group

	Mean expenses (1984 dollars)			Significance test (*t*)	
Plan	Lowest third income group	Middle third income group	Highest third income group	Lowest third vs. middle third	Lowest third vs. highest third
Free	788	736	809	−1.78	0.53
Family pays:					
25 percent	680	588	623	−3.17	−1.47
50 percent	610	550	590	−1.89	−0.49
95 percent	581	494	527	−3.09	−1.41
Individual deductible	609	594	670	−0.57	1.38

Note: The statistics used in the *t* test were corrected for intertemporal and intrafamily correlations. The figure of −3.17 above indicates that, in the case of the 25 percent plan, the null hypothesis that the mean of the middle third income group equals the lowest third can be rejected at the 0.01 level of significance.

The results shown in Table 7-4 are aggregated across the six sites because no differences were found among the sites in the response to insurance plan, despite the differences in the characteristics of the sites shown in Table 7-1. The similarity in the response to plan among the sites gives researchers some confidence that the results can be generalized to other sites.

Effects on Health: Fee-for-Service

Although the evidence was thin and some were skeptical, the predominant opinion when the HIE began was that cost sharing probably did reduce use, although the magnitude of the reduction was highly uncertain.[2] Those on the left who accepted the view that cost sharing reduced use (or, as they put it, that cost sharing was a barrier to care) argued that it reduced necessary use or, in any event, that any gain from a decrease in unnecessary use was more than offset by a decrease in necessary use. By contrast, those on the right argued that the decrease was almost entirely in unnecessary use (or, as they put it, that free care led to abuse of the medical care system). The most direct method for assessing this argument was to examine the health of participants in the various plans at exit. If those on the left were correct, health status should be better on the free care plan, whereas if those on the right were correct, there should be no difference across the plans.

In fact, the results offered some support to both positions. For the average participant, there was little measurable effect of plan on outcome, other than for dental care. Moreover, the results were precise enough that the existence of substantial adverse effects can be ruled out. For those who began the experiment with hypertension or with correctable vision problems, there were adverse effects, and these adverse effects were concentrated among the poor. The remainder of this section describes these results in more detail.

The results of a number of outcome measures for the typical person are shown in Table 7-5. Because one cannot reject the hypothesis of no difference among plans with cost sharing, those plans have been pooled in the column labeled "Total." The five measures of general health include physical health (the first two), mental health, social health, and general health perceptions, that is, a self-assessment of overall health. All these measures are scored on a zero to 100 scale, where 100 is healthiest.

In light of the 95 percent confidence intervals for these measures, the possibility of more than a one- to two-point difference favoring the free plan can be ruled out. How important is such a difference? The meaning of a one-point change in a scale, of course, varies by scale. In the case of the two physical health measures, a ten-point difference in physical functioning, all else being equal, may mean having chronic, mild osteoarthritis, whereas each one-point change in the role functioning scale represents a one-percentage-point difference in the probability of being limited in one's major role. Being fired from one's job causes a three-point difference in the mental health scale, and a one-percentage-point increase in the likelihood of being psychiatrically impaired is associated with a five-point decrease in the social contacts scale. Being diagnosed as hypertensive causes a five-point difference in the health perceptions scale.

The next three measures are of health habits, and they also show no effect of plan. Again, precision is good enough to rule out the likelihood that large effects were not detected because of a too-small sample size. The smoking scale is the risk of mortality based on the amount smoked per day relative to a person who never smoked or an ex-smoker; for example, those who smoked two packs per day would receive a value of 2.07, because their risk of death, all else being equal, is a little more than double that of a non-smoker or an ex-smoker. The measure of weight has been standardized for height in order to measure obesity better.

The two physiologic measures shown, diastolic blood pressure and functional far vision, do show beneficial effects of free care. There is a reduction of 0.8 of a millimeter of mercury in diastolic blood pressure, and a reduction of 0.1 Snellen lines in functional far vision (equal to a change from 20/22.5 to 20/22). These effects, however, are heavily concentrated among those who were hypertensive (or myopic) at enrollment and who were also poor (specifically, in the lowest fifth of the income distribution) (Table 7-6). An examination of 20 additional measures of physiologic health (for example, forced expiratory volume, hemoglobin, urine culture) failed to reveal any other effects except for functional near vision, where effects were similar to those for far vision (Keeler et al., 1987).

The magnitude of the effect for diastolic blood pressure, 0.8 of a millimeter of mercury, may appear small to a clinician accustomed to managing individual cases; however, it causes a nontrivial change in the risk

Table 7-5. Predicted exit values and raw mean differences of health status measures for an average adult, by measure and plan

Health status measures	No.[a]	Cost-sharing plans				Free plan	Predicted mean difference (free minus cost-sharing)[d]	Raw mean difference (free minus cost-sharing)
		Cata-strophic[b]	Inter-med.[c]	Ind. deduct.	Total			
General health (score, 1–100)								
Physical functioning	3,862	86.0	85.0	84.9	85.3	85.3	0.0 (−1.6, 1.5)	−0.3 (−2.3, 1.7)
Role functioning	3,861	95.5	95.0	94.7	95.1	95.4	0.3 (−0.6, 1.2)	−0.3 (−2.2, 1.6)
Mental health	3,862	75.6	75.5	75.8	75.6	75.5	−0.2 (−1.1, 0.8)	−0.1 (−1.1, 1.0)
Social contacts	3,827	69.3	70.2	69.8	69.8	69.4	−0.3 (−2.3, 1.6)	−0.2 (−2.4, 2.0)
Health perceptions	3,843	68.1	68.0	67.9	68.0	67.4	−0.6 (−1.5, 0.3)	−0.9 (−2.1, 0.3)
Health habits								
Smoking (scale, 1–2.20)	3,758	1.28	1.29	1.29	1.29	1.29	0.0 (−0.02, 0.02)	−0.00 (−0.03, 0.03)
Weight (kg)	2,804	72.8	72.6	73.1	72.8	72.8	0.0 (−0.5, 0.5)	0.0 (−1.0, 1.0)
Cholesterol level (mg/dl)	3,381	202	200	204	202	203	1.0 (−1.03, 3.0)	−1.3 (−4.5, 1.9)

Physiologic health							
Diastolic blood pressure (mm Hg)	3,495	79.0	78.5	78.8	78.8	78.0	-0.8 $(-1.5, -0.1)$[e]	-0.9 $(-1.8, -0.1)$[f]
Functional far vision (no. of Snellen lines)	3,477	2.55	2.50	2.51	2.52	2.42	-0.1 $(-0.16, -0.04)$[g]	-0.13 $(-0.21, -0.05)$[h]
Risk of dying (score)	3,317	1.01	0.98	1.03	1.01	0.99	-0.02 $(-0.05, 0.02)$	-0.03 $(-0.08, 0.02)$

a. Numbers of persons in various parts of the analysis are dissimilar because noncompleters were not included for physiologic health, weight, or cholesterol level and because of differences among measures in the number of persons with valid enrollment or exit data. Teenagers aged 14–17 at enrollment and pregnant women were excluded from analyses of weight.

b. 95 percent coinsurance.

c. 25 and 50 percent coinsurance.

d. Numbers in parentheses are 95-percent confidence intervals; an approximate interval is given for role functioning.

e. $t = 2.21$; $p = 0.03$.

f. $t = 2.20$; $p = 0.03$.

g. $t = 3.29$; $p = 0.001$ (persons with normal vision were included and given a value of 2.0).

h. $t = 3.18$; $p = 0.001$.

of death for the poor person with elevated risk factors, though not for the average person (see Tables 7-5 and 7-6). The risk of death is a mathematical function of blood pressure, cholesterol level, and smoking habits. The function comes from epidemiologic studies; all of the effect shown stems from the difference in blood pressure by plan, because there are no effects of free care on cholesterol levels or smoking status. For those who are both poor and at relatively high risk of death, the better blood pressure control results in about a 14 percent reduction in the risk of death (1.00–1.83/2.13).

There was a substantial effect of cost sharing on the use of dental services. The change in the use of dental services resulted in more filled

Table 7-6. Predicted exit values of blood pressure, vision, and risk of dying in high and low income groups at elevated risk

Physiologic measure	Total cost-sharing	Free plan	Difference between free and cost-sharing
Elevated Risk and Low Income[a]			
Diastolic blood pressure	89.3	87.0	−2.3 (−4.9, +0.3)[b]
Functional far vision	3.61	3.30	−0.3 (−0.6, +0.02)
Risk of dying	2.13	1.83	−0.30[c] (−0.6, −0.04)
Elevated Risk and High Income			
Diastolic blood pressure	88.0	88.1	+0.1 (−2.0, +2.2)
Functional far vision	3.21	3.14	−0.07 (−0.4, +0.2)
Risk of dying	2.09	1.96	−0.13 (−0.4, +0.1)

Note: Numbers in parentheses are 95% confidence intervals.

a. The elevated risk for diastolic blood pressure and risk of dying is the least healthy fifth on each measure. For functional far vision, elevated risk in this table refers *only* to the upper one-quarter of the distribution of values for uncorrected natural vision. Predictions in these two columns were made with use of the mean value of the elevated-risk group.

b. $t = 1.72$; $p = 0.08$.

c. $t = 2.23$; $p = 0.03$.

and fewer carious teeth at exit, though there was no measurable effect on the formation of caries. There was also a modest improvement in an index of periodontal health. Space does not permit further discussion of these results here; the interested reader should consult Manning et al., 1985, and Bailit et al., 1985.

All the results presented thus far have been for adults. With the exception of fewer caries and more filled teeth, there were no measurable beneficial effects of free care for children. The interested reader should consult Valdez et al., 1985, and Valdez, 1986 for more details of effects on children.

Because the HIE utilized income-related benefits, something was learned about the administrative issues involved with such benefits. There is, of course, no comparison experiment without income-related benefits, so these lessons cannot be quantified, but they are worthy of a short comment nonetheless. As is clear to anyone who is familiar with the Internal Revenue Service code or with the Aid to Families with Dependent Children (AFDC) program, an income-related benefit is not easy to administer, and there are possibilities for manipulation.

Two lessons were drawn from this experience. First, if there are to be income-related benefits, one should minimize the number of people whose benefits are conditioned on income. In practice, this means relating the back end of the health insurance policy (the stop-loss feature) to income, not the initial deductible or coinsurance, and cutting off the income-related feature at some absolute level of income (for example, the $1,000 ceiling used in the HIE). Such lessons may seem obvious, but a component of the Ford administration plan for national health insurance envisioned an income-related premium, deductible, and coinsurance. Second, one should not alter the household unit whose income and expenses are being pooled until the end of the accounting period. An accounting period of 12 months was used in the HIE (that is, the income-related feature was based on annual income rather than monthly income or some other time period). During the space of a year a household can change: couples separate and divorce; children leave home; single persons marry. Aside from newborn or adopted children, who were recognized immediately, other changes were recognized only when a new accounting period for income began (for example, at the end of the 12-month period). Otherwise there would have been enormous administrative complexity, as when a child, for example, would leave to live with her grandmother and then a few months later return to her mother.

Effects on Use: Health Maintenance Organizations

The findings of the HIE with respect to health maintenance organizations (HMOs) are necessarily less definitive than those with respect to the fee-for-service system because they pertain to only one HMO (the Group Health Cooperative of Puget Sound, Seattle). Moreover, that organization was a well-established staff model HMO. Thus, even if the findings were representative of other group or staff model HMOs, they may well not be representative of Individual Practice Associations (IPAs), not to mention newer Preferred Provider Organizations. Nonetheless, the HIE is the only randomized experiment ever conducted at a well-established HMO, and hence the findings are worthy of attention.[3]

The HMO had a large effect on use, but its effect was entirely on hospital admissions (Table 7-7). Comparisons were made with the free care fee-for-service plan because there is no cost sharing for HMO participants; hence, a comparison with the free care plan is an all-other-factors-equal kind of comparison. Hospital admissions were nearly 40 percent less among the HMO group than in the free care plan, although outpatient visit rates were approximately equal. This translates into a saving of around 25 percent in imputed expenditure. Relative to plans with cost sharing, of course, the saving is lower or even nonexistent. It is not known, however, what use at the HMO would have been had the HMO employed cost sharing.

Because these effects on use were observed among two similar groups, there is a strong implication that the saving observed is attributable to a different, less hospital-intensive style of medical care.[4] Use was also examined among a self-selected group of HMO enrollees, the control group. As shown in Table 7-6, use by the control group was similar to use by the experimental group, implying minimal adverse selection at this HMO.

Effects on Health: Health Maintenance Organizations

Health status results for the HMO bore a considerable similarity to those found for cost sharing, despite the differences in the nature of the reduction in utilization (that is, concentrated in hospital admissions). For the average person there was little measurable effect on outcome, but for those who were poor and sick there was some indication of possible adverse effects (Tables 7-8 and 7-9). The only adverse effects observed for the average person were in two measures, the rate of bed-days due to poor health during a year and the probability of one or more of five serious symptoms, as assessed by a physician panel. (Further details on these measures and other results can be found in Ware et al., 1986, Ware et al., 1987, and Sloss et al., 1987.) In light of the multiple measures being observed, the results for bed-days and serious symptoms may be attributable to chance. The differing qualitative pattern for the sick poor, however, is not likely to be attributable to chance. If one conducts a test of whether the effects of the HMO on health are independent of initial health and income, one can reject the hypothesis at the 1 percent level (see Appendix G of Ware et al., 1987).

Although the HMO's less hospital-intensive style of practice did not measurably affect health status for the average person, patient satisfaction was lower for people randomized into the HMO (Davies et al., 1986). This was not true for all dimensions of patient satisfaction; for example, those randomized to the HMO were more satisfied with office waits than those in fee-for-service medicine (and in fact office waits were shorter at the HMO). But for overall satisfaction, and for the dimensions of satisfaction that seemed to drive cost differences, namely availability of hospitals and specialists, those randomized into the HMO were less satisfied. By contrast, those who had already enrolled at the HMO were, on average, as satisfied as those in the fee-for-service system. Thus, there clearly are a number of individuals who prefer the fee-for-service style of medicine and are willing to pay something for it.

Effects of Findings on Public and Private Policy

Effects on Insurance Plan Design

The effects of any new information on policy are necessarily conjectural. In the case of the Health Insurance Experiment, however, there is a plausible link between the publication of the experimental findings and changes in plan design. In particular, there were substantial increases in cost sharing in private major medical plans in the early 1980s (Table 7-10). The percentage of medium and large companies with first dollar coverage of hospital services declined from 70 to 37 percent between 1982 and 1984 (Goldsmith, 1984). There was also a shift toward comprehensive major medical plans, which are similar to the plans in the HIE (Table 7-11).

What evidence is there that these changes might be attributable to

Table 7-7. Hospital admissions and face-to-face visits, annual rates

Plan	Admission rate/100 persons[a]	Hospital days/ 100 persons	Face-to-face visits[b]	Preventive visits[c]	Imputed annual expenditure per participant[d] (1983 dollars)
GHC Experimental	8.4 (0.67)	49 (9.6)	4.3 (0.14)	0.55 (0.02)	439 (25)
GHC Control	8.3 (1.01)	38 (9.0)	4.7 (0.17)	0.60 (0.02)	469 (44)
Fee-for-service					
Free	13.8 (1.51)	83 (26)	4.2 (0.25)	0.41 (0.03)	609 (66)
25 percent	10.0 (1.43)	87 (28)	3.5 (0.35)	0.32 (0.03)	620 (103)

95 percent	10.5	46	2.9	0.29	459
	(1.68)	(9.9)	(0.34)	(0.04)	(72)
Individual	8.8	28	3.3	0.27	413
deductible	(1.20)	(5.1)	(0.33)	(0.03)	(51)

Note: The sample includes all participants present at enrollment while they remained in the Seattle area. For GHC Controls and Experimentals, the data include both in- and out-of-plan use. Standard errors are given in parentheses.

a. A count of all continuous periods of inpatient treatment.

b. Includes all visits with face-to-face contact with health providers for which a separate charge would have been made in fee-for-service. Excludes radiology, pathology, pre- and postnatal, pre- and postoperative, speech therapy, psychotherapy, dental, chiropractic, podiatry, Christian Science healer, and telephone visits.

c. Includes well-child care, immunizations, screening examinations, routine physical and gynecological examinations, and visits with Pap smears (other than for cancer). Excludes prenatal, vision, and hearing visits. In the case of GHC, includes in-plan and out-of-plan visits.

d. Values include both in-plan and out-of-plan use by GHC participants. The method of imputing expenditure is described in Manning, Leibowitz, Goldberg, et al., 1984. Because of the inclusion of age and sex as covariates, the *t*-statistics are larger than those that would be calculated from the standard errors shown in the table.

The sample consists of all participants present at enrollment while they remained in the Seattle area. Except for decedents, observations or partial years of participation are deleted.

Table 7-8. Predicted health outcomes for a typical person according to health variable and system of care

Variable (direction of better health)	Group health cooperative	Fee-for-service		GHC minus free[a]	GHC minus pay
		Free	Pay		
Health habits					
Smoking	1.28	1.31	1.24	-.02 (-.06, .01)	.04 (.01, .07)*
Weight	72.3	72.4	72.1	-0.1 (-1.1, 0.8)	0.1 (-0.6, 0.9)
Cholesterol level	201.7	205.8	203.6	-4.1 (-10.1, 1.8)	-1.9 (-6.3, 2.5)
Physiologic health					
Diastolic blood pressure	77.0	77.1	77.7	-.06 (-1.6, 1.4)	-.7 (-1.8, 0.5)
Functional far vision	2.7	2.6	2.9	0.1 (-0.1, 0.3)	-0.2 (-0.3, 0.01)
Risk of dying	100	104	96	-4 (-11, 3)	4 (-2, 10)
General health					
Physical functioning	85.6	84.8	86.1	.77 (-2.4, 4.0)	-0.56 (-3.3, 1.9)
Role functioning	94.8	96.6	96.3	-1.8 (-6.7, 3.1)	-1.5 (-6.2, 3.2)
Mental health	75.8	75.7	75.4	.10 (-1.7, 2.0)	.40 (-1.1, 1.9)
Social contacts	69.8	68.8	69.9	1.1 (-2.6, 4.7)	-.07 (-3.0, 2.9)
Health perceptions	69.4	68.1	70.0	1.2 (-0.6, 3.1)	-.65 (-2.1, 0.8)
Bed-days	4.0	3.3	3.4	0.7 (1.4, 0.1)*	0.6 (1.2, 0.04)*
Serious symptoms[b]	16.1	11.6	14.2	4.5 (7.8, 1.1)**	1.9 (4.7, -1.0)

a. Numbers in parentheses are 95 percent confidence intervals.

b. Measured as the number of symptoms.

*$p < 0.05$, two-tailed test; **$p < 0.01$, two-tailed test.

Table 7-9. Predicted outcomes of general health indices according to variable, system of care, income, and initial health status

Variable (direction of better health)	Group health cooperative	Fee-for-service		GHC minus free[a]	GHC minus pay
		Free	Pay		
		Low Income and Initial Ill Health			
Physical functioning	64.1	57.8	60.3	6.3 (−8.4, 20.9)	3.8 (15.7, −8.0)
Role functioning	60.7	64.0	64.2	−3.3 (−29.2, 22.6)	−3.5 (−28.3, 21.3)
Mental health	64.4	67.2	65.5	−2.8 (−8.1, 2.5)	−1.1 (−6.1, 3.9)
Social contacts	46.6	52.6	46.9	−6.0 (−17.5, 5.4)	−0.4 (−14.5, 13.8)
Health perceptions	55.1	57.8	55.9	−2.7 (−7.8, 2.4)	−0.8 (−5.3, 3.7)
Bed-days	9.6	5.9	9.2	3.7 (7.5, 0.5)*	0.4 (4.5, −3.0)
Serious symptoms	34.7	21.8	24.0	12.9 (23.1, 2.8)*	10.7 (22.3, −0.9)
		High Income and Initial Ill Health			
Physical functioning	55.4	52.7	64.7	2.7 (−10.3, 15.7)	−9.3 (−19.2, 0.61)
Role functioning	69.6	70.6	76.6	−1.0 (−24.0, 22.0)	−7.0 (−27.0, 13.0)
Mental health	63.2	67.3	63.1	−4.1 (−10.2, 2.0)	.05 (−4.8, 4.9)
Social contacts	53.1	48.9	46.2	4.2 (−4.8, 13.3)	6.9 (−0.87, 14.7)
Health perceptions	56.6	49.5	55.4	7.1 (2.4, 11.9)**	1.2 (−2.5, 4.9)
Bed-days	7.3	7.7	5.3	−0.4 (2.3, −2.9)	2.0 (4.7, −0.4)
Serious symptoms	25.7	20.3	27.1	5.4 (15.7, −4.8)	−1.4 (8.0, −10.8)

a. Numbers in parentheses are 95 percent confidence intervals.

*$p < 0.05$, two-tailed test; **$p < 0.01$, two-tailed test.

Table 7-10. Comprehensive major medical deductibles among salaried employees (in percentages)

Year	<$50	$50 to <$100	$100	>$100
1982	2	40	46	9
1984	3	8	41	39
1986	3	3	39	55

Source: American Hospital Association, "Digest of National Health Care Use and Expense Indicators," November 1987, mimeo. The data are from The Wyatt Company's 1986 Group Benefits Survey, covering salaried employees of 1,418 U.S. employers. Only a modest portion of this increase could be attributed to inflation since the personal consumption deflator for Gross National Product rose only 3.4 per year between 1982 and 1986.

Note: The 1982 and 1984 numbers do not add to 100%, in part because of rounding errors.

Table 7-11. Prevalence of major medical plans among salaried employees (in percentages)

Year	Basic with major medical	Comprehensive major medical
1982	62	37
1984	40	59
1986	27	72

Source: Same as Table 7–10.

the results of the Health Insurance Experiment? There is little direct evidence. In some cases there is a reference to the HIE results in materials prepared by companies to explain the changes.[5] The changes, however, did coincide with the first major publications of experimental results (Newhouse, Manning, et al., 1981; Brook, Ware, et al., 1983), which were given wide attention in both the general and trade press. Benefits consultants for employers were well aware of the findings. Thus, it is a reasonable surmise that the Experiment played some role in these changes, but there were almost certainly other forces prompting them as well. For example, the sharp recession of the early 1980s clearly motivated employers to find ways to reduce total compensation.

According to the experimental results, the increased use of initial cost sharing should have reduced utilization. In fact, there was a marked decline in hospital days, a decrease of 13 percent between 1982 and 1984 and another 7 percent between 1984 and 1985 among the under-65 group (Manning et al., 1987). Occupancy rates in community hospitals dropped from 75 to 64 percent (American Hospital Association, 1987). Physician visit rates fell between 1982 and 1984 but rose again in 1985 to their 1982 level, perhaps because of a substitution of outpatient for inpatient care (Manning et al., 1987).

The changes in cost sharing described above took place among employees of large and middle-sized companies. The experimental results imply that for this group of persons there would have been minimal or no adverse effects on health status. Indeed, no measurable effects on the health status measures gathered by the National Health Interview Survey have been observed (Table 7-12).

In addition to increased initial cost sharing in the 1980s, many insurance plans increased their coverage of the "back end" of medical bills, analogous to the MDE. Between 1980 and 1984 the number of major medical plans with a maximum coverage limit of $1,000,000 or an unlimited amount rose from 46 percent to 79 percent, and by 1984, 98 percent of employees with a major medical plan had some kind of stop-loss feature, usually between $1,000 and $2,000 (Health Insurance Association of America, 1985, 1987). The degree to which this increase is attribut-

Table 7-12. Selected health status measures from the National Health Interview Survey

Measure	Year		
	1982	1985	1987
Restricted activity day associated with acute or chronic condition (number of days)			
All	14.3	14.8	14.5
Bed-disability	6.4	6.1	6,2
Work- or school loss	4.6	5.2	5.1
Self-assessed health status (%)			
Fair	8.1	7.4	7.3
Poor	3.4	2.9	2.7

Source: National Center for Health Statistics, "Current estimates from the Health Interview Survey, 1982, 1985, 1987," Washington: U.S. Government Printing Office, 1985, 1986, 1988 (series 10, nos. 150, 160, 166).

able to the HIE policies is not known, but the MDE may have served a demonstration effect.

The HIE results also suggested that the poor and sick could suffer from cost sharing. These results may have played some role in tempering the views of those who felt that cost sharing should play a more prominent role in the Medicaid program, although this is difficult to determine. In any event, cost sharing in the Medicaid program did not generally take hold.

The HIE results all apply to the degree of cost sharing within the insured population. They do not necessarily apply to the uninsured, who lie outside the range of variation observed in the HIE. Indeed, there is other evidence that terminating coverage among a poor, sick population had substantial—in some cases even devastating—effects on health status (Lurie et al., 1984, 1986).

Effects on Regulatory and Competitive Initiatives

As noted earlier, the HIE results showed essentially no effect on hospital cost per case, probably because 70 percent of those hospitalized under the cost-sharing plans exceeded their Maximum Dollar Expenditure, with the result that for those hospitalized all plans tended to collapse toward the free plan at the margin.[6] Thus, the HIE results showed that traditional reimbursement insurance would not much affect hospital cost per stay, the component of hospital cost that was accounting for almost all the increase in hospital cost.[7] At the federal level, this became one more incentive to develop the Prospective Payment System for determining hospital budgets, and at the state level it was one more incentive toward rate regulation. In short, if hospital cost increases were perceived as a policy problem, variations in cost sharing would not have a large effect.[8]

During the 1980s there was a substantial growth in the number of HMOs; the number of plans grew from 236 in 1980 to 595 in 1986. Although it is unlikely that the HIE results played an important role in this expansion, the results showing that HMOs pursued a less hospital-intensive style of care with no deleterious results for the average person may have assisted to some degree.[9] There was also a widespread movement to expand the enrollment of Medicaid eligibles in HMOs. Although the HIE results may appear to suggest that fee-for-service medicine might be better for Medicaid eligibles, the HIE free fee-for-service plan is not the same as a Medicaid policy because the Experiment paid physicians at market rates. As is well known, Medicaid plans generally pay physicians well below the rates that both private insurance and Medicare pay. As a result, many private physicians do not accept Medicaid patients. In this situation, a Medicaid eligible may well be better off in an HMO.

Effects on the Policymaking Process within the Government

During the Carter administration, the Department of Health and Human Services constructed a model for estimating the cost of various insurance plans. The early findings from the HIE were incorporated into this model. There was little interest in this subject during the Reagan administration, and the model fell into disuse. Instead, much attention was focused on the Medicare program, a subject about which the Experiment had little to say because Medicare eligibles had not been enrolled. Thus, during the 1980s the major effects of the HIE have probably been on the benefit design of private insurance plans. [10]

Implications of the Findings for Health Services Research

Need to Obtain Outcome Measures

The health status results described above, which showed little or no measurable effect of variation in cost sharing on average health status, were all based on measures of outcome among the individual participants. One inference from these results would be that cost sharing reduced utilization that was primarily inappropriate or that was for treatment of minor or trivial problems.

An alternative strategy for inferring effects on health status is to use data from claims records and charts. Such a strategy produces a markedly different conclusion about the effect of cost sharing.

Data from charts have been used to assess the appropriateness of hospital care in the HIE (Siu et al., 1986). These data showed that cost sharing reduced both appropriate and inappropriate hospitalization by approximately the same percentage. [11] Data from claims were used to appraise the appropriateness of antibiotic prescribing, and they produced a similar finding to that for hospitalization; cost sharing affected the use of antibiotics for bacterial (appropriate) and viral (inappropriate) conditions by approximately the same percentage (Foxman et al., 1987). Data from claims also showed that cost sharing affected medical care use for conditions for which medical care is generally efficacious as much or more as for conditions in which it is not effective (Lohr et al., 1986). Finally, preventive care was lower in the cost-sharing plans. Thus on several fronts cost sharing appeared to reduce not only inappropriate but also appropriate utilization, as judged by data on claims and charts. The only exception was use of the emergency room, in which claims data showed that use for less urgent conditions was notably more responsive to cost sharing than that for more urgent conditions (O'Grady et al., 1985). In sum, one would obtain a considerably more negative view of cost sharing if one had only data from claims and charts than if one had direct measures of outcomes.

There are three possibilities for reconciling the findings based on direct outcome measurement and those based on data from claims and charts. First, the outcome measures could be invalid. In light of the extensive data on the reliability and validity of these measures, however, such a possibility can be dismissed (see Brook et al., 1980 and subsequent; Lohr et al., 1983 and subsequent; Davies et al., 1988). Second, the inferences from the claims and charts could be invalid. Although there is undoubtedly some misclassification of patients from claims data, it seems improbable that the misclassification would be to such a degree as to account for all the various findings just described. Moreover, the inferences on appropriate hospital use come from using the Appropriateness Evaluation Protocol, a well-established method for inferring appropriateness from charts.

If in fact the findings from both the outcome measures and the claims and chart data are correct, then the only possibility is that some people are being made worse off by the additional medical care on the free plan and that this is offsetting the beneficial effects (for example, one can calculate the incidence of side effects from inappropriate prescribing of antibiotics), or that the assumed beneficial effects from the additional appropriate use are small, or both. This inference is somewhat different from what one would obtain from outcome data alone and thus emphasizes the importance of examining both outcome and claims measures. With only outcomes data one could not have inferred that there may well have been both positive and negative effects that offset each other (that is, one might have concluded that all the additional use was for trivial purposes). On the other hand, with only claims data one would have inferred negative health effects.

Follow-on Research

The HIE was an intellectual progenitor of two large research projects: the Health Services Utilization Study (HSUS) and the Medical Outcomes Study (MOS). The HIE showed that both cost sharing and free care left a high (absolute) percentage of inappropriate care. The HSUS study attempted to develop guidelines that would differentially affect inappropriate care (Chassin et al., 1987). The findings of that study have helped bring about a major federal initiative in outcomes research.

Like all research projects, the HIE left a number of questions unanswered. Would the HMO results have been different if it had been possible to include a number of HMOs? Would the results be different among the aged? The HIE suggested that there were beneficial effects of additional care among the poor and the sick, but because it had sampled a general population, it had rather few people who were both poor and sick. Would it have detected more important beneficial effects among this subgroup if they had been more numerous? The MOS (Tarlov et al., 1989) was directed at these issues. Although it was not an experimental study, it did seek to compare outcomes among those enrolled in different kinds of delivery systems (including three HMOs, as well as the fee-for-service system), it did oversample the chronically ill, and it did include the aged.

The Role of Randomized Experiments in Health Services Research

Although there is and will continue to be a large role for nonexperimental studies, one can clearly have greater confidence in the findings of randomized studies. A striking example of the difference comes from comparing the HIE results on coverage of outpatient services with those of the so-called California Medi-Cal "experiment," which showed that coverage of outpatient services appeared to reduce costs. Specifically, the California results appeared to show that instituting a $1.00 per visit charge in the Medicaid program in California increased total expenditure;

although the copayment caused a reduction in office visits, there appeared to be an increase in hospitalization that more than offset the saving from fewer outpatient visits (Roemer et al., 1975; Helms et al., 1978). The increase in hospitalization was interpreted as a consequence of the copayment's inducing patients not to seek care at an early stage ("penny-wise and pound-foolish"). Effects on outcomes were not measured. The California experiment was, however, not a true experiment in that the group that had to pay for visits was not similar to the group that did not; in particular, the former group had relatively higher income, because the poorer portion of the Medicaid population was exempted from the copayment.

The HIE result is, of course, exactly the opposite (see Table 7-3), and it is similar to the result of the other true experiment on this issue, which was conducted in Kansas in 1970 (Hill and Veney, 1970; Lewis and Keairnes, 1970). What might explain the different results in California?

The California experiment inferred an effect of cost sharing by comparing hospital use before and after the copayment was instituted in the groups subject to and exempt from cost sharing. If in fact the copayment deterred people from seeking care until they had to be hospitalized, one should have seen a rise in hospitalization rates among the group in which the copayment was instituted and a flat rate among the group that continued to be exempt from the copayment. Instead, there was a fall in hospital admissions among the group with no cost sharing, while the group with cost sharing had a flat pattern. The fall in use may have been an artifact if those who were hospitalized in the "before" period had a transitory fall in income and therefore were differentially assigned to the group exempt from copayment. Whether or not this explanation is correct, there is certainly a dramatic difference between the findings of the two randomized studies and the one nonrandomized "experiment."

Perhaps because they come from a randomized experiment, the results from the HIE on the effects of cost sharing have been generally accepted. Indeed, their acceptance appears to have gone beyond the research community; the relevant nonexperimental work did not lead to changes in benefit design, whereas the HIE arguably did. There could have been several reasons for this. The nonexperimental studies diverged substantially in their findings, and they contained no outcome results. Even had the nonexperimental studies found similar results, however, nonrandomized studies may not be as readily accepted. Thus, one can make a case that more definitive studies are worth their cost.

Cost is an often cited drawback of a large randomized experiment. Although experiments are without question expensive relative to retrospective observational studies, they are not necessarily expensive with respect to prospective observational studies, such as the MOS, because much of the expense of an experiment is connected with data collection, not with randomization. [12]

More fundamentally, the cost of the experiment has to be compared with its benefits. In light of the knowledge gained from the HIE, a good case can be made that institutions supporting research, such as the government and foundations, should have some of their portfolio in large, long-term projects. This is not easy to do, however. In the case of government there is a natural tendency not to look past the next election and hence to focus on projects that will produce results in the short term. There is also a tendency not to concentrate funding because of Congress's desire to see federal monies spent in each congressional district. Both factors tend to lead to small projects, but such projects are often simply on too small a scale to lead to major advances in knowledge. In the case of many foundations, the scale required may simply be too great for their resources.

Although controlled experiments have many obvious advantages, they also have drawbacks. The expense of the experiment means that there are many dollars in one basket if the design or execution of the experiment turns out to be flawed. Because the experiment is prospective, it necessarily takes time. If there are relevant nonexperimental data available, it will certainly be faster to analyze them.

Moreover, during the time the experiment is being conducted, the policy environment may change. For example, there was no interest in the executive branch in national health insurance when the HIE ended, although there was great interest when it began. Conversely, there was little or no interest in changing Medicare when the Experiment began, but the year after the field work ended, the Prospective Payment System was implemented. The moral is that any experiment needs to focus on enduring questions: in this case, what services to cover and how well to cover them, questions that must be answered by any private as well as public insurance plan.

In conclusion, one might ask how the design of the HIE would have changed if the changes in the policy environment had been anticipated. Three such changes might have been made. First, there has been much greater interest in the HMO findings than was originally anticipated, largely because HMOs are now a much more prominent part of the delivery system. The HMO portion of the experiment was distinctly secondary to the fee-for-service portion and necessarily was less precise. The HIE was designed at the same time when the initial HMO Act of 1973 was enacted. What I have been terming fee-for-service remained for many years after 1973 the dominant delivery system. Today, however, managed care is on the ascendancy, and it appears as if the "unmanaged" fee-for-service system that was studied in the HIE will play a smaller role in the future. If this had been anticipated, more HMOs might have been included in the Experiment. Within the constraint of a given budget, however, including more HMOs would have reduced the size of the fee-for-service sample. It is not clear that the resulting loss of precision would have been acceptable.

Second, Medicare is no longer sacrosanct. For example, the cost-sharing arrangements in Medicare have changed. Hence the elderly might have been included in the HIE, although in this case as well it is not clear that the reduced precision among the nonelderly sample would have been acceptable.

Third, the HIE was designed at a time when the major policy interest was in a comprehensive national health insurance program, and thus it was important to determine effects of alternative health insurance plans for the general population. In view of the finding that the outcome effects are concentrated among the poor and the sick, there would have been a strong case for oversampling such individuals.

A final lesson from the HIE is not restricted to experiments but rather applies to many health services research projects, namely that such projects are best done with an interdisciplinary team. The HIE, for example, needed researchers with expertise in medicine, economics, statistics, measurement psychology, survey methods, and data base management, as well as overall project management, in order to succeed. It was essential to the conduct of the project that individuals trained in those fields not only were part of the project but had day-to-day interactions. Without such interactions, the project would not have produced much of value.

8

Alternative Delivery Systems

Harold S. Luft and Ellen M. Morrison

While some American health policy analysts look abroad for examples to implement in the U.S. environment, analysts from other countries often come to the United States to learn about health maintenance organizations (HMOs) and other alternative delivery systems. These alternative forms of financing and delivery of medical care still represent a relatively small part of the whole system, but they are important examples of the pluralistic approach common to most U.S. policies. Furthermore, just as the states have been seen as laboratories for the testing of social policies that may eventually be adopted nationally, alternative delivery systems are often seen as demonstrations of what may be implemented eventually as national health policy.

The general term *alternative delivery system* (ADS) is used to include a wide range of approaches to the financing and delivery of medical care. The most widely known type of ADS is the health maintenance organization, or HMO, which traditionally takes on responsibility for providing medical care to a clearly defined population which has enrolled voluntarily. Furthermore, there are economic incentives for the providers to exercise some controls over the costs of the services delivered (Luft, 1981). The HMO is distinguished from the traditional system of medical care providers working on a fee-for-service basis, with payments made either directly by the patient or through a third-party insurer which pays for services rendered. (As will be discussed below, the distinctions among various types of payment-delivery systems are becoming blurred.) Other types of alternative delivery systems include preferred provider organizations (PPOs), which take a wide variety of forms but generally have incentives for patients to selectively use some providers who agree to accept specified fees and utilization review systems (Gabel, Ermann, et al., 1986).

Perhaps because of the nature of HMOs as alternative systems for the provision of medical care, the study of HMOs has incorporated many of the key issues addressed by health services research. For example, the initial policy interest in HMOs arose from the observation that medical care use and costs for HMO enrollees were lower than for people with conventional insurance. To assess the validity of this observation, researchers had to explore the factors underlying medical care use and control for differences in both health status and preferences for different styles of practice. The exploration of differences in hospital use pointed to variations in both length of stay for a given condition and different propensities to hospitalize a patient for a given problem. Following the cost issue a step further led to an examination of the costs of "producing" a physician office visit or a day in the hospital. That is, are HMOs more efficient producers of medical care, rather than more effective in containing utilization of service?

Cost, however, is only one measure of a system. If HMOs had lower costs but worse patient outcomes and were unable to satisfy their enrollees, there would be little interest in them. Thus, the more complete analyses of HMOs required the development of quality measures and the application of consumer satisfaction measures. Furthermore, health policy concerns in the United States focus on issues not only of cost but also of equity and performance in a complex environment. Thus, if HMOs are satisfactory providers only for the middle class, they would be at best a partial solution, particularly since public policy is generally more directive when it comes to the poor. The combination of employer-based health insurance and tax incentives used for the working population means that an assessment of HMOs must be done in the context of a pluralistic system rather than as a laboratory experiment, leading to research on the functioning of HMOs in a competitive market.

We have two major goals in this chapter. One is to offer a brief review of the evidence concerning the performance of alternative delivery systems, and in particular, HMOs. The second is to illustrate how health services research in this area has been responsive to policy concerns about HMOs and how this research has more general applicability. This area of research has broader implications largely because HMOs and their market environments are a microcosm of the larger medical care system. Because of the need to understand HMOs and ADSs in context, we present in the next section a brief overview of the changing medical care environment and patterns of ADS growth. In the following section we focus on various aspects of HMO performance by discussing policymakers' hopes and fears with respect to a series of questions. For example, what is the record of HMOs in promoting health and improving access for the underserved? How effective have they been at containing costs and promoting competition? Have they jeopardized the quality of care or behaved irresponsibly? Are they being overpaid or underpaid relative to the risks of their enrollees? In the final section we attempt to lay out a policy-oriented research agenda by focusing on the areas in which there are major gaps in our knowledge and discussing how filling those gaps with respect to ADSs will also benefit the larger health services research and health policy field.

The Changing Market and Policy Environment

Some HMOs can trace their roots back to the mid-nineteenth century, when various immigrant and laboring groups formed associations to provide for their health care (Trauner, 1977). These groups typically remained local and were open to a relatively small fraction of the population. Some of the largest current HMOs, including Kaiser, Group Health Cooperative of Puget Sound, and Health Insurance Plan of Greater New York, began their "public" marketing phase in the period after World War II. They were called prepaid group practices (PGPs) or group practice prepayment plans and had two key characteristics in common. For a fixed monthly premium, a wide range of preventive and acute care services was provided. Furthermore, these services were delivered by physicians practicing either as a group contracting with the health plan or as employees of the health plan.

The combination of group practice which threatened the "normal" referral relationships among independent practitioners, and prepayment, in an era when the vast majority of Americans had no health insurance, was clearly a radical innovation. Not surprisingly, there was vigorous opposition to these health plans by organized medicine, which at the time was still opposing even third-party reimbursement (American Medical Association, 1934; Numbers, 1978).

The underlying rationale behind these plans was that if the enrollees paid a small amount each month, enough money could be collected to cover the average health care costs of employed individuals and their families. Furthermore, many of the physicians involved in these plans saw the group practice model, pioneered by the Mayo brothers and others in the Midwest, as a way to provide better-quality care. The routine sharing of medical records provided an implicit form of peer review, and consultations could be obtained in an easy, informal process. The responsibility for all the care needed by an enrolled population led to a natural concern for "population-based" measures of utilization and cost, such as hospital days and physician visits per 1,000 enrollees. (Even today insurance plans do not have reliable data on such basic measures of utilization.) The responsibility of the plan for future medical care may also have assisted those with a focus on preventive measures, such as immunization and prenatal care. Thus, the group practice plans in the 1950s were organizations whose primary focus was on the expansion of benefits and the enhancement of quality. There was relatively little attention paid to cost containment.

The Health Insurance Plan in New York was noteworthy for its internally supported research department, which included Sam Shapiro, Paul Densen, and Marilyn Einhorn. They produced a series of research papers in the 1950s and early 1960s which indicated that HIP members utilized significantly fewer hospital days than comparable people in conventional insurance plans (Densen, Deardorff, and Balamuth, 1958; Densen, Shapiro, and Einhorn, 1959; Densen, 1960, 1962). They were also able to show that perinatal outcomes were better for enrollees in HIP (Shapiro, Weiner, and Densen, 1958, 1960). Not only were these studies classics in terms of their design and execution, but they began to move the concept of prepaid group practices into the research and policy arena.

The early 1960s saw the development of an activist policy agenda in the health field. One perception which arose out of early research was that there was an impending physician shortage (Fein, 1967). This led to attempts to estimate how many physicians and other health professionals would be required by the nation, particularly given the expansion of health insurance coverage brought about by the passage of Medicare and Medicaid. The National Advisory Commission on Health Manpower (1967) undertook a series of analyses to estimate the likely supply and demand for health care personnel. An important piece of their work was an analysis of the Kaiser Foundation Health Plan. Given Kaiser's responsibility for providing care to a large enrolled population of known age and sex, its staffing ratios could be used to set a bound on the possible national needs. Use of the Kaiser data by the Commission may have increased the plan's national visibility.

Through the latter part of the 1960s, as the federal costs of the Medicare and Medicaid program grew far more rapidly than anticipated, there was increased interest in PGPs as additional studies were published suggesting lower hospitalization rates for their enrollees (Dozier et al., 1968; Hastings et al., 1970; Perrott, 1971;). PGPs, however, were still a very small part of the health care delivery system. The major plans of the 1940s and 1950s still dominated what could hardly be called an "industry." A new generation of plans was established in the 1960s and early 1970s, often by medical schools (Harvard Community Health Plan, Community Health Care Center Plan [Yale], Medical Care Group of Washington University, Columbia Medical Plan [Johns Hopkins], Georgetown University Health Plan, George Washington University Health Plan). The Office of Economic Opportunity supported Neighborhood Health Centers to establish delivery systems in poverty areas, and some of these were modeled on PGPs.

Under the Nixon administration there was a pulling back from the activist strategy of the Kennedy-Johnson years toward a more competitive, market-oriented approach. The idea that PGPs could take care of a population at lower cost than conventional insurance plans was very attractive. Even more appealing was the notion that the health plan assumed responsibility for providing the necessary services within a fixed budget, thus avoiding the unpredictable cost overruns of the Medicare and Medicaid programs. The notion of group practice, however, was still anathema to organized medicine. Thus, the concept of prepaid plans was broadened to include those which would contract with individual physicians or associations of physicians. These contracts would put the providers somewhat at risk financially—a key point in the PGP model—but not require that they practice together or relinquish the bulk of their patients who would still be fee-for-service. A model for such plans already existed in the Central Valley of California, where Foundations for Medical Care were established to help monitor utilization and costs in an effort to prevent Kaiser from entering the area (Harrington, 1971). Paul Ellwood and Lewis Butler then coined a new name for the expanded notion: health maintenance organization, or HMO. This name focused on health enhancement rather than cost containment, and it bore no reference to either prepayment or group practice. President Nixon's

White Paper on Health brought forth the concept of HMOs in 1971 (U.S. Office of the White House Press Secretary, 1971).

The HMO Act (P.L. 93–222) which followed this interest in HMOs by the administration and the Congress was intended to help promote the development and growth of HMOs. Grants and loans were made available for the planning and development of new HMOs, restrictive state legislation was superseded, and federally qualified HMOs were given the right to request that employers offer them as an alternative to conventional health insurance. Employers were also prevented from contributing more to conventional health insurance plans than to HMOs. These provisions were intended to establish a "level playing field" on which HMOs could prove their greater efficiency and thereby grow and prosper. However, the HMO Act also included several provisions that HMOs found to be quite burdensome, such as a minimum benefits package which was often far more extensive than that offered by conventional insurers.

The Nixon administration also encouraged state Medicaid programs to contract with HMOs or similar prepaid plans to provide services for Medicaid beneficiaries on a capitated basis. Several states, including California, Michigan, Hawaii, and New York, developed major programs along these lines. In some instances the health plans were outgrowths of the OEO Neighborhood Health Center models, and in other cases they were new organizations. HMO involvement in the Medicare program was minimal because the government required that the HMO share the potential saving but cover all the losses under risk-based capitation contracts.

The various incentives and infusions of development funds led to the rapid growth of HMOs in the mid-1970s. Between 1970 and 1975, the number of HMOs increased fivefold (Gruber, Shadle, and Polich, 1988). The failure rate of these new plans, however, was also quite high. One of the major reasons for this was the lack of administrators skilled in running a complex organization such as an HMO. A reason for the allegedly higher failure rate among federal grantees was the program's preference for allocating money to organizations that were unable to raise private funds, and thus were at greater risk of failure. It is not clear, however, whether the failure rate for HMOs was notably higher than that experienced by small businesses in general. In addition to the business failures of some HMOs, there were also a series of scandals, notably in California among plans contracting with the state's Medicaid program (MediCal). These scandals involved fraudulent marketing, excessively high administrative costs to milk profits from purportedly nonprofit firms, and poor quality of care (Goldberg, 1975; California Department of Health, 1975; Chavkin and Treseder, 1977). New legislation tightened the extent of oversight, especially in California through its Knox-Keene Act.

The 1980s brought major changes to the HMO industry and the medical care sector. The Reagan administration took an active stance in encouraging competition and reducing the government's role in all sectors, including medical care. The HMO grant and loan program was terminated; instead, private investors were encouraged to finance growth and development in the industry (NICHMOD National Industry Council for HMO Development, 1984). Not surprisingly, this change led to a decreased role for locally sponsored HMOs and a rapid growth in the proportion of plans sponsored by national firms and insurers.

A program was developed to test risk-based contracting under Medicare. (There had already been a much smaller study of four HMOs with risk-based contracts—Marshfield Medical Foundation, Fallon Community Health Plan, Kaiser-Portland, and Health Central and Interstudy (acting as an administrative agent for four Minneapolis plans) (Galblum and Trieger, 1982). The new study was to include 27 sites (Langwell, Rossiter, et al., 1987). However, before the study was fully under way the Tax Equity and Fiscal Responsibility Act (TEFRA) of 1982 changed the rules under which HMOs could contract routinely with Medicare (Langwell, Rossiter, et al., 1987). These new rules established a rate based upon the local fee-for-service costs of Medicare beneficiaries adjusted for the age, sex, and disability status of the enrollees. HMOs could receive a premium equal to 95 percent of this rate, called the Adjusted Average Per Capita Cost (AAPCC) (GHAA, 1989). While losses would be borne by the HMO, savings could be retained to offer additional benefits or reduced premiums for enrollees, thus providing incentives to attract new enrollees. Most of the demonstration sites converted to TEFRA status and the study subsequently provided and continues to provide a wealth of information on HMO coverage for Medicare beneficiaries.

Specific legislative and regulatory changes directed at HMOs, however, were but a small part of the changing medical care environment of the 1980s. Medical care costs were rising very rapidly in the first third of the decade, leading to increased attention by policymakers and employers, who bore a substantial fraction of the premium cost. In some parts of the nation HMO premiums tended to be somewhat lower than those of conventional insurance plans. Enrollment growth in HMOs was very rapid, and conventional insurers began to respond by increasing copayments and deductibles and requiring second opinions and preadmission certification for certain types of cases. More important, the Prospective Payment System (PPS) using Diagnosis Related Groups (DRGs) was implemented for Medicare in 1983. Although this system was phased in over several years and, except in a few states in which insurers adopted DRGs, only affected Medicare beneficiaries directly, it had a much wider impact. Hospital length of stay fell for Medicare beneficiaries (as expected) and for the non-elderly (which was not expected). Moreover, admissions fell for both groups, in contrast to the simple economic incentives of the program (Gutterman, Eggers, et al., 1988). Although tighter utilization review may account for some of these changes (Feldstein, Wickizer, and Wheeler, 1988; Scheffler, Gibbs, and Gurnick, 1988), another explanation is that PPS signaled health care providers that a major change in medical care was beginning. PPS shifted medical care from a system in which all plausibly necessary and "reasonably priced" services would be *reimbursed* to a *payment* system in which there would be fixed amounts of money for certain purposes, such as an inpatient admission. While an HMO focuses on a fixed amount of money for a group of enrollees per year, both systems have within them the notion of fixed budgets rather than blank checks.

There also seems to have been a shift in the acceptability of entrepreneurial behavior by physicians, although this is still controversial (Relman, 1980; Gray, 1983). To some degree, this may have been encouraged by PPS through its incentives to treat patients on an outpatient basis. These indirect incentives, in conjunction with new medical technology and direct efforts by other payors, led physicians to establish free-standing surgery centers and other outpatient services such as chemotherapy clinics and imaging centers. The first effect of these changes was to have shifted services from the inpatient to the outpatient setting, often at a significant saving. In the longer run, however, some view these new outpatient procedures as cost-increasing because more services are provided than would otherwise have been the case. While these interpretations are still controversial, it is undoubtedly true that the line between inpatient and ambulatory care has been blurred. This makes it almost impossible to compare HMOs and other delivery systems using the traditional measures of hospital admissions, inpatient days, and physician office visits.

Not only have lines between inpatient and outpatient services been blurred, but it is no longer possible to talk about HMO versus fee for service (FFS). The classic FFS situation involved a third-party payor who imposed certain deductibles and copayments on its insureds, but otherwise reimbursed providers for services rendered as long as fees were not too far out of line. Moreover, the insureds had the same coverage when treated by any licensed provider. The situation now is quite different. Roughly 32 percent of people with insurance coverage also have various types of utilization management built into their policies (Gabel, Jachich-Toth, et al., 1988), including requirements for preadmission certification, mandatory second opinions, lack of coverage for certain procedures on an inpatient basis, and concurrent review of hospital length of stay. Approximately 50 million people are enrolled in a preferred provider organization (PPO). PPOs typically include utilization management and also provide economic incentives for people to use selected providers who agree to negotiated fees and utilization management and who may have been selected because they are more efficient. In extreme forms of PPOs, called exclusive provider organizations or EPOs, there is no coverage for providers not contracting with the plan. At the same time, HMOs have backed away from the classic model offering comprehensive benefits with nominal copayments, but with a restricted set of providers. Some now have significant copayments for all services, although still far smaller than those in insurance plans. Others are addressing the negative aspects of limited freedom of choice by offering a package of traditional HMO benefits and coverage if the enrollee uses the plan's providers and by requiring coinsurance and deductibles for out-of-plan services. From the patient's perspective, this arrangement is similar to a PPO. Thus, the relatively clear discussions of the past about two distinct models are now replaced by fuzzy comparisons of plans and coverage packages which cannot be clearly identified as FFS or HMO, regardless of the labels of the sponsoring organizations (Feldman, Kralewski, and Dowd, 1989).

Policymakers' Hopes and Fears: A Review of the Evidence

As indicated earlier, although HMOs and other alternative delivery systems are the result of innovations and developments in the private sector, they have been strongly influenced by various state and federal policies. Furthermore, in the pluralistic medical care system of the United States, entities such as HMOs are often seen as potential solutions to problems which are not addressed at a national level. Thus, HMOs and similar systems have been touted as models for health promotion, vehicles for delivering services to the poor, effective means of cost containment, and promoters of increased competition (Enthoven, 1980, 1988; Enthoven and Kronick, 1989a, 1989b). The HMO model also has a large number of critics, who claim that its advantages will be unfulfilled and that there are significant risks associated with HMOs. These risks include the possibility that the fixed budgets will lead to undertreatment and poor quality of care (Schwartz, 1978; Levinson, 1987; Hillman, 1987), that injecting large sums of money and a business orientation into the medical care environment will lead to fraud, abuse, and politically embarrassing situations, and that HMOs will attract the low-risk people but be paid average risk premiums, thereby destroying the risk pooling system (Luft, 1986).

Given the differences between the two polar models of delivery—unrestricted choice of fee-for-service provider with third-party reimbursement and capitation to a selected set of providers—one would expect a great deal of controversy over the likelihood that HMOs would be better than the status quo. The disputes first occur on the basis of polemics in political settings and "theory" in academic settings. Over time, however, evidence accumulates on how well HMOs are able to meet the high expectations of their advocates, or create the disasters predicted by their detractors.

There is still very little evidence on the performance of PPOs and the more recent hybrid plans combining HMOs with some freedom of choice and utilization management. In fact, the usual pattern is that the "trade press" carries articles on the announcement of new plans to be offered in the marketplace; then during the next few years some of these plans are put into place, enrollment grows, and financial performance is usually glowing (at least in part because of the rapid growth). At this point the first research projects may be designed, but grant proposals usually take about a year to be reviewed and funded, and then several years to execute if substantial data collection and analysis are undertaken. Publication of results then takes another year or two, given the usual review and publication process. Thus, the first real research results will often lag the initial trade reports by six or more years, by which time the industry may have changed substantially. Over time, however, as the industry stabilizes and the amount of research grows, one can develop a more reliable picture of what is happening in the field, both because it is more stable and because there are enough studies of various settings to be able to avoid the problems of overgeneralizing from limited amounts of data. The evidence on HMOs is far more solid now than it was in the late 1970s (Luft, 1981) and is easier to interpret. The evidence on PPOs and some of the newer ADS models, however, is still far from the equivalent depth available for HMOs a decade ago.

HMOs for Health Promotion and Disease Prevention

To some extent, the expectations of HMOs as engines for health promotion arise from the new name given to capitated arrangements and prepaid group practices in the early 1970s as a political "marketing" device. Regardless of the name, there is some logic behind the expectation that HMOs will attempt to keep their enrollees healthy *if* prevention is less expensive than cure. It is important to note, however, that the decision must be evaluated from the HMO's perspective, rather than a social one (Luft, 1976). For example, certain types of prevention may be socially desirable because they prevent premature death. If these deaths are sudden and are associated with minimal medical care costs, then an HMO may have little reason to "invest" in ongoing preventive treatments to avert these deaths. If preventive costs are incurred now but reduced medical care expenditures occur much later, as with estrogen replacement therapy which may prevent hip fractures decades later, the probability that those individuals will still be enrolled in the HMO must be taken into account. Finally, many of the interventions which can promote health and prevent disease are social and behavioral rather than medical and thus are difficult for a medical care organization to implement.

An early review of the evidence on whether HMOs actually provide more preventive services suggested that, without controlling for differences in benefits and coverage, enrollees in some HMOs received more "preventive services," such as immunizations and checkups, than did people in conventional insurance plans (Luft, 1978). For other HMOs there was no evidence of increased consumption of such services. However, when one recognized that all the HMOs offered comprehensive coverage for such services and only some of the FFS plans did so, and then controlled for this difference in coverage, the inconsistent findings were explained. That is, when people with FFS reimbursement insurance were not covered for preventive services they used fewer such services than did the HMO enrollees, but when one compared people with comprehensive FFS coverage that included preventive services to those in HMOs, there were no differences.

These findings support the notion that coverage and financial costs are important factors in medical care use, especially for the more discretionary and patient-oriented decisions. One should note, however, that some of these findings may be outdated by changes in public policy concerning certain preventive services such as the mandatory immunization of school children. Such laws essentially guarantee uniform immunization rates in the eligible population, although some of the poorest children will not be immunized. Those children, however, would be in families unable to afford to enroll in an HMO.

It is generally the case, however, that HMOs will offer far more complete coverage of routine physical examinations than conventional insurance plans. Recognizing this difference leads to the question of whether people with a greater desire for preventive services may prefer to enroll in HMOs. For example, suppose there are two people in good health, one of whom likes to have a periodic checkup just to "make sure" nothing is wrong while the other prefers to see a doctor only in response to symptoms. If each is offered the choice of an HMO and a conventional insurance plan at comparable prices, the HMO will tend to be more attractive to the first person. If one then observes more preventive services being consumed by the first person, it would be incorrect to attribute all that difference to the HMO. There is substantial evidence that in some cases preferences for certain types of coverage and services, as well as orientation to medical care, differs between HMO enrollees and those choosing FFS coverage (Bashshur and Metzner, 1967; Garfield, 1970; Garfield et al., 1976; Berki and Ashcraft, 1980; Feinson, Hansell, and Mechanic, 1988).

The best way to measure a "pure HMO effect" independent of such self-selection effects is to assign people randomly to HMO and FFS settings. The RAND Health Insurance Study incorporated this type of random assignment and therefore provides valuable information on this question as well as others in which selection bias may be a problem. It is important to recognize that the RAND study compared one HMO, Group Health Cooperative of Puget Sound, with a set of different FFS insurance coverages. One of these was essentially complete coverage for a wide range of services and is referred to as the "free" plan, while the others incorporated a series of copayments and deductibles. The free plan offered coverage comparable to that of the HMO, that is, no out-of-pocket costs for the enrollee, while the other plans were more comparable to conventionally available insurance plans, although none had the "modern" forms of utilization management (for example, preadmission certification, second surgical opinion, concurrent review).

The RAND studies indicate few differences in the overall use of ambulatory services between the HMO and free plan enrollees. The HMO enrollees did have a somewhat higher rate of preventive service utilization than did those with either some or no copayments. Fortunately, the RAND experiment included measures of health status on enrollment and at the end of the study, so it is possible to determine whether the differences in coverage and utilization had any measurable effect on health (Ware et al., 1986). In general, however, the health status of the HMO enrollees was comparable to that of the enrollees in the free plan, even though the latter consumed approximately 35 percent more medical care. Few differences were apparent between the free and copayment groups in health status, so it appears that the additional preventive services had little measurable benefit. One may argue, however, that the sample sizes were too small to be able to detect what might still be clinically relevant differences.

Although the RAND study is a "gold standard" experiment in terms of its design and execution, its major weakness in terms of its results concerning HMOs is that the one HMO included is a large, well-respected, staff model plan with strong consumer control. Thus, it is difficult to know how generalizable the results would be to other HMOs and settings. It should be noted, however, that the question of HMOs was only one of many studied by the Health Insurance Experiment, and that when the study was begun in the early 1970s, there were few HMOs and even fewer willing to participate in such a study (Newhouse, 1974). More important, in the climate of the 1970s there was considerable concern that all the lower costs reported by HMOs were due to favorable selection of low-risk enrollees (see below) and that HMOs might really offer poorer quality care (Schwartz, 1978). If this was found to be true for a "Cadillac" plan such as Group Health, one could assume that other HMOs would be even worse. The RAND study was able to reject that important hypothesis, but it could not exclude the possibility that some plans did not perform as well as Group Health Cooperative.

There are some additional studies addressing the question of increased health promotion and disease prevention in HMOs. In one, work loss days of California Department of Transportation employees enrolled in HMOs, predominantly Kaiser, were found to be the same as those of employees in FFS plans, even though the HMO members had higher risks of sickness (Roemer, 1982).

Many HMOs provide periodic newsletters to their enrollees with hints about healthy life-styles and recommendations concerning when to seek attention for certain problems. It may well be the case that such consumer/patient education is a major factor in reducing medical care costs in the long run, but the evidence on this is relatively weak. Interestingly, some FFS plans provide similar types of services (Blue Cross and Blue Shield Association, 1989). The financial structures of the two systems may actually encourage FFS carriers to do more of this type of work than HMOs. Most HMOs quote a premium which is the same for all enrollee groups, although there may be some adjustments for differences in age composition. The costs associated with health promotion are borne by the HMO and either passed on through the premium or recaptured through lower medical care costs. Savings through reduced work loss and lower disability costs are captured directly by the employer. In the FFS setting the insurer can bill the employer specifically for the health promotion activities, and since many insurers also carry the disability and workers' compensation policies for the employer, these savings can be highlighted as an offset against the health insurance premium surcharge.

One potentially important development is an ongoing project funded by the Hartford Foundation. A consortium of HMOs and the RAND Corporation are attempting to develop a set of quality measures which can be used to compare plans. Several of these measures focus on health promotion, such as a target reduction in cigarette smoking. If such quality measures are adopted widely, then HMOs may give even more attention to health promotion activities.

Access for the Underserved

When considering the potential of using HMOs to deliver services to the poor, it is important to remember the context of the problem—that is, the poor cannot afford to pay for medical care by themselves, and public programs are often underfunded. Clearly, HMOs by themselves cannot solve these problems. However, HMOs might be able to address certain other difficulties faced by the poor. Since they are organized systems with a total budget that can be reallocated internally, HMOs may be able to provide a more appropriate mix of services than the FFS reimbursement system under Medicaid. For example, HMOs may encourage access to primary care physicians and pay for this by reducing the inappropriate use of emergency rooms and hospital outpatient departments. HMOs may also institute formal case management to constrain the use of resources by the small number of very high cost cases.

HMOs seeking to serve the nonworking poor, however, must contend with a series of problems quite different from those faced by plans serving employed populations. First, the poor often live in different parts of the community than do the working and middle classes. Clinics and other provider sites are generally not well located to serve both Medicaid and employed populations. If a clinic is established in a low-income neighborhood, its revenues may be almost entirely dependent on the Medicaid contract, which increases the risk of financial failure. Second, Medicaid programs are typically only willing to pay an HMO as much as the average FFS recipient costs, and Medicaid beneficiaries are unable to supplement the state's contribution (in contrast to employees supplementing an employer's contribution). Thus, HMOs with higher costs (that is, those that require enrollee contributions) exclude themselves from the Medicaid market. Third, Medicaid FFS payments have typically lagged behind general FFS costs, forcing an implicit subsidy by Medicaid providers. Medicaid HMO contracts can in effect make a subsidy explicit as well as larger, resulting in an unattractive business venture. Finally, the issue of continued Medicaid eligibility is a major problem. If eligibility is dependent on income, then people whose incomes are close to the cutoff point may move in and out of eligibility. This can cause enormous problems for the HMO, both because of the administrative burdens associated with tracking enrollment and because of the inadvertent provision of services to ineligible individuals.

It is also important to recognize that the Medicaid population is actually composed of several important subpopulations based on their reasons for eligibility. Mothers (and sometimes fathers) with dependent children are covered under the Aid to Families with Dependent Children (AFDC). A family's eligibility within the AFDC program is sensitive to the parents' work patterns, ongoing communication to the case worker, and in a single mother's case, any relationship to the father of any of her children. A major problem with this group is the lack of prenatal care, a problem exacerbated by cultural and language barriers. Within FFS

Medicaid, especially in rural areas, few obstetricians are willing to accept Medicaid payment. Some states provide Medicaid coverage to a "medically indigent" population of families or individuals that do not qualify (because of income or family composition) for AFDC but are unable to afford health care coverage from private sources. This group, however, is the most likely to move in and out of eligibility quickly, which results in administrative difficulties for HMOs. The disabled are another group of categorically eligible persons, but their medical care costs are often quite high and they may have strong preexisting attachments to FFS providers, reducing their willingness to join an HMO. A very expensive group of Medicaid recipients is the elderly in nursing homes, but few HMOs have been interested in the long-term care sector. (There are some demonstrations of "social HMOs" which combine coverage for traditional medical care services and long-term care [Newcomer and Harrington, 1986; Greenberg et al., 1988].) Finally, a small number of Medicaid recipients become eligible because of extremely high medical care costs relative to their income. Although these might be the type of people who could benefit the most from HMO-style care, they are not eligible until they have already incurred high costs; then some will continue to do so and others will recover and be relatively low utilizers of care in subsequent periods. Since it is generally impossible to know beforehand what future costs will be, this is a group for whom premium setting is extraordinarily difficult.

It is also important to examine the HMO "option" from the perspective of the Medicaid recipient. Although it is difficult to become eligible, once eligible the Medicaid recipient has freedom of choice of any physician and other health care provider willing to accept Medicaid payments. These often include the area's major teaching hospitals and clinics in low-income areas. Moreover, there are no copayments or deductibles. If the Medicaid recipient joins an HMO, the choice of providers may be far more restricted and less convenient. Furthermore, those individuals the Medicaid program may be most interested in having join the HMO—the high utilizers of services—are generally the ones least willing to give up their existing providers, particularly since they face no copayments or deductibles.

Given these problems, it is not surprising that HMOs have played a relatively small role in most state Medicaid programs. It is possible to identify several major periods of HMO involvement with the poor. The first began in the mid-1960s with the Great Society programs and the establishment of Medicaid. The Office of Economic Opportunity contracted with a number of HMOs as Neighborhood Health Center sites (Sparer and Anderson, 1973), while certain Medicaid programs contracted with large HMOs to enroll recipients as part of demonstration projects. In other instances, states contracted with HMOs that concentrated on serving the poor (Gaus, Cooper, and Hirschman, 1976). Many of the latter were in California, where former governor Ronald Reagan encouraged the development of prepaid health plans (PHPs) as well as budget cutbacks for the fee-for-service Medicaid program. Subsequently, a series of scandals was uncovered concerning marketing abuses, excessive administrative costs and profits, and poor quality of care in many of the PHPs (California State Legislative Analyst, 1973; Goldberg, 1975). Some studies indicated that those PHPs with a high proportion of non-Medicaid enrollees had fewer quality problems (Louis and McCord, 1974). These findings led to both much more stringent regulation by the state, and federal requirements that no more than 50 percent of a plan's enrollment be Medicaid or Medicare patients. In the latter part of the 1970s there was a major falloff in the number of HMOs with Medicaid contracts.

In 1981 the Omnibus Budget Reconciliation Act allowed much greater flexibility for states to contract for services for their Medicaid recipients. Some states, such as California, used this flexibility to contract selectively with specific hospitals at reduced rates (Johns, Derzon, and Anderson, 1985). Other states, including Wisconsin and Michigan, greatly expanded their Medicaid contracts with HMOs. A key feature of some of these second-generation Medicaid contracts is a forced choice among plans for the recipients in a certain area. This is designed to reduce the problem of biased selection which was thought to leave the states' FFS option with the highest-cost people and "overpay" the HMOs (DesHarnais, 1985). A more complete discussion of the biased selection issue is given in a later section.

Although there has been some recent research on these new Medicaid-HMO programs, they do not seem to have been a major focus of either research or policy. Much more attention has been given to problems of covering the uninsured poor who are not eligible for Medicaid and to the relatively slow enrollment of Medicare beneficiaries in HMOs, which are quite different problems. The shift in focus may reflect the recognition that the cost-containment problems of most Medicaid programs are associated with nursing home costs and social/cultural issues that HMOs cannot address. It may also reflect the fact that 50 state-based programs are more difficult to study than those with major federal involvement.

Cost Containment

Although the early HMOs were not specifically designed to contain costs, that is the primary reason for the current policy interest in HMOs. When the HMO strategy was first proposed in the early 1970s, there was substantial controversy over whether HMOs really could provide medical care of comparable quality and at lower cost than the FFS sector. Many traditional practitioners believed that all of the reported differences in hospital use and cost were due to the enrollment of healthier people by the HMOs. A substantial body of comparison studies provided strong evidence that the differences in hospital use and cost were not just attributable to differences in the age and sex composition of the enrollees in various plans (Luft, 1981). Further evidence came from the RAND Health Insurance Study, in which it was clearly demonstrated that people randomly assigned to an HMO had approximately 28 percent lower medical care use than those in the free FFS plan (Manning, Liebowitz, et al., 1984). Thus, there is now relatively little disagreement about the contention that HMOs *can* contain costs relative to open-ended fee-for-service with minimal copayments. There is, however, substantial controversy about their effectiveness relative to some of the more aggressive forms of cost containment in FFS settings and about whether these cost savings are realized and to whom they accrue.

Most of the studies of the cost and utilization of medical care under various plans were done using data from the pre-1983 period. Even in the RAND study, the enrollees in the FFS plan with substantial copayments and deductibles also had total medical care use of about 32 percent below that of the free FFS plan. In other words, one could contain costs to about the same degree using either the structured system of a large group practice HMO or the price incentives of substantial deductibles. The effects of these two systems, however, were not the same. Relative to the free FFS enrollees, those in the HMO had lower hospital use but comparable ambulatory care use, while those in the large deductible plan had lower ambulatory use but comparable hospital use. Clearly, the two patterns of care are not equally attractive to all people, and many observers are concerned that skimping on ambulatory or primary care may lead to more health problems in the long run.

There are several reasons to question the generalizability of the RAND and other older data to the current policy situation. First, the FFS sector has become much more cost-conscious since the early 1980s. Increased concern about costs is reflected in increased deductibles and copayments in conventional insurance plans. (These still, however, are far below the "high deductible" plan tested by RAND.) More direct approaches to contain costs include preadmission certification, concurrent review, mandatory second opinions, and the transfer of many inpatient procedures to the outpatient setting. Although it is difficult to determine the relative importance of each of these approaches, since many are implemented simultaneously, there is substantial evidence that together they have helped to contain costs (Feldstein, Wickizer, and Wheeler, 1988; Scheffler, Gibbs, and Gurnick, 1988). Thus, while it is clear that the well-managed HMOs of the late 1970s could contain costs relative to the "bloated" FFS sector, we do not know whether the modern HMO has as substantial an advantage relative to the "trimmed-down" FFS providers of the late 1980s.

The much greater diversity of HMOs and FFS cost-containment plans makes it far more difficult to develop estimates of the costs in different settings and to know how broadly generalizable such results will be. For example, it is no longer possible to discuss HMOs in terms of two basic models—prepaid group and individual practice association. Instead, there is a wide range of plans with differing organizational structures and financial arrangements. A recent study indicates that, across a sample of 283 HMOs, paying the physicians by salary or capitation was associated with lower hospitalization rates. None of the more complex payment schemes, such as withholding accounts or bonuses based on productivity, had a significant effect (Hillman, Pauly, and Kerstein, 1989). Hospitalization data are far easier to acquire than total cost data, but the shift of a vast number of procedures and diagnostic tests to an outpatient basis makes comparisons based on hospital use less meaningful because the data are more sensitive to plan-specific decisions about treatment site.

While the problem of generalizability is a crucial one for the research community, much of the concern by policymakers about cost containment in HMOs really focuses on the appropriation of the saving. To understand this, it is important to recognize that the term *cost* is used in quite different ways by different parties in the health care field. From a global perspective, the total cost of a health care system is the cost of all the medical care used within the system, as well as the cost of administration and any profits earned by providers and insurers in the system. This cost is typically borne by consumers and sponsors such as employers and the government. In the typical employer-sponsored health plan, the insurance carrier or HMO quotes a premium for the enrollee and the employer or union pays a certain amount up to the total premium cost. The employee is responsible for any remaining premium and for copayments for services offered by the plan as well as services not covered by the plan. While copayments have the indirect effect of giving consumers an incentive to use fewer health care services, they have the direct effect of shifting the burden of cost from premium to out-of-pocket payments, that is, from employer to employee. (If the employer had been paying the full premium cost, then such a shift would reduce his cost. If, at the margin, the employee had been paying the premium, then such a shift would change the cost burden from a payroll deduction to a point-of-service obligation.)

This conceptual framework becomes important when one considers two major differences between HMOs and FFS reimbursement plans. First, HMOs typically rely on copayments and deductibles to a minor degree, and their benefit packages tend to be broader than those offered by conventional plans. Therefore, if an HMO and an FFS plan had comparable total expenditures, as in one of the cases in the RAND study, the cost burden could be quite different because the costs for the HMO enrollees would be totally included in the premium whereas the costs under the FFS plan would be split between the premium and out-of-pocket costs. If the total costs for the HMO are lower than for the FFS plan, it can easily be the case that the premiums are comparable but the out-of-pocket costs for the FFS enrollees are higher. The employer who provides an equal contribution to both plans, as required by the HMO Act, is then paying a larger share of the total costs for the HMO enrollees. Put another way, by bundling its lower total cost into its premium rather than spreading it between premium and out-of-pocket payments, the HMO is able to offer its enrollees a more comprehensive benefit package at no additional cost. The employer, however, sees the HMO as offering it no saving in spite of the often substantial administrative costs associated with offering both FFS and HMO options.

Employers' discontent with HMO cost saving is often exacerbated by differences in how HMOs and insurers set premiums. For large employers, conventional insurers either experience-rate their policies or provide administrative services only, so lower medical care expenditures are almost immediately translated into lower premiums and potentially lower contribution levels. Many HMOs use community rating so that premiums are set based upon the experience of all enrollees, regardless of their sponsor. Some employers believe these premiums reflect not the cost of delivering services but the price the HMO thinks the market will bear, so that lower costs *within* the HMO may be translated into higher HMO profits rather than lower premiums. (If the HMO actually attracts a lower-risk set of enrollees, these concerns are even greater. The issue of biased selection will be discussed in more detail below.) Until the 1988 amendments to the HMO Act, an HMO was required to community-rate in order to be federally qualified. Now that the amendments have changed that requirement, HMOs have more options, such as remaining federally qualified *and* using experience rating.

Promotion of Competition

Although the early proponents of the HMO strategy in the 1970s predicted extremely rapid growth for HMOs and a subsequent conversion of the U.S. health care system, these changes would affect both those who enrolled in HMOs and those who did not. Alain Enthoven in his 1980 book outlined a model of a competitive medical care environment in which competition from the rapidly growing HMO sector would lead to a growth of cost-containing programs by FFS providers. Thus, even people who never left their FFS physicians would experience a slowing in medical care costs from the growth of HMOs.

There have been changes instituted in the FFS sector that tend to reduce costs, but there is little evidence that these changes occurred in response to competition from HMOs. (It is possible that the observation that HMOs were able to contain costs without noticeably sacrificing quality may have made it easier for payors to institute such changes without overwhelming provider opposition, but it is more likely that the implementation of Medicare's Prospective Payment System had a much greater impact.) A substantial number of investigators have searched for evidence that HMO growth in an area leads to slower growth in costs or utilization among non-HMO enrollees (Goldberg and Greenberg,

1981; McLaughlin, Merrill, and Freed 1984; Luft, Maerki, and Trauner, 1986; Hay and Leahy, 1987; McLaughlin, 1987, 1988, 1989). In general, there is little reason to believe that a strong competitive effect exists, and there are substantial empirical problems in testing for such an effect (Zellner and Wolfe, 1989).

A more detailed consideration of the local medical care environment may offer some insight into why major competitive effects have not been noticed. First, one must note that although there has has been substantial growth both in the number of HMOs and in the number of people enrolled in HMOs, this growth has been far from even. In a few areas, for example, Minnesota and California, HMOs account for over 20 percent of the population, but in most places their collective market share is quite small. Furthermore, with the exception of the Minneapolis–St. Paul area, most of the high-penetration markets have had substantial HMO presence for decades. This makes it impossible to determine whether characteristics of the local environment were conducive to HMO growth *and* low hospitalization rates or whether the growth of already large HMOs had a further competitive effect. For the vast majority of the other areas, HMO market share is relatively low, so it is possible that market share must exceed a certain threshold to have a measurable effect on the FFS system.

A second consideration is that the market for medical care is primarily a local one, and even if a metropolitan area has several HMOs, they may be in geographically segmented markets, so the extent of between-plan competition is smaller than one would think from examining metropolitan area statistics. The complexity of HMO competition is further compounded by the fact that broadly based independent practice associations (IPAs) may be in competition with FFS insurers and PPOs rather than with other HMOs. Models of oligopoly or monopolistic competition may be more appropriate to the HMO industry. These models suggest that product differentiation and advertising are the primary modes of competition, rather than price competition. It is also possible that tacit collusion among HMOs could occur within local markets. For example, the major plan in the area could set its premium at a "comfortable" level and all the others would follow suit. In Minneapolis–St. Paul, the relative lack of community-rated premiums (because most plans did not seek federal qualification) may have made it possible for such pricing even to be employer-specific.

One could argue that even if competition among HMOs did not lead to premium reductions in the short run, they would still have strong incentives to pressure their medical care providers to be more efficient. In a premium competitive setting, conventional insurers would have to exact similar price reductions from FFS providers in order to stay in business. There are many anecdotal reports of increased pressures by HMOs on their physician providers and some research on HMO-hospital contracts. One problem in the hospital arena is that strong patient preferences for hospitals can reduce an HMO's bargaining power (Appel and Acquilina, 1982; Kralewski, Countryman, and Shatin, 1982). Furthermore, long-standing relationships may well be preferred over short-run price reductions. On the physician side, the insurers have attempted to negotiate lower fees through PPOs, but it is still difficult for them to control the volume of services. Without the ability to tie physician incentives to total medical care expenditures for a group of enrollees—essentially forming an HMO—it is difficult for the FFS insurer really to control costs in the long run. The problem arises from the fact that reductions in overall medical care costs can only be accomplished by reducing the number of providers, their incomes, or both.

HMOs and Quality

The assessment of quality of care in HMOs must be considered in the context of uncertainty about the measurement of "quality." Objective evaluation of quality in the medical care system is only beginning to occur. Although there is a broad literature on various ways to assess quality, the approaches have usually been applied in experiments or demonstrations rather than on a cross section of providers (Donabedian, 1982, 1984, 1988a, 1988b; Lohr and Brook, 1984; Williamson, 1988). One useful classification of quality problems focuses on problems of overuse, underuse, and poor technical quality. An example of overuse is the case of carotid endarterectomy, in which it is estimated that 32 percent of the procedures do not meet reasonable indications for appropriateness and put the patient at too great a risk of a poor outcome (Winslow, Solomon, et al., 1988). An example of underuse is the failure to undertake a diagnostic test when it is indicated, thereby placing the patient at risk for undetected and treatable disease. Poor technical quality refers to procedures and services done when appropriate, but which are carried out in such a way that the patient's well-being is unnecessarily threatened. In each case, it is important to take into account the patient's preferences for the extent of intervention and his or her evaluation of the process of care as well as the health care professionals' assessments of the level and adequacy of care.

The economic incentives of various systems would suggest that underuse is a potential in HMOs and overuse a potential in the fee-for-services setting (Pauly, 1970). Poor technical quality could occur in either setting. Much of the early fear of poor quality in HMOs was attributable to the assumption that FFS provided the best quality, and anything less was skimping. In fact, there are countervailing incentives in each system. Since FFS almost always includes substantial copayments and deductibles, these financial barriers could deter patients from seeking care in certain situations, thus leading to underuse. Furthermore, since these problems may result in the person never seeing a physician, the problem might not be detected by the usual methods of chart review. In the HMO setting, some people feel that the list of covered benefits represents an entitlement rather than services that are to be provided when medically necessary (Freidson, 1973). Thus, some HMO enrollees may overuse certain services. It should be clear, therefore, that quality should be established independent of delivery system.

The fact that an HMO is supposed to be an organized system for medical care delivery suggests that it may be able to monitor quality somewhat better than in the nonorganized FFS sector. For example, group and staff model plans often have routine sharing of medical records, and IPA models have the ability to use claims data to develop profiles of their practitioners' practices. More important, since the HMO is potentially liable for poor quality of care in ways that a reimbursement plan is not, the organization has a much greater incentive to police itself. (The liability of the organization is far from settled, and some plans even believe that attempting to monitor and improve quality is an admission of responsibility. IPAs can attempt to claim that each contracting physician is solely liable, but group and staff model plans are less able to use this defense.)

Most of the earlier studies suggest that the quality of care in HMOs is comparable to that in the fee-for-service setting (Luft, 1981). In general, the more recent evidence supports this view. For example, studies of cancer treatment suggest that there are either no differences or a more rapid diagnosis among HMO enrollees but a somewhat longer interval from diagnosis to treatment (Greenwald, 1987). Of course, one problem in all of these comparisons is the potential for the results to be influenced by self-selection. Thus, if people who are prone to seek medical care and establish strong physician relationships stay in FFS while those who tend to avoid care join HMOs, then this may affect the likelihood that a symptom is reported or a recommendation for treatment is pursued.

The RAND study provides some very useful but not generalizable results. Not only were enrollees randomized, but their health status was assessed systematically both at the beginning and the end of the trial. As mentioned earlier, overall there were no differences in health status for enrollees in the HMO and in the FFS plan. However, low-income people with health problems at the beginning of the study who were assigned to the HMO had worse outcomes than comparable people assigned to the free FFS plan. Middle-income healthy people in the HMO did better than members of their cohort assigned to FFS (Ware et al., 1986). However, it is important to note two caveats to these findings. First, the free FFS plan was substantially more expensive than the HMO and far more expensive than the Medicaid programs usually made available to the poor. Second, Group Health, the HMO in the study, had ongoing contracts with the state of Washington Medicaid program to care for low-income populations which included special outreach services and transportation to the Group Health sites to encourage access, but these special services were not included by RAND for the low-income enrollees in the experiment.

Given the sensitivity of data concerning quality of care, it is reasonable to assume that the HMOs willing to participate in research studies are probably not among those with the most problems. (This is also true for studies of quality in the FFS sector.) Thus, it is probably most accurate to say that the large, mature HMOs can offer care comparable to that of the FFS system, but we have little evidence on whether this is also the case for the newer HMOs and for HMOs of other forms. It is reasonable to assume there will be some variability in the quality of care across HMOs, but there is no reason to believe this variation will be any greater than one would find in the FFS sector.

The lack of evidence concerning poor quality may, in fact, be evidence of generally good quality. Given the antipathy of many physicians in traditional practice to prepaid arrangements and the ease with which a disgruntled patient can switch out of an HMO during open enrollment season, one would expect a large number of malpractice cases and headline-grabbing allegations if HMOs were, in fact, frequently providing poor quality care. Although there certainly are such cases, they are relatively few in number.

HMOs and Payor Responsibility

A sponsor, such as an employer or the government, may be under pressure to expand coverage or benefits in an FFS setting, but any quality of care problems are likely to be focused on the individual physicians or other providers who have delivered the care, not on the sponsor. As sponsors develop more direct interventions, such as utilization management techniques which may deny payment for some services in certain circumstances, the sponsor becomes more subject to criticism for making the wrong decisions. In the context of HMOs, the sponsor may be faulted for the selection of the choice of plans, for example, the selection of an HMO with quality problems. In addition to quality of care problems, a sponsor may be perceived as responsible for intrusive marketing techniques used by certain plans and even for the plan's solvency. If an HMO suffers financial difficulties, enrollees who find themselves being billed by providers (because the HMO has not paid the bills) may seek payment from the sponsor. In extreme cases a plan may close and leave its enrollees without coverage, leaving the sponsor liable for the health coverage of those enrollees.

The notion of a "sponsor" suggests that the employer or public agency has some responsibility for its employees or program beneficiaries (Enthoven and Kronick, 1989a, 1989b). It is certainly reasonable to assume that a health benefits department or a public agency would be better able than individuals to evaluate plan offerings and make sure they meet certain basic standards before presenting them as potential choices. On the other hand, it is not reasonable to expect even sophisticated sponsors to anticipate problems that are not yet detectable. If sponsors were only to offer the biggest and most reputable plans, new and potentially better options would be excluded from the market. On the other hand, it is reasonable to expect that sponsors will act quickly to demand corrective actions or to terminate contracts when problems are found.

Two cases illustrate this issue. In 1987 it became clear that Maxicare was in financial difficulty (Kenkel and Palm, 1988; Kenkel, 1988a, 1988b; Gardner, 1988a, 1988b; Larkin, 1989a, 1989b). Maxicare terminated some of its contracts with California's Medicaid program and began some restructuring. Some employers, such as the University of California, took this as a signal that Maxicare might have to institute further cutbacks or even declare bankruptcy. If this happened, the university would have to negotiate a special open season to allow its Maxicare members to enroll in other plans, and there would be potential problems with providers seeking payment from university enrollees for services which should have been paid by Maxicare. To avoid this problem, the university decided to drop Maxicare as an option in its open season in October 1988, thereby forcing those enrollees to choose other plans. The forced switching was not appreciated by those Maxicare members who were happy with their providers, and there was some protest. When Maxicare declared bankruptcy in the spring of 1989, the university's withdrawal appeared to have been a good strategy, although it could be criticized as further weakening the HMO by cutting away its enrollment base—the "run on the bank" phenomenon.

It is important to note that substantial losses and even bankruptcies, such as those incurred by Maxicare, do not necessarily reflect problems in the system, or a failure of policy. One could even argue that a provider system that did not have occasional losses and failures was not being pressured enough to be efficient. However, there is a need to be concerned about the impact of failures and bad debts on the enrollees. If providers seek to recover fees from the former enrollees, or if a history of business failures makes it impossible for new plans to enter the market because providers are afraid of future problems, then there is a role for public policy. Some states have developed guaranty pools which levy a fee on all HMOs to establish a fund to pay off the debts of those who fail (Davis, 1989). Although this may make it easier for new plans to enter the market, the approach is opposed by the stronger plans, who argue that it forces them to subsidize their poorly managed competition. This is analogous to the arguments made by some of the stronger savings and loan institutions about the cost of the federal bailout being borne by the stronger firms.

A second set of embarrassing situations is exemplified by the scandal surrounding International Medical Centers Inc. (IMC) of Florida. In 1987 IMC had more Medicare beneficiaries enrolled in a risk contract than any other HMO in the nation. The plan was alleged to have poor quality of care and to have used fraudulent marketing techniques. The president of IMC was ultimately indicted on charges of bribery, obstruction of justice, and conspiracy (Baldwin, 1987). A similar series of scandals erupted in the early 1970s among Prepaid Health Plans contracting with California's MediCal program (Goldberg, 1975; Chavkin and Treseder, 1977). Although it would be ideal if problems could be avoided that result in enrollees being misled or, more important, put at risk by poor quality care, it is important that bad outcomes such as these be distinguished from the alleged failure of the public agency in policing the system. In each of these situations there were also charges that regulatory agencies were not sufficiently vigilant in detecting problems and pursuing complaints (California State Legislative Analyst, 1973; U.S. General Accounting Office, 1986). For example, if problems were identified quickly and corrective action taken, then it would be apparent that even though not all health care providers are altruistic and there may be some "bad apples," the regulatory system is capable of assuring the public safety. In fact, it is probably noteworthy that the California and IMC cases are identified as scandals because of the allegations of *insufficient regulation,* rather than just health plan malfeasance. There is a substantial history of health plans being forced to undertake corrective actions, and while these may achieve some brief news coverage, they are evidence of a well-working system rather than a scandal.

It is also important to note that there is an increasing concern about the role of financial incentives in the FFS system. Some of this debate has focused on the role of for-profit entities, but the issue is more sharply drawn when it comes to the question of physician ownership of entities to which they may refer patients, such as laboratories or imaging centers (Gray, 1986; Hyman and Williamson, 1989). Likewise, direct dispensing of pharmaceuticals by physicians is a growing policy question (Relman, 1987). When viewed in this context, the regulation of HMOs to support care in the best interest of the patient is merely one part of a governmental role in the entire health care system.

Biased Selection and Equitable Payment

Health insurance actuaries rely on the assumption that in addition to a random component there are certain factors, such as age and gender, that influence the need for medical care in predictable ways as well. If a large enough group of people is in the insurance pool, the underlying need can be predicted with a fair degree of accuracy. A health insurer can influence the amount of care demanded through benefit design that determines what services are covered and what copayments and deductibles need to be paid by the enrollee. HMOs can also influence demand through decisions concerning coverage as well as decreased accessibility. Given a benefit design and a delivery system with known provider costs, it is not too difficult for a health plan to estimate the total costs of care to be used by a reasonably large group of people, such as all the employees of a given company.

If people within the group have a choice among several health care options, such as an FFS reimbursement plan and several types of HMOs, then the actuarial approach described above is severely threatened. For example, suppose that people who anticipate using medical care in the next year are more likely to enroll in one plan, perhaps because its coverage is more complete or because it offers a wider range of specialists. If this occurs, then the usual adjustments for age and gender may be insufficient to determine at a reasonable estimate of use if some plans attract (intentionally or not) a disproportionate share of the high-cost users of care while others have more than their share of the low utilizers.

One solution to biased selection is experience rating, whereby the premium quoted to each subgroup of enrollees reflects the group's past costs. Experience rating reduces the incentive to attract only low utilizers of care. That is, if high utilizers pay high premiums and low utilizers pay low premiums, then biased selection doesn't matter. This type of pure experience rating has two difficulties. First, many would argue that it is inequitable and that it is contrary to the notion of spreading risk across both the healthy and the sick. In fact, in the extreme case, it obviates the need for insurance because the premiums actually exceed the cost of care as a result of administrative and marketing costs. Second, HMOs argue that they are more efficient, and therefore should be offered more nearly *what it would have cost the FFS system to provide the same coverage.* They argue further that if they are merely paid what they spend, then there is no reason for them to try to be more efficient.

Even without these arguments against the use of experience rating, there are several legal and practical problems involved with using it as a solution to biased selection. Until recently, federally qualified HMOs were required to use community rating, a system under which all enrollee groups were charged the same premium. This meant that from the employer's perspective, the FFS premium would often be experience-rated and therefore reflected the experience of only those employees choosing that option, while the HMO premiums bore little relation to the costs of the firm's enrollees. At the same time, the HMO Act required the employer to make the same dollar contribution to both FFS and HMO plans. If the FFS plan attracted the relatively high cost enrollees and the HMOs the relatively low cost enrollees, then an average contribution level might be far less than the FFS premium and would more than cover the HMO premium. When the employer contribution rises above the premium cost, enrollment is free for some plans but requires out-of-pocket spending for others, with the free plans tending to attract the lower cost enrollees (Luft and Trauner, 1985). This situation is exacerbated by the common use of the FFS premium as the guidepost for employer contributions, so if the FFS plan suffers adverse selection over time and its premiums reflect the increased costs, then the employer contribution is forced up even more rapidly than would otherwise be the case.

There is a growing body of evidence to support the contention that biased selection does occur in certain situations (Wilensky and Rossiter, 1986; Luft and Miller, 1988). It appears that favorable selection is somewhat more likely to be present among enrollees in PGPs than in IPAs. However, there is also evidence that PGPs sometimes are recipients of an adverse mix of enrollees. Furthermore, one cannot even identify consistent patterns for specific HMOs. That is, a given HMO may attract the less risky people from one enrollee group and the more risky ones from another group. There is also evidence to suggest that, while some HMOs may attract the less risky people on enrollment, the ones who leave the HMO are the relatively low utilizers of services, implying adverse selection on disenrollment for the HMO (Buchanan and Cretin, 1986; Luft and Miller, 1988). In any event, the mere presence of data supporting the notion that adverse selection exists provides employers with a basis for claiming that the current use of community rating by HMOs is unfair and costs them money.

The situation is somewhat different in the public sector. Medicare risk contracts are based on the Adjusted Average Per Capita Cost (AAPCC), which is calculated by HCFA for each county. It is meant to represent the cost to Medicare for FFS services used by beneficiaries living in that county, adjusting for age, gender, and disability status. HMOs are offered contracts based on 95 percent of the AAPCC with adjustments based on the mix of enrollees they attract (GHAA, 1989). Plans cannot charge beneficiaries more than the AAPCC unless they offer services not included in the basic Medicare package. If their costs are less than the AAPCC, they are required to offer additional benefits. Not surprisingly, a key determinant of the willingness of HMOs to enter into risk contracts is the size of the AAPCC in the local area (Adamache and Rossiter, 1986). Thus, one could argue that biased selection is occurring at the macro level, because HMOs are not willing to participate in the areas in which FFS costs to Medicare are relatively low. More important, there is some evidence that the AAPCC does not adjust sufficiently for the differences in risk not captured by age, gender, and disability status (Beebe, Lubitz, et al., 1985; Thomas and Lichtenstein, 1986; Epstein and Cumella, 1988). HCFA is now pursuing a means of further adjusting rates to reduce the potential for biased selection.

The policy problems arising from the presence of biased selection are many. First, people choose health plans in a nonrandom manner, with the result that there are some selection differences. If these differences become substantial, and particularly if some people are very much more expensive to cover than others, then health plans will focus their attention on selecting the low-risk people and avoiding the high-risk people. This could leave some people without coverage; and these will be the ones who need it the most and can probably least afford it. It will also divert the attention of managers from improving efficiency to selective marketing. Second, some plans will be overpaid because they benefit from favorable selection. If the overpayments are small and the excess revenue is returned in additional benefits, this is a lesser problem than if it is siphoned off in profits. In extreme cases, the ability to select enrollees favorably may attract disreputable "fast buck" plans rather than organizations designed to deliver health care effectively—a situation likely to result in public scandals. Finally, if policymakers, in both the public and private sectors, develop the perception that biased selection is a costly and insoluble problem, this will erode their support for HMOs and other competitive options that encourage efficiency in medical care.

A Policy-Oriented Research Agenda

A decade ago there was great debate about HMOs, but this debate focused on whether they actually could save money without jeopardizing quality of care. There was a common perception that all their alleged cost saving was due to favorable risk selection and that any increased involvement of physicians in HMOs would only be by poorly (often foreign) trained physicians. It is quite clear now that HMOs can offer health care coverage at lower total cost with comparable quality. Furthermore, HMOs have been able to attract a broad cross section of physicians (Trauner, Luft, and Hunt, 1986). In spite of knowing much more about HMOs than was the case a decade ago, it is even more difficult now than before to offer useful policy advice about HMOs and ADSs. A major reason for this is the change in the medical care environment. It is no longer correct to discuss HMOs in terms of IPAs and PGPs, as if these were homogeneous sets of plans; nor is there a uniform "open-ended FFS" system. Instead, there is a bewildering array of cost containment and utilization management approaches used in varying degrees by organizations across the spectrum (Feldman, Kralewski, and Dowd, 1989). Any policy changes should take into account the underlying structure and organization of plans, rather than arbitrary categories that are no longer meaningful. In addition, the last decade has demonstrated how rapidly the medical care system can adapt to policy changes and economic incentives. Using currently available data systems, it takes time for new delivery systems to be captured in the data, for data to reach the researchers' attention, for the analysis to be done, and for results to be published. New data collection systems could shorten the inherent lags in this process.

Developing Better Measures of Benefits and Categories of Health Plans

It is currently almost impossible to compare the performance of health plans or even their premiums because there are no uniform ways of measuring benefits, patient incentives, and provider incentives (Feldman, Kralewski, and Dowd, 1989). It is meaningless to compare trends in premiums when some plans are increasing coverage through new benefits and others are reducing coverage by increasing copayment and deductibles. Furthermore, it is important to measure effective coverage rather than just "book" coverage. For instance, if outpatient mental health benefits are offered but must be obtained through one overworked provider with long waiting lists, the coverage is less than what it appears. Likewise, some "second opinion" programs offer very low barriers while others essentially block all requests for certain types of services. If providers learn that certain requests are always denied, they may cease to make them, so the absence of denials is not evidence of an ineffective program (Ham, 1989). Thus, it is necessary to develop measures of coverage and benefits which take into account not only the "legal" coverage, but effective coverage as well. Effective coverage may also exceed legal coverage because health benefits officers sometimes make exceptions and pay for services not covered by the plan.

It is also important that a new set of labels and categories be developed to characterize the range of health care delivery systems in terms of the types of financial and organizational relationships they incorporate. A new nomenclature is required to focus the attention of researchers on the important factors which may distinguish plans and help in our understanding of why some work better than others. Advances of this type are also necessary to guide policymakers in drawing regulations and laws concerning health plan behavior. For example, states sometimes have different regulations for insurance companies and HMOs and entirely separate sets of rules with respect to the "individual behavior" of physicians and other providers. As the lines disappear between the role of financing and organizational incentives, these regulations become increasingly unable to address new behaviors.

Methods for Assessing HMO/ADS Quality of Care

It is likely that consumer decisions in the future will be increasingly sensitive to differences in quality of care rather than just price differences. As major sponsors for publicly funded enrollees in HMOs, the federal and state governments must be able to monitor and assess the quality of care in various settings. If this is not done, then the potential for scandals concerning the lack of public oversight is substantial. It is difficult to develop measures of quality within the FFS environment, but it is far more problematic to develop measures appropriate to both FFS and prepaid settings (U.S. Congress Office of Technology Assessment, 1988; Luft, 1988). The difficulty arises from differences in the types of data being collected and in the nature of the interactions between the individual and the health care system.

The FFS system is built around the notion of paying for each service that is rendered. There is a "paper trail" of bills for each procedure which makes it possible to document what was and what was not done, at least for services paid by the insurer. Although there are serious problems in using such administrative data bases for the assessment of quality of care, it is possible in some circumstances to use these routinely collected data as a guide to identify situations in which more careful investigation is necessary (Roos, Roos, and Sharp, 1987). Some HMOs, on the other hand, pay their providers on a salary or capitation basis and thus have little need for detailed billing records. Even if "dummy bills" are required, it is likely that the quality of the data recorded through this process will be inferior to those which are used to determine payment.

In the longer run, data to assess quality of care should go beyond that collected in routine administrative data sets. However, this will not address a more fundamental problem in assessing quality in FFS and prepaid systems. It is important to recognize that the overall quality of care depends on the person with a problem getting into the health care system and the system providing the appropriate services with sufficient technical expertise and in a manner which meets the expectations of the patient. The primary focus of attention in the FFS system has been on whether the services have been of appropriate technical quality, and this can often be evaluated by examining the medical records and other data. Suppose, however, that it is determined that the patient delayed seeking treatment and that this led to a poor outcome. If this occurred in the HMO setting, questions might be raised about the use of barriers to entry in order to reduce utilization. If it occurred in the FFS setting, perhaps because of high deductibles and copayments, it is unlikely that the blame would be directed toward anyone. Likewise, if HMOs develop programs to help their members avoid lower back problems or cease smoking, the improved quality of life would be difficult to assess without population-based measures since these people may be prevented from ever becoming patients.

It may also be the case that quality assessment measures will have to be multidimensional. For example, it is conceivable that the nature of the various systems may allow HMOs and other capitated, organized arrangements to offer better quality in terms of preventing problems and assuring early intervention, but their closed-panel nature may not be as well designed to assure the very best in technical expertise in certain clinical areas. It is not clear that one can develop a single scoring system to combine such different types of quality. Instead, it may be appropriate to provide different measures so that consumers can decide among various options. At the same time, policymakers may decide to set minimum quality levels for all plans offered to publicly sponsored enrollees.

Understanding Differences in HMO Performance

While some types of HMOs may, on average, have lower hospital use or costs than other types, even if the typology is appropriate, we do not know how those differences arise. For example, is it the case that certain organizational and financial structures lead physicians to change their decisions concerning the necessity of hospitalization or the desirability of certain tests and procedures? If so, do their decisions still reflect reasonable choices within the context of high-quality patient care, or are they forced or enticed into compromising quality for financial reward? (This concern is equally applicable to HMO and FFS settings.) If incentives and structures matter, what is the appropriate balance to achieve both efficient and high-quality care? This last question is far more difficult to answer because it requires that one go beyond the mere detection of a problem to determining when that problem must be addressed in the public policy arena. This is comparable to the distinction between knowing that excessive speed is a factor in highway accidents and deciding precisely what should be the maximum speed in various areas.

It may also be the case that economic incentives and organizational structures have little impact on changing the behavior of physicians but instead just reinforce the behaviors of those who choose to work in prepaid settings. That is, some physicians may be inherently aggressive and others conservative in their practice styles, and prepaid settings may merely attract a disproportionate share of the latter. If so, then there may an effective limit to the number of conservative practitioners available to HMOs, and further changes in medical practice may have to occur in medical training programs and or in the selection of medical students.

Incentives for Health Promotion and Disease Prevention

The organized delivery systems that form the core of HMOs and their financial incentives to keep people healthy provide a natural setting for efforts to promote health and prevent disease. The evidence to date on the extent of such activities is not overwhelming, and there are some reasons to believe that HMOs are deterred from aggressive actions by high rates of enrollee turnover and a desire not to appear too avant-garde. Substantially more research is needed to explore what is currently done by various plans and what appears to work in terms of actually changing behavior and improving health and preventing disease.

Investigations should be undertaken at several levels. First, are there factors to explain why some ADSs are more oriented toward health promotion and disease prevention (HPDP) activities than others? For example, does greater enrollee stability have an impact on a plan's willingness to invest in programs which may pay off in reduced medical care use several years later? Alternatively, are HPDP programs used largely as marketing tools, both to improve the image of a health plan and, possibly, to attract the more health-conscious individuals who may also be lower users of medical care? (For example, committed smokers may avoid plans in which they are bombarded with smoking cessation programs.) Second, which programs seem to work better and which are less effective? If the reasons for success and failure are independent of the nature of the HMO, then these findings may also be useful for more general HPDP programs. Third, do some of the current financing arrangements impede the development of innovative programs? For example, some HPDP activities may have only nominal effects on medical care use but substantial effects on work loss days. If a health plan is able to link those two features, it may be far more willing to undertake certain programs than if the costs of the intervention appear in the health insurance premium and the benefits accrue directly to the employer.

Biased Selection and "Fair" Rates

There is currently sufficient evidence to reject the null hypothesis that biased selection never occurs. What is not known, however, is the relative importance of various factors in encouraging favorable or adverse selection. For example, how important is the mix of choices available to the potential enrollee? Does it matter if there are many HMOs of different forms or if there is merely the choice of one HMO and one FFS plan? How important are differences in the specific coverages offered by the various plans? For example, if only one offers *dental* coverage, does this attract people with low or high expected *medical* expenditures? What is the impact of premium differences of various amounts? How important are employer decisions in determining the contribution level? For example, is it better to tie the contribution to the employee-only option or to an amount based on family size? Does the short lock-in period under Medicare (30 days) worsen the selection problem, and, if so, what alternatives are possible that will protect consumers if there are quality problems?

Little is known about the dynamics of biased selection. For example, does biased selection always feed upon itself, so that premiums rise in the plan with adverse selection, leading to an exodus of the less sick and further increases in premiums? If this does not always occur, then what factors encourage or forestall such a spiral, and are these subject to implementation by public and private policymakers? Does the presence of selection lead to a diversion of a plan's interest from increasing efficiency to courting low-risk enrollees? Is it possible to design a system to adjust either premiums or contributions to reflect differences in risk across plans? Will such adjustments be sufficient to reduce selection biases to a manageable level without eliminating incentives to increase efficiency?

Marketplace Rules for Viable Competition

Most research to date has focused on individual organizations or classes of organizations. However, these entities are located in different locations, each with its own medical care structure and history. Even if exact clones of the HMOs present in Minneapolis–St. Paul were established in other communities, it is unlikely that they would perform in the same fashion because the medical care environments and the people within them would be different. Much more work needs to be done on the role of such environmental and personal factors in the performance of specific plans and the functioning of the health care system at the community level.

Once we know more about the working of the medical care market, it may be possible to establish ground rules for acceptable behavior in the market, analogous to antitrust guidelines. Some rules may relate to the ways in which risk differentials are evaluated and offset; others may relate to the acceptability of financial incentives for physicians and other key decision makers. For example, there are already prohibitions against certain types of kickbacks and fee-splitting arrangements. Should these apply to all types of incentive payments, or should they be limited to only certain types? What is the appropriate balance of governmental regulation of minimal quality standards versus the provision of information to the public about the scores of various providers on quality assessment scales?

In general, it is clear that although we have learned a great deal about the performance of the medical care system and alternative delivery systems, there is still much more to be investigated. Unlike most biomedical problems, the medical care system is a moving target composed of man-made systems and incentives which adapt to changing social, economic, and policy factors. This means that it will probably be impossible to design a set of policy measures that will always be optimal. However, if we increase our understanding of how the medical care system and its components work, then it will be easier to identify policy changes to continually improve the system.

The Link Between Health Services Research and Research on Alternative Delivery Systems

To a substantial degree, one cannot develop an understanding of alternative delivery systems without understanding the primary components of the U.S. health care system. This means that research on ADSs will both depend upon the larger research enterprise and contribute to it in major ways. For example, the increasing attention to developing valid and reliable measures of quality will help in the comparison of various types of HMOs and other alternative delivery systems. At the same time, those who try to apply such measures of quality to ADSs will make clear the necessity of designing measures that neither incorporate assumptions that certain patterns of care which may reflect financial incentives are necessarily the "gold standard" nor require data available only in certain payment systems. A likely important outcome of this interaction is the development of quality measures that are population-based rather than just patient-care-based. Such measures will allow the assessment of quality for various segments of the population, such as the poor, racial and ethnic minorities, and people in various states.

Recent attention to questions of variations in medical practice and appropriateness of certain types of care stems, in part, from the observation that HMOs seem to use fewer services for their enrollees yet have comparable outcomes. Similar patterns of variation are seen across geographic areas, yet little is known about why these variations occur and whether they can be influenced by external factors. For example, research on the practice patterns of physicians joining HMOs may help to identify whether they had a cost-conscious practice type before joining the HMO or whether they learned a new practice style "on the job." If the latter is true, then more detailed studies would be necessary to explore the relative importance of education, economic incentives, and other factors. The answers to such research could guide potential efforts to alter inappropriate practices in the FFS environment.

Research on the problem of biased selection is important for the management of the "mini-markets" for health insurance coverage that occur within employer health benefit plans. Lessons from such research may also be applicable for public policy approaches to the problems of the uninsured at the state and federal level as well as to the role of various delivery systems within the Medicare program. Careful analyses of the nature of local medical care markets can also be extremely valuable. While it would be interesting to know how hospitals react to HMO contracting and how various health plans compete with each other in local environments, there are much larger lessons to be learned from such studies. Each can provide evidence on how various actors behave in certain situations. As policymakers at the national level attempt to address problems in the health care system, they are faced with the reality that it is impossible to experiment in the "real world" with various potential policies. Lessons from the natural growth and development of alternative delivery systems can help identify those strategies that should be avoided and those that seem most promising.

9

Health Manpower Forecasting:
The Case of Physician Supply

Uwe E. Reinhardt

The supply of physicians has long been a concern of public policy in this country. During the four decades preceding World War II, it was widely believed that the nation suffered from a surplus of physicians. Following World War II and until about the mid-1970s, it was generally assumed that there were too few. The nation then had about 160 active physicians per 100,000 population. The conventional wisdom since about the mid-1970s has been that the United States is moving, once again, toward a sizable physician surplus; the physician-population ratio has risen to 211 active physicians per 100,000 population in 1985 and is heading for a projected level of 250 by the year 2000. The view that this high ratio will then constitute a physician surplus, however, is by no means universally shared (see, for example, Schwartz, Sloan, and Mendelson, 1988).

This perennial concern over the nation's supply of physicians has spawned one of the oldest branches of health services research in this country: health manpower forecasting and the allied research supporting such forecasts. The objective of this chapter is to review the evolution of this research enterprise and to assess its role in the formation of health policy.

The first section of the chapter sets forth a theoretical framework that illustrates the difficulty of forecasting in this area. Models designed to overcome these difficulties at the practical level are described in the second section. The third and fourth sections are focused on the interplay between health manpower forecasting and the formulation of public policy on the nation's supply of physicians. Some suggestions for future research are presented in the concluding section.

A Theoretical Framework for Health Manpower Forecasting

The basic steps in forecasting the future supply and requirements of physicians are always the same. The forecast begins with a projection of changes in the size and sociodemographic composition of the population that is to be served by the manpower in question—in the present case, physicians. Next, the population forecast is translated somehow into a projection of that population's "need" or "demand" for physician services. On the basis of an assumed physician-productivity ratio (defined as the average number of physician services procured per year per physician), the projected service requirement is then translated into the corresponding number of full-time-equivalent physicians needed to produce the required services. Finally, the projected requirement of physicians can be compared with the supply of active physicians likely to be yielded by the projected population and by additional physicians recruited from abroad. This comparison points up potential future imbalances that may require remedial public policy.

Figure 9-1 illustrates this research task at a highly conceptual level. In that scheme, the vector $\{L_{1t}, L_{2t}, \ldots, L_{mt}\}$ represents the entire array of health manpower needed to attain a chosen target health status for a given population at a future point in time t. For example, L_{1t} may denote the number of full-time *physicians* needed for that purpose, L_{2t} the number of full-time *nurses*, L_{3t} the number of full-time *cytotechnologists,* and so on.

In each setting for health care—be it a medical practice, a hospital, a nursing home, or any other setting—a particular combination of health manpower, supported by other inputs, is used to produce health services. In Figure 9-1 the quantity of each type of health service is denoted by the notation S. Thus, S_1 might represent the annual output of a particular service rendered in the hospital. The symbol f_1 denotes the so-called *production function* (a mathematical relationship to be described later) that describes the transformation of the services of health manpower and of other inputs into that particular hospital service. Similarly, S_{k+1} might represent the annual volume of, say, patient visits at physicians' offices and f_{k+1} the production function for that type of service, and so on for all of the other services rendered by the health system. Finally, a particular combination of *health services* constitutes the *medical treatment* prescribed to respond to a particular medical condition. As indicated in the figure, the medical treatments dispensed by a health

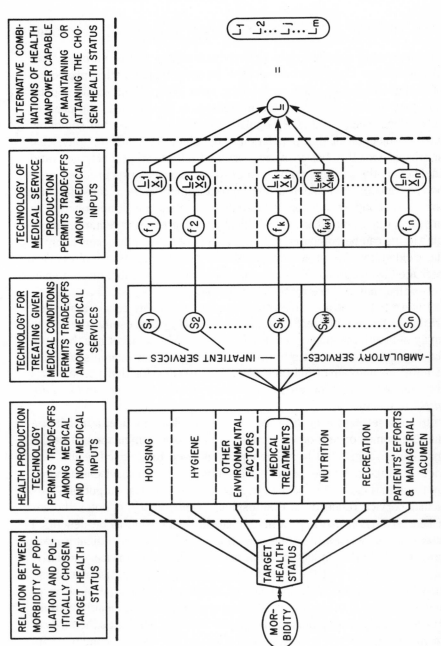

Figure 9-1. Potential trade-offs in the production of health. (From Reinhardt, 1975b.)

system should be thought of as only one of many inputs determing the health status of the population, a point commonly overlooked by pundits who are quick to blame international differences in health status indicators—such as infant mortality rates—strictly on the associated health systems.

It is emphasized in this scheme that, in principle, one ought never to look at just one type of health manpower in abstraction from other types, because many of them can act as substitutes for one another. In practice, this means that acceptable levels of health care can come forth from a great variety of different health manpower-to-population ratios—for example, from quite different physician-population ratios. To economists and other health services researchers, that supposition may be instinctive. Remarkably, the notion is still being resisted at the practical level of policy, where policymakers often act as though the production of health care were ruled by technically determined, fixed health manpower-to-population ratios.

In Figure 9-1 it is assumed that one can project the morbidity likely to be suffered by a given population at some future time and that it is also possible to define and quantify a technically feasible level of health status that policymakers would like to achieve for that projected population. Although this idea seems bold, it is not just theory. In the fall of 1980, the U.S. Department of Health and Human Services announced very specific health status targets to be achieved by 1990 in its *Promoting Health/Preventing Disease: Objectives for the Nation* (1980). Progress toward these objectives was reported in the department's *1990 Health Objectives for the Nation: A Mid-Course Review* (1986). It may be noted in passing that, according to the report, many of the midway goals had been surpassed at that point.

Potential Substitution among Different Inputs into the Production of Health

The health status achieved for a given population is the output from a multifactor health production process managed, in the first instance, by individuals themselves as they choose a particular life-style. To be sure, the most powerful determinants of an individual's health status tend to be congenital and environmental factors beyond the individual's managerial control. Even so, the individual almost always does have some influence over positive or negative changes from his or her natural health endowment.

Only occasionally are physicians drawn into the individual's health production process. In such instances physicians act as diagnosticians who provide information on the patient's health status, as management consultants and agents who help compose the patient's demand for health services, and, typically, also as the providers of at least some of the recommended medical procedures. How physicians perform their dual role of agent for the patient and supplier of health care—particularly how financial incentives bear on that performance—has long been a matter of controversy in health manpower forecasting. The issue will be discussed later in this chapter.

Researchers have traditionally found a rather low linear correlation between the per capita use of health services or health care resources per capita, on the one hand, and observable health status in the relevant populations, on the other (see, for example, Fuchs, 1974; McKinlay and McKinlay, 1977). That low correlation should not be surprising. First, as noted, since health care is but one of many inputs into the production of health, simple first-order correlations do not control for the influence of many other factors. Second, although *other things being equal* the use of health services may well have a powerful positive impact on measurable health status, the input of health services is likely to be subject to rapidly diminishing marginal returns. Third, *measurable* health status indicators do not usually capture all positive contributions made by health care. For example, simply providing patients with accurate information on their health status may be viewed by them as a valuable contribution to the quality of life, particularly if that information confirms a good health status.

Although there have been numerous studies of the effects of particular environmental, socioeconomic, demographic, and behavioral factors on measurable health status, only a few studies have sought to embrace all these variables formally within the framework of a full-fledged health production function (see, for example, Auster, Leveson, and Sarachek, 1969; Silver, 1972; and, notably, Hadley, 1982). These studies generally have found a positive incremental association between the use of health services and measurable health status (usually, mortality rates), after control for all other factors affecting health status. For example, Hadley found that over the empirically relevant range of his observations and for the bulk of the population, a 10 percent increase in the per capita use of medical care tended to be associated with a 1.5 percent decrease in mortality, other things being equal (1982, p. 169). Furthermore, studies of this sort do support the hypothesis that the input of medical care into the health production process is subject to rapidly diminishing marginal returns in terms of measurable health status.

As Figure 9-1 suggests, full-fledged, empirical health production functions would be the logical starting point for health manpower projections. Unfortunately, none of the empirical estimates available so far have been sufficiently detailed and precise for that purpose. Were such estimates available, one could derive from them normative levels of health care utilization per capita within a larger optimization model in which other inputs into the production of health—for example, housing or nutrition—would be traded off against medical care in a manner that minimizes the total social resource costs of attaining the desired level of health status.

Even without that formalism, however, it is increasingly being appreciated by policymakers in both the private and public sectors that such trade-offs ought to be made—that, for example, the rate of infant mortality among low-income families could, in principle, be vastly reduced with means completely outside the medical model. Sadly, these insights are not easily translated into coherent policy action within the fragmented budgetary processes typical of modern democracies. In that setting, the production of *better health* (as distinct from *health care*) is likely to be economically efficient solely by happenstance. More typically, health care will be either overused or underused relative to the economically efficient combination of all the factors going into the production of health.

Potential Shifts in the Setting of Health Care Production

As suggested in Figure 9-1, any target level of medical interventions used in the production of better health could be produced in a variety of different settings, and with a variety of different methods within each setting. Each possibility implies a different requirement of health manpower.

Shifts in the setting of health care, or changes in methods of delivery, can make earlier health manpower forecasts highly uncertain *ex ante* and seem widely off the mark *ex post*. During the 1960s and 1970s, for example, it was generally not foreseen how massive a shift from the inpatient to the outpatient setting would occur during the 1980s for a great variety of medical treatments. Table 9-1 illustrates this shift with data from the Blue Cross plans. This shift was made possible in part by technological developments that made the transfer of treatments to the outpatient setting clinically safe; but it was also accelerated by a significant increase in the degree of external, regulatory control over the utilization of inpatient health care instituted by both public and private third-party payors during the 1980s.

The ultimate impact of this shift from the inpatient to the outpatient setting on overall health manpower requirements deserves more careful investigation than it has hitherto received, because that impact may be substantial. With the empirical insights gained from such studies, a health manpower forecasting model could be used to simulate the effect of future potential shifts in the setting of health care on future requirements of physicians or other types of health manpower.

Shifts of care from the traditional fee-for-service medical practice to health maintenance organizations (HMOs) also are known to have substantial effects on the requirement for medical manpower. The factor driving health manpower requirements in that shift is not so much the setting per se, but the distinct *financial incentives* that accompany the delivery of health care. Under the HMO insurance contract, these incentives encourage economy in the use of medical care inputs in the production of health and also in the use of real resources in the production of health services. Chiefly by virtue of these incentives, staff or group model HMOs tend to be able to serve more than 800 patients per full-time-equivalent physician. In their recently published study of practice patterns in large prepaid group practices, Mulhausen and McGee (1989) found that a closed panel HMO appears to be able to operate with a ratio

Table 9-1. Shifts in the locus of health care delivery: Blue Cross and Blue Shield Plans, 1983–1988

Service	1983	1988	Percentage change, 1983–1988
Hospital inpatient admissions per 1,000 members	107	85	−21%
Hospital outpatient visits per 1,000 members	350	490	+40%

Source: Blue Cross and Blue Shield Association (1989), pp. 5 and 7.

as low as an average of 111 physicians per 100,000 population, which implies about 900 patients per physician. Even if that number did not fully reflect differences in the mix of patients served by current HMOs and the fee-for-service sector, a fully adjusted ratio would still remain far below the overall ratio already attained in the United States. Tarlov (1986) posits a ratio of 120 physicians per 100,000 enrollees for a staff model HMO, a ratio also accepted by Schwartz, Sloan, and Mendelson (1988, p. 892) in their recent manpower projection. The comparable ratio for the traditional fee-for-service sector is now closer to 450–500 patients per physician, but it is falling steadily, reaching levels below 200 in some cities.

To illustrate the effect a shift from the traditional fee-for-service setting to a staff model HMO setting would have on total physician requirements, let us denote by H the physician-enrollee ratio needed in an HMO, by F the corresponding ratio needed in the fee-for-service sector, and by T_r the overall physician-population ratio required for the nation as a whole. Then if x denotes the percentage of the population served by staff model HMOs, the overall required physician-population ratio can be calculated from the expression

$$T_r = F - x\,(F - H). \tag{1}$$

If H were 120, for example, and F 200, then the overall required ratio of physicians per 100,000 population would be 184 if 20 percent of the population were in HMOs, but only 160 if 50 percent of the population were in HMOs.

Conversely, if one lets the variable T_a denote the overall supply of physicians per 100,000 population actually available at some point in time, and F_a the number of physicians per 100,000 population left over for the fee-for-service sector after subtracting the physicians needed for the HMO sector, then, in terms of the variables defined above, we can express the ratio pressing in on the fee-for-service sector as

$$F_a = \left(\frac{1}{1 - x}\right)(T_a - x\,H). \tag{2}$$

In Figure 9-2, F_a is plotted on alternative values of x on the assumption that the required physician-enrollee ratio for HMOs is $H = 120$ per 100,000 enrollees and that the overall average physician-population ratio available to the population as a whole is $T_a = 230$ physicians per 100,000

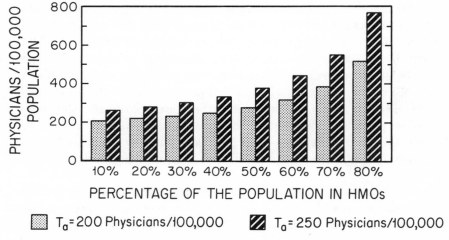

Figure 9-2. Physicians per 100,000 population left over for the fee-for-service sector as a function of HMO enrollment.

population (the ratio of *patient care* physicians per 100,000 population certain to be available in the year 2000). Clearly, with a given overall supply of medical manpower, a major shift of patients from the traditional fee-for-service sector to staff model HMOs could exert enormous economic pressure on the fee-for-service sector. For example, if half the American population were in staff model HMOs operating at a ratio of 120 physicians per 100,000 enrollees, then there would be 340 physicians left over per 100,000 population remaining in the fee-for-service sector. This implies that physicians in that sector would have to earn their gross income (currently an average of about $250,000 per year) from an average of only 295 patients, or about 100 families if one posits an average family size of about three. Physicians would either have very low incomes or would have to be able to charge very high fees, which would be improbable given the competitive presence of the HMO sector.

Potential Health Manpower Substitution within a Given Setting

Even within a given health care facility—a hospital, a nursing home, or a medical practice—one type of health manpower can often be traded off against another in the production of given sets of services. These trade-offs can be represented analytically with the aid of health service production functions. A production function is a mathematical relationship indicating the rates of output technically attainable with alternative combinations of productive inputs. In a medical practice, for example, these inputs are the time spent by physicians and their support staff, the floor space available to them, the number of examination rooms at their disposal, and so on.

At the level of theory, a production function is generally understood to define the *maximum* rates of outputs technically attainable with alternative combinations of inputs, which implies that the production processes are operated as efficiently as is technically feasible. In empirical estimation, however, it is usually not known which producers in one's sample are perfectly efficient technically and which are not.[1] An empirically estimated production function therefore usually reflects the *average* observed rates of output obtained with alternative combinations of inputs by a sample of different producers at one point in time.

A reliable production function estimate for a particular production process is a powerful analytical summary of that process. Such an estimate can be used to calculate the incremental contribution to output made by additions of one input to a given set of other inputs. For example, in the context of medical practice, the function allows one to calculate on average how many more patients per week a physician can see in the office if his or her support staff is increased by one person of a particular skill, or if the number of examination rooms is increased. Alternatively, the function can be used to identify the alternative combinations of physician time and the time of physician support staff capable of producing a given number of patient visits per week. In other words, it can be used to gain information on technically feasible trade-off curves between any two types of health manpower. Figure 9-3 illustrates such trade-off curves for physician-patient office visits in private medical practice.

If reliable production function estimates for all major categories of health services and all alternative health care settings were available to manpower forecasters, the latter could use these estimates to simulate alternative combinations of manpower—that is, the alternative manpower combinations $\{L_1, L_2, \ldots, L^m\}$ of Figure 9-1—that are capable of delivering a required set of medical treatments which, in turn, are deemed necessary to treat a given projected morbidity. Such numerical exercises would make it clear to policymakers that there does not exist just one ideal, technically determined manpower-population ratio, deviations from which, ipso facto, denote either a surplus or a shortage of

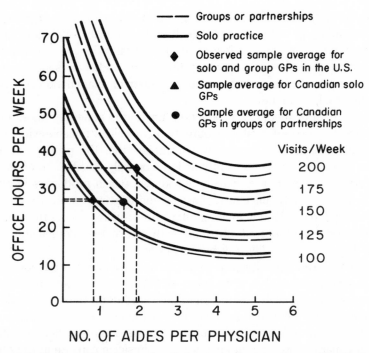

Figure 9-3. Estimated feasible trade-offs between physician time and auxiliary personnel, general practitioners. (From Reinhardt, 1975a.)

that type of manpower. For example, research of this sort on the use of health manpower in the hospital sector may possibly reveal that current fears of a chronic nursing shortage are based on the assumption of fixed nurse-to-bed ratios, totally in abstraction of the potential for health manpower substitution or capital-for-labor substitution within hospitals.

With the aid of empirical production functions, manpower forecasters could also identify the least-cost combination of manpower capable of supporting a desired set of medical treatments. Figure 9-4 illustrates that method hypothetically. In that diagram, the curved line represents an assumed, empirically estimated trade-off curve between two types of health manpower—for example, physician time and time of physician-support staff. In the technical jargon of economists, such a curve is known as an *isoquant,* that is, it traces out the alternative combination of these two types of manpower input capable of producing the *same quantity* of output. The straight lines in Figure 9-4 represent so-called

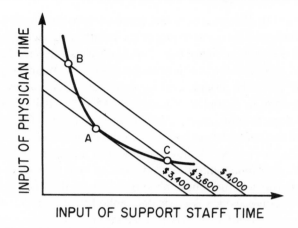

Figure 9-4. Potential trade-offs between types of health manpower: The concept of economic efficiency.

isocost curves, that is, each line represents alternative combinations of the two types of manpower inputs that cost the same.[2] Combinations A, B, and C in the diagram all are capable of yielding, say, 100 patient visits per week. Combination B is relatively more intensive in its use of physician time than are combinations A and C. It is also the most expensive manpower combination, because it lies on the isocost line for $4,000 per week. Combination C, which costs $3,600 per week, is relatively more intensive in its use of physician-support staff than are combinations A and B. Finally, combination A, costing $3,400 per week, lies in between these extremes; it represents the least-cost manpower combination just capable of yielding 100 patient visits per week. Deviations from that least-cost combination would connote degrees of economic inefficiency in the use of human resources. Although it would be *technically* feasible to produce 100 patient visits per week with even fewer physicians than are implied by combination A, that extreme degree of economizing on the use of physician time would not be *economically optimal.*

Full-Fledged Behavioral Models of the Health Care Sector
Even under the best of circumstances, however, such simulation exercises would only reveal what would be technically feasible and economically desirable. By themselves, they would not provide one with a clue to the manpower combination likely to be used by the health system in

future years. For that purpose, the forecaster really ought to have at hand a full-fledged *behavioral* model of the health care sector, one example of which is shown in Figure 9-5. This figure illustrates the bare-bones structure of a behavioral health-sector model as it might be perceived through the particular prism used by economists. An arrow from one block in the diagram to another should be read as "partially determines." The figure depicts four distinct, interrelated markets: the market for health services (centered on box 11), the market for health manpower (box 23), the market for health manpower training (box 25), and the markets for other inputs into the production of health services (box 14). Not shown in the scheme, but implied by box 6, is the market for health insurance coverage, which is intricately linked to the market for health services because health care and health insurance coverage are typically jointly chosen.

The future supply of medical manpower is determined in the domestic market for health manpower training (box 25 in Figure 9-5) and the inflow of foreign medical graduates (box 29 for fully trained physicians and box 30 for physicians still requiring residency training). The inflow of foreign medical graduates (FMGs) is really the export of foreign-produced medical education to the United States. In the absence of borders and immigration laws, the latter flow would be determined in the foreign markets for health manpower training and by the decisions of the FMGs themselves. In effect, however, the binding constraint on that flow has been U.S. government policy on immigration, which needs to be anticipated to project the future flow of FMGs to this country.

Ever since World War II, the flow of graduates from the domestic market for health manpower training has been determined effectively by the supply side of that market (box 26), notably by federal and state policies on the financing of medical schools. Although the ratio of qualified applicants to available medical school places has fallen substantially during the 1980s, the market can still be said to be in a state of disequilibrium. In spite of the typically high tuition now charged by American medical schools, the demand for medical school places among intrinsically qualified candidates at this time still appears to exceed the supply of available places. In Figure 9-5, that situation would be described as one for which $E_{id} > E_{is}$, where subscript i denotes a particular type of health manpower, in this case, physicians.

In his earlier work, Sloan (1970, 1971) had investigated the determinants of the demand for medical education (box 20 in Figure 9-5). He

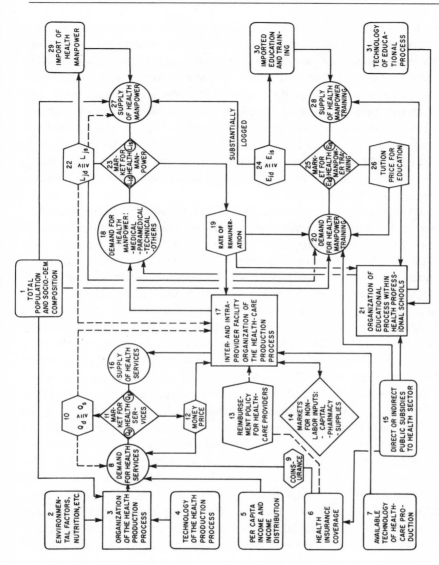

Figure 9-5. A market-based health care system. (From Reinhardt, 1974.)

had found that demand to be somewhat sensitive to economic factors, such as tuition charges and expected earnings in medical practice and in rival professions. But probably because the supply of American medical graduates had been fully determined by the available capacity of medical schools for so long, there have been only a few studies since then on the factors that drive young Americans to enter medical school in favor of alternative professional careers (Bazzioli, 1986) or that drive the choice of a medical specialty (Hadley, 1977; Marder, Kletke, et al., 1988). In light of the falling ratio of medical school applications to available places, however, these facets of health manpower warrant more intensive study in the years ahead.

Among the numerous factors driving occupational choice there surely must be the pecuniary dimension, usually represented in economic analysis by the internal rate of return to medical education (roughly, the annual rate of profit a medical education returns on the investment it requires in terms of monetary outlays and forgone earnings in the next best professional alternative). Sloan (1970) found that candidates entering medical school during the later 1960s faced an annual rate of return of somewhere around 25 percent to their investment of money and opportunity costs in four years of medical school and one year of internship. More recent work (Burstein and Cromwell, 1985; Marder, Kletke, et al., 1988) suggests that the rapidly growing physician-population ratio in the meantime has served to depress these rates, although not to unattractive levels. For example, if one measures the opportunity cost of a medical career by the forgone average income that would have been earned with a career in law, then the estimated annual rate of return to a decision to enter the profession of medicine rather than of law was 9.1 percent in 1974 and 14.2 percent in 1985. Table 9-2 presents these and alternative estimates with opportunity costs measured by still other careers. In short, so far a medical career is by no means a low-yield investment in human capital. Incidentally, if one measures the opportunity cost of a medical career strictly by the average forgone earnings yielded by a baccalaureate degree, then the return to medicine would appear to be 16.8 percent in 1974 and 16 percent in 1985, although the investment *base* on which these rates would be earned is, of course, much smaller than the base implied by the forgone earnings of a lawyer (Marder, Kletke, et al., 1988).

Finally, it must be emphasized that, although pecuniary factors have been found to enter the decision to become a physician and to choose a particular medical specialty, it is also clear from the available research that many other noneconomic factors enter that decision as well. Successful future research on these choices is therefore is likely to be interdisciplinary.

The total supply of medical manpower (box 27 in Figure 9-5) feeds directly into the markets for health manpower in general (box 23), where it confronts the demand for health manpower (box 18). The demand for health manpower emerges from the market for health services (box 11) by the interaction of the demand for health services (box 8) with their supply (box 16), which, in turn, is shaped by the organization of the health system in general (box 17). The market for health insurance (boxes 6 and 9) obviously also has a strong influence on the market for health services.

Part of the market for health services is the market for *physician services* proper. Just how that market clears (that is, what factors make the quantity demanded, Q_d, equal the quantity supplied, Q_s, after sudden changes on either the demand or supply side of that market) has remained a mystery and, hence, a controversy among health services researchers. At issue are the questions of whether, how, and to what

Table 9-2. Estimated annual rates of return to the decision to enter the medical profession rather than a competing profession

Measure of opportunity cost	Estimated annual rate of return to medicine above the competing profession[a]	
	1974	1985
The stream of earnings that could have been earned in:		
Law	9.1%	14.2%
Accounting	13.9%	13.8%
Engineering	11.6%	9.9%
Other postgraduate education	20.5%	18.3%

Source: Marder, Kletke, et al. (1988), table 6.1.

a. This is the estimated average rate of return to the investment represented by the money spent on tuition and other incidental costs of medical school and by the earnings forgone by not pursuing the other professional career listed under the heading "Measure of Opportunity Cost."

extent physicians on the supply side of that market (box 16) can manipulate the demand for their services (box 8).

In a normal, competitive market, for example, suppliers can seek to increase the quantity of their goods and services demanded by the rest of society either by lowering prices or by enhancing the quality of these goods and services, or by both means. Of course, in many markets suppliers can also seek to induce additional demand simply by persuading potential customers through truthful or deceptive advertising, although there are limits to that mechanism. The question in connection with physician services hinges on the degree to which physicians can increase the demand for their services through the analogue of advertising (see Reinhardt, 1985b, p. 190) simply by persuading their patients to accept such services, rather than through the more traditional equilibrators operating in normal markets: reductions in prices (fees) or enhancements of quality. If physicians had a fairly high degree of discretion in this respect, then a growing physician surplus would tend to be at least partially camouflaged by the delivery of added health services whose benefit-cost ratio might be trivial or even negative. I shall return to that question in a later section.

During the past two decades, much of the work of health services researchers in general, and of health economists in particular, has sought to identify empirically the nature and strengths of the causal flows in Figure 9-5. To attempt even a cursory overview of this vast body of research would go much beyond the limits of this chapter and is not my objective. Suffice it to note that this research has no parallel elsewhere in the industrialized world at this time, either in terms of its sheer volume or in terms of its technical sophistication. Much is now known with reasonable precision about the behavior of at least some parts of the American health care sector that could only be guessed at one or two decades earlier.

Alas, despite this impressive research record, it is as yet too early to fashion from this considerable wealth of empirical information one reliable, behavioral model of the entire health care sector that could be used to project health manpower shortages or surpluses decades hence.[3] (It may be added, of course, that *reliable* long-run forecasting models of this sort do not yet exist for any other sector of the economy, nor even for the economy as a whole.)[4] The nature of such a comprehensive health sector model is illustrated here only to emphasize that a health manpower forecast will pinpoint, at best, the most likely physician requirements and supplies of an entire probability distribution of possible numbers that may actually obtain in the future. These probability distributions of possible future numbers always exhibit some dispersion of possible values about the most likely value being projected by the forecasters. That dispersion, of course, increases rapidly with the length of the forecast horizon. Thus, the very best any forecaster could ever do would be to estimate the parameters of the probability distributions that describe the range of possible future values of the projected variable.

It follows that one cannot fairly cast aspersions at health manpower forecasters if, say, the physician supply or requirement projected for a point in time ten or twenty years hence turns out, *ex post,* to have been wide of the mark, just as one should not ridicule those who seek to forecast bond yields or foreign exchange rates only several months hence. First, the forecasted variables themselves usually are functions of a host of other variables whose future time path is uncertain at the time the forecast is made. Second, and more important, the forecasts themselves often trigger policy actions designed to close gaps between the forecasted numbers and preferred targets. As will be seen later, this has certainly been the case in health manpower forecasting.

Pragmatic Models for Health Manpower Forecasting

Because an operational, full-fledged, behavioral model of the health sector has never been available to health manpower forecasters, they have traditionally made do with more compact models that can be viewed as rough-and-cut summaries of the larger model sketched out in Figure 9-5. Figure 9-6, which is largely self-explanatory, illustrates the more compact models that have been used in recent decades. All the variables in this figure have time subscripts, which implies that each of them should, in principle, be projected separately. The most difficult variables to project, and also the most crucial ones, are (1) the projected per capita demand for physician services at time t (variable D_t) and (2) physician productivity, defined here as the projected average output of physician services per full-time-equivalent physician at time t (variable Q_t). If one writes out the ratio D_t/Q_t as

$$D_t/Q_t = \frac{\text{Projected Number of Physician Services/Population}}{\text{Projected Number of Physician Services/Physician}} \quad [3]$$

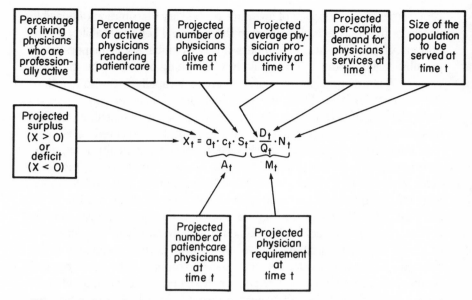

Figure 9-6. A simple forecasting equation for physician manpower.

then the ratio will appear as nothing other than the physician-population ratio deemed necessary to provide the projected service requirements D_t.

Figure 9-7 illustrates this forecasting equation diagrammatically. The diagram represents a construct often used by economists to illustrate the interaction among variables. It is not a regular Cartesian coordinate; instead, it contains four positive quadrants pasted back-to-back so that every axis measures a positive direction for the variable in question. The heavy, solid, upward-sloping line labeled A in Quadrant I of the figure represents the projected supply of patient care physicians (the term $a_t c_t S_t$ in the forecasting equation). Quadrant II depicts the growth of the total population (N_t) as a function of time. Because that quadrant is upside down, the curve slopes downward. Quadrant III depicts the total demand (need) for physician services as a function of the population size. That line also slopes down because the quadrant is upside down. The slope of the line is the per capita demand for physician services (the variable D_t in the forecasting equation), here held constant over time to facilitate the graphic illustration. Quadrant IV depicts the total number of physician services available as a function of the total number of patient

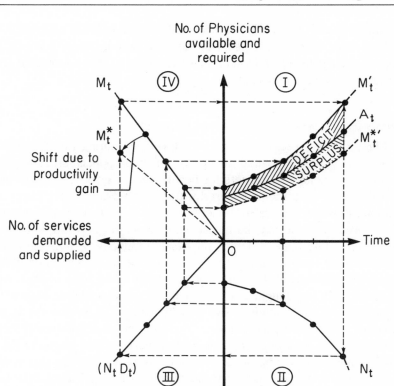

Figure 9-7. A rudimentary health manpower forecasting model.

care physicians. The slope of that line represents physician productivity (the variable Q_t in the forecasting equation), once again held constant here for ease of graphic representation.

Figure 9-7 is a convenient pedagogic device to make the entire process of health manpower forecasting graphic. One starts with a point on the time axis (some future year), reads off the projected population for that year in Quadrant II, reads off the corresponding demand for physician services in Quadrant III, translates that demand into the corresponding required number of physicians in Quadrant IV, and then compares that projected requirement of physicians with the projected supply of patient care physicians in Quadrant I to assess the supply-demand balance. Shifts in any of the curves in the diagram directly translate themselves into changes in the projected surplus or deficit of physicians. For example, the indicated shift of the input-output line in Quadrant IV represents a gain in physician productivity; it could turn a projected physician shortage into a surplus.

Needs-based versus Demand-based Forecasts

Many of the forecasting exercises developed during the first half of this century simply posited normative physician-population ratios that were recommended as targets for health manpower policy. These normative ratios were then compared with projected actual physician-population ratios at future dates to identify probable shortages or surpluses. Such forecasts generally did not attempt to project separate series for per capita utilization (D_t) and physician productivity (Q_t) explicitly. Instead, they assumed implicitly that per capita demand and output per physician would grow at roughly the same rate over time. More recent work typically has sought to project each of the variables in Figure 9-6 separately. In these studies, the utilization series D_t is either a *needs-based* or a *demand-based* estimate. Because the choice between these two bases remains rather controversial, it merits added comment here.

The needs-based approach to health manpower forecasting is the purely epidemiological approach illustrated earlier in Figure 9-1. Under that approach, an attempt is made to project the morbidity to be treated in future years and to estimate the medical services that will be needed to respond adequately to that projected morbidity. The projected need for medical services is then translated into the number of full-time physicians required to produce the needed service, a procedure that either explicitly or implicitly assumes a projected time path of physician productivity (Q_t). Classic illustrations of that approach are Lee and Jones (1933) and the Final Report of the Graduate Medical Education National Advisory Commission (1980), hereafter referred to simply by its famous acronym, GMENAC.

Under the needs-based approach, no attention is paid to the question of whether society will actually be willing to finance all of the treatments deemed to be "needed," or whether future medical manpower will actually locate itself in accordance with the geographic distribution of the projected need for medical care. Nor is allowance made for the possibility that, within limits, physicians in surplus may seek to eliminate that surplus by artificially stimulating the demand for their services beyond a level justifiable on purely medical grounds. In short, the approach is normative and not predictive. It merely yields recommended targets.

The virtue of needs-based forecasting is that it reflects an informed consensus among medical experts on the task that will have to be achieved in the future if society wishes to own up to the much-mouthed maxim that every citizen should have access to "needed" medical care and, furthermore, if society does not deploy the available medical manpower wastefully—for example, by devoting it disproportionately to the wealthy, worried well rather than to critically ill members of, say, uninsured low-income families. A major shortcoming of the approach is that it remains, essentially, organized, wishful, expert thinking that may be quite removed from the real world.

The demand-based approach typically seeks to project the *effective future demand* for medical care, that is, perceived need backed up by ability and willingness to pay for that care. On that approach, the time path of future utilization is an extrapolation of observed current utilization patterns, adjusted where possible for projected changes in the sociodemographic composition of the population and for changes in insurance coverage. In effect, such forecasts seek to simulate what a full-fledged behavioral model of the health-care sector would project, without actually going into the guts of such a model. Recent examples of this type of forecasting are Schwartz, Sloan, and Mendelson (1988) and Marder, Kletke, et al. (1988).

In contrast to the needs-based approach, which is purely normative in the sense that it suggests what *ought* to happen in the future, the demand-based approach is purely positive in the sense that it merely seeks to *predict* the future. The demand-based approach implicitly allows for the possibility of physician-induced demand for health services since, in its purest form, it does not even distinguish between medically necessary and unnecessary procedures. It tacitly regards treatments *accepted* by patients as treatments *demanded* by them.

For example, a needs-based forecast would project a surplus of a given specialty of physicians if the projected supply of these specialists exceeded the number required to meet the projected need for their services. By contrast, if it could reasonably be conjectured that these specialists are likely to spend a significant part of their time on medically dubious or outright unnecessary procedures—a conjecture entirely justified within the American context (Brook and Vaiana, 1989)—then a demand-based forecast might characterize that very same situation as a projected physician shortage, if the supply of physicians is judged inadequate to meet the projected demand for both appropriate and inappropriate procedures. Similarly, if the projected supply of physicians is judged to be inadequate to meet the need for medical intervention projected by medical experts, then the needs-based approach would project a physician shortage. The demand-based approach, on the other hand, might well characterize that very same situation as a projected physician surplus if some of the projected need of care is not likely to be backed up by a willingness to finance that care, and if the projected supply of physician services exceeds the projected demand for those services (that is, perceived need of care that *is* backed up by a willingness to finance that care).

This difference in methodology—the purely *normative* versus the purely *positive* basis of forecasting—has caused much confusion in the debate of health manpower policy, and it is likely to have contributed to the current controversy over the question of whether or not the United States now faces a physician shortage or a surplus. Those who, like the GMENAC Report, point to a sizable future physician surplus tend to lean on the needs-based approach, while those who, like Schwartz, Sloan, and Mendelson (1988), doubt the emergence of a surplus tend to rely on a demand-based approach.

In fact, of course, neither approach is inherently superior to the other, nor are they mutually contradictory. The two approaches merely respond to quite different policy questions. One seeks to yield normative targets, and the other seeks to predict what would be likely to happen if policy were not geared deliberately to move the health sector toward the normative target. Ideally, a comprehensive health manpower forecast ought to embrace both approaches.

Early Health Manpower Forecasts and Their Impact on Health Manpower Policy[5]

Probably the first formal attempt to assess the adequacy of the nation's physician supply was undertaken, during the period 1908–1910, by the Carnegie Foundation for the Advancement of Teaching. The final report of that study, known today as the Flexner Report, noted in its introduction that "taking the United States as a whole, physicians are four or five times as numerous in proportion to population as in older countries like

Germany" (Flexner, 1910, p. x). Implicitly, the Flexner Report took Germany's lower physician-population ratio as more nearly the proper ratio. The Flexner Report subsequently became the blueprint for a major reform of medical education in the United States, which led, *inter alia,* to a substantial reduction in the number of American medical schools.

The notion that the United States was beset by a physician surplus continued into the 1930s. In a report written by the Commission on Medical Education, organized by the Association of American Medical Colleges and supported by a number of prestigious foundations, it was concluded that

> if the United States had the same ratio of physicians to the population as England and Wales, there would be about 82,500 doctors in this country. If the ratio were the same as in Germany, the total would be 79,000; France, 73,000; Norway, 70,000; Sweden, 42,500. The actual number at present in the United States is 156,440 . . . An adequate medical service for the country could probably be provided by about 120,000 active physicians . . . On such an assumption there is an oversupply of at least 25,000 physicians in this country. (Final Report of the Commission on Medical Education, 1932, cited in Ginzberg, 1987, p. 6)

Very shortly thereafter, however, Roger Lee and Lewis Jones argued in *The Fundamentals of Good Medical Care* (1933) that as of that year the United States actually had 13,000 *fewer* physicians than could be considered adequate on medical grounds. This study is the first attempt at a proper needs-based approach, relying upon detailed assessments of morbidity and expert opinion on the care needed to address that morbidity properly. The study sought to alert policymakers that, in spite of the prevailing protestations over physician surpluses at the time, millions of Americans actually went without financial or physical access to adequate health care.

The Lee-Jones study was followed, after World War II, by the Ewing Report in 1948, the Mountin-Pennell-Berger report in 1949, the President's Commission on the Health Needs of the Nation in 1953, the 1958 report of the Department of Health, Education, and Welfare consultants, known as the Bayne-Jones report, and the report of the Surgeon General's Consultant Group on Medical Education in 1959, more commonly known as the Bane Report. Each of these reports based their forecasts on some normative physician-population ratio, which typically was the ratio prevailing in the more richly endowed regions of the country. Alternatively, it was recommended that, within the forecast horizon, every region in the United States be brought to at least the average national physician-population ratio prevailing at the time of the forecast. Given that approach, it is not surprising that each report continued the theme first sounded in the Lee-Jones Report, namely, that the nation was facing a severe physician shortage.

Each of these reports called for a major expansion of medical school capacity, and each called for direct federal assistance to both students and institutions to facilitate that expansion. The Bayne-Jones report, for example, had called for an increase in the number of first-year medical school places from 6,800 in 1955 to 8,700 in 1970. The subsequent Bane Committee report called for an expansion in first-year places from 7,400 in 1959 to 11,000 in 1975. Little thought appears to have been given in these reports to the long-run effects of large increases in medical school capacity on the supply of active physicians, since, for decades to come, the number of entering practitioners would continue to outnumber vastly the number exiting from medical practice.

The Political Response to the Predicted Physician Shortage

Neither the Eisenhower administration, on receiving the bulk of these reports, nor the Congress was willing to embark upon the bold new direction recommended by the forecasters. Hitherto, the federal government had supported medical education only indirectly and stealthily through the awarding of research grants, a time-hallowed method in higher education. The sundry manpower commissions recommended the direct and open intrusion of federal financing into medical *education,* which was vigorously opposed by organized medicine (Ginzberg, 1987, p. 19).

The dire forecasts therefore collected dust until the years of the Kennedy-Johnson administration, when they became the analytic foundation for the pathbreaking Health Professions Educational Assistance Act (HPEAA) signed into law in 1963. The HPEAA provided the substantial, direct federal assistance called for by the postwar health manpower commissions. It offered matching federal grants for the construction of medical schools as well as loans and grants to students of medicine, osteopathy, and dentistry. Together, the original act and its subsequent amendments of 1965, 1968, and 1971 helped literally to double the capacity of American medical schools within a very short time, in part with the powerful incentive of capitation grants, which made each school's federal grants directly proportional to the size of its student body.

This massive expansion in the capacity of American medical schools was accompanied by an equally massive influx of foreign medical graduates, who were eagerly invited into the country not only to augment the overall supply of physicians quickly but also to staff hospitals and clinics in locations shunned by American physicians—for example, in rural areas or in the low-income sections of major cities. Throughout the first half of the 1970s, close to a third of the 50,000 to 60,000 residency positions in graduate medical education in the United States were filled by foreign medical graduates. By the mid-1980s, that percentage had declined once again to about 17 percent, although of a larger total of 75,000 residencies (Marder, Kletke, et al., 1988, fig. 4 and table 4).

Passage of these generous HPEAA amendments was undoubtedly facilitated by yet another round of health manpower forecasts coming forth during the latter part of the 1960s, each forecasting sizable shortages of physicians as of the mid-1970s. In 1967, for example, the prestigious National Advisory Commission on Health Manpower issued a much-publicized report recommending a continued expansion of first-year enrollments in existing medical schools and the establishment of new schools. Close on its heels followed a forecast by the U.S. Department of Labor, Bureau of Labor Statistics (1967), which offered similar advice. That forecast, in turn, was followed by a U.S. Public Health Service (1967) report recommending that the United States attain, by 1975, the physician-population ratio attained by the best-endowed region in the United States in 1966. Using this standard, the Public Health Service projected a shortage of 50,000 as of 1969, a figure that was cited also in the *1970 Manpower Report of the President,* whence it found its way into the Carnegie Commission's highly influential report *Higher Education and the Nation's Health: Policies for Medical and Dental Education* (1970).

The Carnegie Commission posited a direct linkage between health manpower and better health and, on that thesis, recommended that the number of medical school entrants or their equivalent be increased by 50 percent, from the 10,800 estimated for 1970–71 to about 15,300 by 1976 and about 16,400 by 1978 (1970, pp. 2 and 43). That bold recommendation had been fully realized by 1980. Between 1966 and the early

1980s, the number of American allopathic medical schools (conferring the M.D. degree) increased from 89 to 127, and first-year enrollments in these schools from 8,900 to 17,300. In 1987 there were still 127 allopathic schools, with 16,779 first-year places and 15,872 graduates (Marder, Kletke, et al., 1988, tables 2.11 and 2.12). In addition, enrollment in osteopathic schools (conferring the D.O. degree) increased rapidly as well, from 623 first-year places in 1970–71 to 1,724 in 1986–87 (Council on Graduate Medical Education, 1988, vol. 2, table 3, p. 18).

Second Thoughts among Policy Analysts

As policymakers opened the floodgates to American and foreign-trained would-be entrants into medical practice in the United States, health services researchers began to wonder whether there could be too much of a good thing (see, for example, Dickinson, 1948; Ginzberg, 1960, 1966). Protected from the relentless political pressure to produce quick solutions to perceived social problems, the research community had the luxury of taking a long-run perspective. Figure 9-8 illustrates that perspective.

The lower of the two curves in Figure 9-8 represents the projected physician-population ratio likely to be generated by projected graduations as of 1973. It assumes a gradual expansion of medical school capacity from about 10,000 graduates in 1973 to about 16,000 in 1990. The curve includes foreign-trained medical graduates (FMGs) already practicing in the United States as of 1973, but it *excludes* all FMGs entering thereafter. In effect, the curve significantly underestimates the physician-population ratio that would actually obtain under a sustained influx of FMGs. The upper curve in the figure projects the physician-population ratio that would obtain if the annual number of graduates were increased to 25,000 by 1990, as was occasionally being proposed at the time (see, for example, Gerber, 1967). Once again, that supply projection excludes any influx of FMGs after 1973, which is, of course, not realistic. The point of the graph, however, is not to make projections of the actual physician-population ratio likely to obtain, but merely to illustrate the long-run implications of policies that sought to meet a perceived physician shortage quickly through vast increases in the capacity of American medical schools (and by opening the borders to large numbers of FMGs).[6] In the longer run, such a policy may overshoot the target by a wide margin.

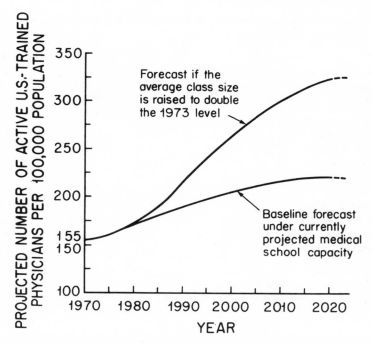

Figure 9-8. Long-run impact of medical school expansion on the supply of active U.S.-trained physicians, United States, 1970–2020. (From Reinhardt, 1975a.)

Aside from the long-run implications simply of medical school expansion, researchers also pointed to the enormous differences one observes across the United States in prevailing physician-population ratios (see Table 9-3). It was noted that these differences were substantially offset by differences in the number of annual physician-patient visits in medical practices and hospitals, which, in turn, appeared to be explained in part by more extensive reliance on physician support personnel in areas with low physician density and high annual rates of patient visits per physician (see Table 9-4). Although differences in the quality of the physician-patient visit might explain some of the observed differential in weekly visits, it was reasonable to attribute a good part of it to genuine differences in physician productivity.

The notion that the physician shortage projected for the 1970s might be partially solved by encouraging greater physician productivity had been put forth as early as 1949 by the economist Frank G. Dickinson in his critique of the Ewing Report of 1948.[7] This idea was formally incor-

Table 9-3. Physician-population ratios, patient loads, and medical fees by size of county, United States, 1970

Demographic county classification[a]	Physician-population ratio[b]	Weekly patient visits		Fee for an initial office visit (in dollars)
		Total	Office	
Non-metropolitan:				
10,000–24,999	51	223	167	7.15
25,000–49,999	64	217	164	7.13
50,000 or more	87	192	153	7.96
Metropolitan:				
50,000–499,999	107	194	150	8.65
500,000–999,999	141	167	140	9.33
1,000,000–4,999,999	150	138	114	9.00
5,000,000 or more	191	124	109	10.34

Source: Reinhardt (1975a), table 2–6.

a. Numbers refer to inhabitants.

b. Number of nonfederal physicians in patient care per 100,000 resident population as of December 31, 1970.

porated into the analysis of the National Advisory Commission on Health Manpower (1967) and was the central theme of Rashi Fein's *The Doctor Shortage* (1967).

Figure 9-9 illustrates the sensitivity of projected physician requirements to assumptions about the future growth in physician productivity. The vertical axis in that diagram represents the required future physician-population ratio 10 and 20 years hence, under varying assumptions about the future ratio of the per capita demand for physician services at future time t (variable D_t) to the number of physician services produced per physician in year t (variable Q_t). As noted earlier in connection with Figure 9-6, this ratio (D_t/Q_t) *is* the projected required physician-population ratio.

Now suppose initially that the forecaster had assumed the future growth in physician productivity to be just offset by future growth in the per capita demand for physician services and that, on this assumption, a ratio of 185 full-time physicians per 100,000 population was deemed adequate to serve the projected needs of the population. If, however, the future growth in physician productivity outpaced the growth in per capita

Table 9-4. Relationship between number of aides per M.D. and practice hours, hourly patient visits, and expenditures on medical supplies per visit

	Number of aides per M.D.[a]				
	0 to 0.5	0.51 to 1.00	1.0 to 2.00	2.01 to 3.00	More than 3.00
Total practice hours/week[b]					
General practitioners (N = 371)	54	55	59	60	62
Pediatricians (N = 133)	49	50	50	56	55
Obstetricians/gynecologists (N = 101)	49	51	55	53	61
Total patient visits/practice hour[c]					
General practitioners	2.2	2.6	3.2	3.8	4.0
Pediatricians	1.8	2.6	3.3	3.8	3.9
Obstetricians/gynecologists	1.7	1.9	2.5	2.8	3.2
Medical supplies/office visit[d]					
General practitioners	$0.55	$0.45	$0.56	$0.55	$0.66
Pediatricians	.56	.33	.49	.50	.66
Obstetricians/gynecologists	.41	.48	.43	.62	.78

Source: Reinhardt (1975a), table 4–9.

a. Includes solo practitioners only. N denotes number of respondents.

b. Excludes time spent on reading, research, and teaching.

c. Patient visits include visits to patients in the home or in hospitals.

d. Reported expenditures on medical supplies and drugs and small instruments per visit at the physician's office.

demand by one percentage point per year, only 167 physicians per 100,000 population would be needed ten years hence, and only 151 twenty years hence. On the other hand, if physician productivity lagged growth in per capita demand by one percentage point, then about 203 physicians per 100,000 population would be needed ten years hence and 226 twenty years hence. It may be noted that, during the late 1960s and early 1970s, health services researchers estimated the annual growth in physician productivity[8] during the period 1945–1968 to have been anywhere between 2 percent and 4 percent, a range that bracketed the estimated annual growth in per capita demand (Reinhardt, 1975, chap. 3).

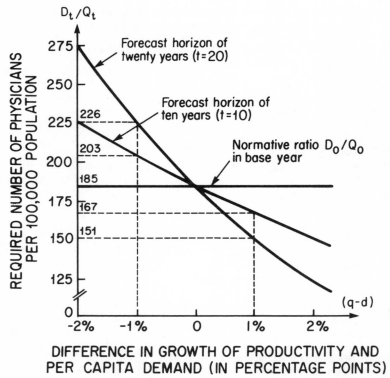

Figure 9-9. Sensitivity of future physician requirements to growth in physician productivity. (From Reinhardt, 1975a.)

Research on Physician Productivity

In the late 1960s, the available empirical information on physician productivity was very rough indeed. It consisted in the main of long-term trends in the average real annual gross billings per physician or in average annual patient visits per physician. Such estimates, however, were considered treacherous by the research community, because there is never any assurance that historical trends will replicate themselves in the future. For example, it might have been thought in the midst of the perceived physician shortage during the 1960s that all potential sources of gains in physician productivity would by then have been fully exploited by the health sector. To gain a better idea of the potential for future increases in physician productivity, researchers deemed it essential to explore the determinants of that important parameter more formally. Work on that issue began in earnest toward the end of the decade.

As noted earlier, empirical information on the determinants of physician productivity is obtained most easily through econometric estimation of physician-service production functions. Such estimates were first published by Smith, Miller, and Golladay (1972) and by Reinhardt (1972). The former researchers styled the physician's practice as a multi-product firm and based their estimates on linear activity analysis, that is, a so-called *discrete production function* model. That model allowed them to represent the output from a medical practice as an entire array of some 40 distinct physician services. On the other hand, the model forced them to estimate empirically a separate input-output coefficient for each pair of some 7 types of health manpower and some 40 types of physician services. They accomplished this task through work sampling techniques, a variant of time-and-motion studies. Once the large set of input-output coefficients was estimated in this way, the model was then manipulated with linear programming techniques to identify the degree of health manpower substitution that seemed technically feasible within a modern medical practice,[9] and also to identify least-cost combinations of health manpower for given sets of output of the 40-odd physician services embraced by their study.

Reinhardt (1972, 1975) used a continuous production function specification whose parameters were estimated empirically from the data yielded by a large, nationwide cross section of medical practices. In that production function specification, the output from the physician's practice was represented by a single index: the number of weekly patient visits at the physician's office.[10] That output index, of course, is much cruder than the multidimensional representation used by Smith, Miller, and Golladay (1972). On the other hand, the method is easier to implement in practice and also much less sensitive to errors in measuring particular observations. As already illustrated in Figure 9-3, a continuous production function can be used both to identify technically feasible trade-offs among types of health manpower and to identify the economically most efficient health manpower combination capable of producing given rates of patient visits.

Both of these production function studies indicated that there was much more leeway than had traditionally been thought by health manpower planners for substituting nonphysician labor for physicians within medical practices. Both studies also suggested that this potential did not appear to have been fully exploited by the representative American physician at that time—that, from a strictly economic point of view, the prevailing pattern of medical practice in the United States appeared to ' be wasteful in the use of medical manpower.

Indeed, the research suggested further that, had American medical schools not been expanded so rapidly during the late 1960s and early 1970s, even rather large future increases in the per capita demand for patient visits—increases far in excess of those that actually obtained by the mid-1980s—could easily have been met simply through greater reliance on physician substitutes within medical practices (see, for example, Reinhardt, 1975, chap. 7). Rumors of a pervasive physician shortage during the late 1960s seem to have been much exaggerated, just as the current nursing shortage may one day be found to have been exaggerated, once research identifies the full potential for health manpower substitution within the hospital.

Unfortunately, the very swiftness of the expansionist health manpower policy during the late 1960s had rendered these research insights on the physician shortage moot. Had these insights been available half a decade earlier, they might well have given policymakers pause and altered the course of health manpower policy in the ensuing years. To be sure, those expansionary policies cannot fairly be characterized as an uninformed overreaction on the part of policymakers to the dire health manpower forecasts pouring forth during the 1950s and 1960s. These policymakers were not reacting solely to the forecasters. Additional political pressure for a major expansion of medical schools came from two other sources which might well have overpowered even earlier warnings of a potential physician surplus.

First, the passage of the Medicare and Medicaid programs in 1965, after years of vehement political debate, must have made policymakers nervous. No sensible politician, having voted for these ambitious programs, would have wanted to stand accused later on of having promised vastly expanded health care benefits to the aged and the poor without thinking about the health manpower needed to realize this grand promise. In part the rapid expansion of medical school capacity during this period simply reflected normal risk aversion in the political arena.

A second source of political pressure for a major expansion of medical school places, however, undoubtedly came from the parents of the large and relatively well educated baby boom generation. These parents desperately sought lucrative career opportunities for their numerous offspring, not only in medical schools but in all areas of higher education. This parental pressure, incidentally, was not confined solely to the United States; it was manifest in every other country beset by a postwar baby boom. Most of the European nations, for example, expanded their medical schools during the 1970s even more rapidly than did the United States (see Schroeder, 1984; Reinhardt, 1985a), and they now report physician-population ratios far in excess of ours. Unlike Amercians, who still enjoy the luxury of debating whether or not the United States actually does face a physician surplus, European policymakers are now anxiously exploring how to cope with the massive physician surpluses that everybody agrees they now face.

From Physician Shortage to Surplus: The GMENAC Report

Long before the ratio of active physicians to population actually began to rise in response to the massive expansion of medical school capacity during the late 1960s, the writings of health services researchers persuaded policymakers that the gates leading to the practice of medicine might have been opened too far, with possibly undesirable consequences for health care in the United States. Sometime toward the mid-1970s, talk of an overall physician shortage gave way to talk of a physician surplus, and interest in physician productivity gave way to concern over a perceived maldistribution of American physicians across geographic regions and across medical specialties and concern over the prospect that a physician surplus might drive up the cost of medical care beyond levels justifiable on purely medical grounds.

As early as 1973, Assistant Secretary for Health Charles Edwards had warned Congress that the nation faced the prospect of a major physician surplus (Ginzberg, 1987, p. 33), and in April of 1976 the Secretary of Health, Education, and Welfare appointed the Graduate Medical Education National Advisory Committee (GMENAC) with the mandate to review the state of American graduate medical education and to assess the supply of and demand for medical manpower in the United States.

Long before the GMENAC issued its report in late 1980, however, this shift in perceptions of the health manpower situation had already influenced federal legislation. The 1976 amendment of the Health Professions Educational Assistance Act, for example, explicitly mentioned the prospect of a physician surplus. The act curtailed the capitation grants for medical schools and the flow of foreign medical graduates into American medical practice, and it provided instead direct financial incentives designed to redistribute physicians both geographically and across specialties. Chief among the new policy instruments was the National Health Services Corps (NHSC), an imaginative scholarship program designed to direct graduating physicians into rural areas or urban institutions characterized by a shortage of medical manpower in return for federal financing of their medical education.

In the meantime, under the leadership of Alvin R. Tarlov, and with the active support of the Carter administration, the GMENAC launched what is surely one of the most ambitious health manpower forecasting exercises ever undertaken in the history of American health services research. The product of that research effort was reported in September of 1980. In a nutshell, the report predicted an overall surplus of 70,000 physicians by 1990 and one of 145,000 physicians by 2000, although for some primary care specialties the GMENAC actually projected future shortages.[11]

Not surprisingly, Congress and the rest of the nation greeted the GMENAC report with very little interest. Although the prospect of a physician shortage tends to strike fear into the hearts of the public—and hence of politicians—it is just not clear to anyone then and now whether a physician surplus actually is harmful to anyone other than physicians' financial health. Indeed, it has been argued, notably by neoclassical economists (Harris, 1986; Rossiter and Wilensky, 1987; Feldman and Sloan, 1988), that from the patient's perspective, the greater the supply of competing physicians, the better. Furthermore, by the early 1980s the nation had persuaded itself of the view that the best public policy in most matters is for the government not to do anything at all—to let the private markets work out whatever imbalances might develop in the economy.

On the other hand, the GMENAC report quickly triggered a passionate debate among stakeholders in American medical education and in the research community. One would have expected opposition to the report from the medical education establishment, whose flow of public subsidies might be reduced by Congress on the strength of the report. Remarkably, however, the American Medical Association and some medical specialty societies (particularly the American College of Surgeons) also sharply attacked the report, although one would have thought that they might welcome any policy to reduce the number of physicians seeking their income from a patient pool projected to grow much less rapidly than the supply of physicians. Perhaps, in setting their policies, the leaders of organized medicine trade off the size of their members' average income against the size of their organizations' political base, which finds strength in number. Perhaps there may have been yet other, and possibly loftier, reasons for organized medicine's reaction to the GMENAC report, reasons not easily grasped by an economist's one-track mind.

In American political debate, it is customary never to couch one's reaction to a particular study in terms of its potential impact upon one's own economic or political position. Instead, the proper etiquette is to phrase that reaction strictly as a seemingly objective, scientific evaluation of the *methodology* used in the study.[12] And thus it is that the GMENAC study, easily the most imaginative and sophisticated health manpower forecast ever produced in the United States, has been subjected to an unusual onslaught of vehement criticism on purely methodological grounds, an onslaught that continues to this day (see, for example, American College of Surgeons, 1989).

To develop its forecast, the GMENAC simultaneously launched three distinct modeling efforts: (1) a Physician Supply Model; (2) a Graduate Medical Education Model; and (3) a Physician Requirements Model. In its principal structure, the Physician Supply Model was standard issue. It went beyond the state of the art mainly in its attempt to break down the overall supply of physicians into numerous specialties and subspecialties, which, incidentally, required the development of a separate Graduate Medical Education Model. Unfortunately, the finer the forecaster's breakdown into medical specialties, the more visible will be forecasting errors that would wash out in less disaggregated forecasts. By its bold attempt to travel down that route, the GMENAC obviously enhanced the probability of being proved wrong, *ex post,* by actual events. Even so, one should not fault the GMENAC for taking this bold methodological step; one could at most fault it for setting perhaps more store by the accuracy of its supply forecasts than was warranted at the time.

The GMENAC's Physician Requirements Model represents a classic needs-based approach, although an unusually elaborate one. Through a lengthy interplay of its own analytical staff with a set of Delphi panels composed of clinical experts, the Committee projected (1) the future population of the United States, broken down by sociodemographic groups, (2) detailed information on the morbidity likely to emerge from that population, (3) the set of medical services likely to be required to respond to that morbidity *effectively* and *efficiently*, and, finally, (4) the number of physicians in each specialty implied by a proper clinical response to the projected morbidity. On the basis of the requirements model, the GMENAC projected a requirement of 498,250 full-time-equivalent physicians by the year 2000. Its Physician Supply Model had projected supplies under four different scenarios, yielding numbers ranging from a low of 573,000 to a high of 684,000 physicians by the year 2000, suggesting an overall physician surplus anywhere between 75,000 and 186,000 physicians in that year (see GMENAC, 1980, fig. 2, p. 10).

Although the use of Delphi panels is sometimes frowned upon by purists in the scientific community—and they are an easy target for critics who are adversely affected by recommendations emerging from such studies—one may alternatively laud the technique as an attempt by researchers to reach out to the users of scientific research. A standing complaint among these users has been that, in structuring their analyses and in extracting policy recommendations from them, researchers too often are insensitive to the constraints, irrationality, and other imperfections said to beset the so-called "real world." A judicious use of carefully chosen Delphi panels can go a long way toward meeting that objection.

If one seeks fault with the GMENAC's Physician Requirements Model, however, one can find it in two major areas. First, in the translation of the projected need for medical services into the number of physician hours needed to meet these needs, the GMENAC implicitly assumed fixed input-output coefficients. To be sure, the Committee sought to use for this purpose what it thought of as *optimal* input-output ratios. Even so, the use of a fixed set of such ratios tends to obscure from view the enormous flexibility that a health system really has in responding to the health needs of a nation, a point made at length in earlier sections of this chapter. Within fairly broad limits, one can actually be more relaxed about the future health manpower situation than seems widely assumed among policymakers. Second, although the GMENAC study went boldly into the area of disaggregating the supply of physicians by specialty, it failed to extend that disaggregation to gender. Perhaps that omission is understandable within the context of a time period—the late 1970s—in which any allusion to possible differences between men and women immediately triggered charges of sexism. A disaggregation of the future supply of physicians into gender, however, *is* important.

The proportion of women physicians in the overall supply is growing rapidly. In 1969–70, only about 8 percent of medical school graduates were women. By 1986–87, that proportion had reached 32 percent (Marder, Kletke, et al., 1988, table 2.12). It is likely to rise further in the future. Moreover, there appear to be sizable differences in the practice patterns of men and women physicians. These differences had been noted as early as the mid-1970s (see, for example, Kehrer, 1976). In her analysis of hourly rates of patient visits among American physicians, Langwell (1982) found that, after adjusting for specialty, women physicians saw an average of only 60 to 70 percent as many patients per practice hour as did their male counterparts. Using data from the AMA's annual survey of 1981, Reinhardt (1985a) found that, on average, women internists tended to see only 81 percent as many patients per practice hour as did their male counterparts, devoted about 92 percent as many weekly hours to medical practice, and practiced only 92 percent as many weeks per year. Overall, women internists in the sample saw only about 70 percent as many patients per year as did their male counterparts.

Incidentally, similar tendencies are manifest elsewhere in the world. In their study of physicians in the Canadian province of Quebec, Berry and colleagues (1978) found that, after controlling for other practice inputs, female physicians saw 20 to 30 percent fewer patients per hour than did their male counterparts. Similar results were reported in a study of women physicians in France published by the *Centre de Recherche pour L'Etude et l'Observation des Conditions de Vie* (see CREDOC, 1983). Table 9-5 presents some rather striking data adapted from that study. It should be noted that physician fees are uniform across France, so that differences in patient billings cannot reflect gender-driven differences in professional fees.

The factors that have driven these observed differences in practice patterns are not yet well understood, nor is it known how stable these differences are likely to be over time. That question should receive sustained attention in health services research in the future, as the proportion of women in American medical practice grows. In the meantime, some health manpower forecasters have begun explicitly to adjust their projections for these differences. In their paper "The Projected Physician Surplus Reevaluated," for example, Jacobsen and Rimm (1987) assert on the basis of an earlier study (Jussim and Muller, 1975) that, *during their lifetime,* female physicians will be only 60 percent as pro-

Table 9-5. Differentials in workload of men and women physicians in private
practice, France, 1981

Specialty and age	Patient billings/year (in francs)		Visits and consultations/year	
	Men	Women	Men	Women
General practice				
Age 35 or less	262,000	138,000	3,863	1,919
35 to 44 years	358,000	187,000	5,280	2,412
45 to 54 years	349,000	183,000	5,105	2,340
55 to 64 years	303,000	171,000	4,234	2,099
65 years or older	201,000	113,000	2,818	1,448
All general practitioners	305,000	157,000	4,452	2,087

Source: Adapted from CREDOC (1983), table 46, p. 93.

ductive as male physicians. Combined with an assumed increased proportion of female physicians by the year 2000 (they seem to have
assumed 16 percent), they conclude that the physician supply projected
for the year 2000 by the GMENAC must be multiplied by a factor of
0.937 just to account for the increasing proportion of female physicians
in the pool. After further adjustment for an unanticipated decline in physicians entering practice and a general decline of physician productivity
(calling for a further multiplicative adjustment factor of 0.940), the
authors reduce the physician surplus projected by the GMENAC from
145,000 to 39,000, and even further to 6,000 if foreign medical graduates were barred from entering American medical practice after 1986
(see their Exhibit 2, p. 53).

Similarly, in their recent reevaluation of the GMENAC forecast,
Schwartz, Sloan, and Mendelson reduce the projected *effective* number
of physicians in the year 2000 by 4,000 on the assumption that women
physicians will work an average of 8 percent fewer hours per year than
men physicians (1988, p. 895). Remarkably, these authors do not make
any adjustments for the often observed differences in the *hourly* visit
rates of male and female physicians. Perhaps they assumed that this
particular differential would vanish over time. As Frank A. Riddick, Jr.,
a member of the AMA's Council on Medical Education, remarked before
the Council on Graduate Medical Education (established by Congress in
1985 under Public Law 99-272): "AMA data indicate that female physi-

cians have lower productivity than male physicians, working 90 percent as many hours per week in patient care activities and having 75 percent as many patient visits . . . *However, recent studies indicate that differences in the productivity of male and female physicians have decreased in recent years"* (Riddick, 1987, p. 163; italics added).

The Lingering Controversy over Medical Manpower

Since the GMENAC Report appeared in 1980, two questions have dominated the debate on health manpower policy. First, does the United States actually face a surplus of physicians? Second, even if there were such a surplus, who would actually be harmed by it? Research has not been able to answer either of these questions conclusively, although not for want of trying.

Does the United States Face a Physician Surplus?

At this time, policymakers sincerely interested in obtaining a bearing on the future supply of and demand for medical manpower in this country could forge their perceptions from a wide range of forecasts, spanning the set from a predicted overall shortage of physicians by the year 2000 to a massive and growing surplus. One of the key factors driving the differences among these forecasts has been the assumed growth in enrollment in health maintenance organizations (HMOs). As noted earlier, HMOs are able to operate with much lower physician-to-population ratios than does the rest of the health system (see especially Figure 9-2). A second major variable surrounded by great uncertainty is future growth in the demand for physician services, which, of course, depends significantly on society's willingness to continue financing the large increase in outlays on physician services experienced in the past two decades.

In a revisit of the GMENAC forecast that he directed, for example, Alvin R. Tarlov concluded in 1986 that the physician surplus in the year 2000 would be likely to exceed even the earlier alarming forecast of a massive physician surplus (see Tarlov, 1986). Noting the rapid enrollment of the population in HMOs during the 1980s and assuming such plans to be able to operate with some 120 physicians per 100,000 enrollees (versus 225 or more in the traditional fee-for-service system), Tar-

274 • Uwe E. Reinhardt

lov projected a surplus of about 180,000 physicians if 20 percent of the population were enrolled in HMOs by the year 2000, and a surplus of 220,000 physicians if as many as 40 percent of the population were then enrolled in HMOs.

A similar prediction was made in the same year by Steinwachs and colleagues (1986). The authors concluded that, as a result of the deeper penetration of HMOs into the American health system than had been assumed in the GMENAC study, 20 percent fewer primary care physicians than projected by GMENAC would be needed for children and 50 percent fewer for adults.

At the other end of the spectrum is the recent forecast authored by Schwartz, Sloan, and Mendelson (1988), who project an impending *shortage* of physicians by the year 2000. These authors' forecast is summarized most easily with the help of the simple forecasting equation illustrated earlier in Figures 9-6 and 9-7. That equation is reproduced here for easier reference; its variables are defined in Figure 9-6.

$$X_t = a_t c_t S_t - (D_t/Q_t)N_t. \tag{4}$$

$$\begin{array}{ccc}
\text{projected} & \text{effective} & \text{physician} \\
\text{surplus/} & \text{physician} & \text{requirement} \\
\text{shortage} & \text{supply} &
\end{array}$$

First, the authors quite properly define the projected supply of physicians not just as those who will be professionally active in the target year (the product $a_t S_t$ in equation [3]), but only as those likely to be active in *patient care* (that is, the product $a_t c_t S_t$). This adjustment results in a deduction of 112,000 physicians from the 700,000 or so physicians projected to be *professionally active* by the U.S. Bureau of Health Professions (1988b). Apparently, according to the authors, the parameter c_t (the proportion of professionally active physicians actually engaged in patient care) has been tacitly and erroneously set equal to 1 in most other forecasts.

Next, Schwartz, Sloan, and Mendelson apparently differ with others on the projected increase in the per capita demand for physician services (the growth in variable D_t of equation [3]). Most other studies posit much lower growth rates in that variable than do these authors (see, for example, the U.S. Bureau of Health Professions, 1988b).

In order to sidestep the possibility that data from the fee-for-service sector reflect utilization induced by physicians for purely pecuniary reasons—that is, in order to get as close to a true needs-based approach as they can—the authors base their projected physician requirements on the historical experience of the Kaiser Foundation Medical Plan in Southern California, which, presumably, offers physicians no incentive to provide patients any but truly needed health services. Furthermore, in order to avoid having to make explicit assumptions about future physician productivity (the variable Q_t in equation [3]), the authors simply project the future growth in the physician-to-population ratio (that is, in the ratio D_t/Q_t in equation [3]). In other words, they simply proceed with the more compact forecasting equation

$$(D/Q)_{2000} = (D/Q)_{1983} (1 + g)^{17}, \qquad [5]$$

where $(D/Q)_{2000}$ denotes the required physician-to-population ratio in the year 2000, $(D/Q)_{1983}$ the physician-to-enrollee ratio in the Kaiser Plan in base year 1983 (1 physician per 840 patients or 119 physicians per 100,000 enrollees), and variable g is the projected growth rate in the required physician-to-population ratio.

Clearly, the estimated future growth of the required physician-population ratio (variable g in equation [5]) is *the* crucial driver in this forecasting exercise. It is, in effect, the difference between the projected future growth in the per capita demand for physicians' services and the projected future growth (positive or negative) of physician productivity.[13] As such, it is a highly problematic variable, one for which it is not easy to acquire an intuitive grasp.

Using data from the period 1965–1983, and after eliminating the effect strictly of increases in the percentage of enrollees aged 65 and over in the Kaiser Plan, the authors estimate the baseline growth rate g for Kaiser to have been 1.03 percent per year over the period 1965–1983 (versus 2.20 percent for the fee-for-service sector). The authors then assume that this rate of growth in Kaiser's physician-enrollee ratio will persist until at least the year 2000 and, moreover, that this growth experience will be representative of all HMOs in the United States. Finally, the authors adjust that baseline growth rate further for the growth in the percentage of the aged in the U.S. population and assume that this percentage will apply to the HMO sector as well as to the rest of the health sector. This adjustment for the aging of the population per se brings the estimated growth rate in the required physician-enrollee ratio in HMOs (variable g in equation [5]) to 1.60 percent per year. In other words, Schwartz, Sloan, and Mendelson project that by the year 2000, HMOs in the United States will require a ratio of

$$156 = 119 (1 + .016)^{17} \qquad [6]$$

physicians per 100,000 enrollees, or about 1 physician for 640 patients.

Like Tarlov (1986), the authors assume that, by the year 2000, 44 percent of all Americans will be in tightly managed, competitive health plans—possibly an overly conservative assumption. In contrast to Tarlov, however, the authors assume that only about 20 percent of the population will be in staff model HMOs like Kaiser, and that the rest will be in independent practice associations (IPAs) and preferred provider organizations (PPOs). The latter type of arrangements are assumed to use 10 percent more physicians per enrollee than a bona fide staff model HMO, a quite reasonable and possibly conservative assumption. Finally, it is assumed that the remainder of the population will be served, in the year 2000, by the traditional fee-for-service system at a rate of 480 patients per patient care physician (or 208 patient care physicians per 100,000 population). On that basis, and after adjusting further for overall population growth (the variable N_t in equation [4] above), they project a requirement of 592,000 patient care physicians by the year 2000, against a supply of 585,000. In other words, the authors project a physician *shortage* of 7,000 for the year 2000.

Schwartz, Sloan, and Mendelson observe that, depending upon the particular set of assumptions one makes about the future growth in per capita demand, the number of persons enrolled in HMOs, and a number of other factors, the future supply of physicians could either fall short of projected demand by as many as 83,000 physicians or exceed that demand by as many as 40,000 physicians. This, of course, is a rather disturbing range of possibilities for a forecasting horizon of only 10 years and for a projected overall supply of somewhere around 600,000 physicians. In reacting to that wide range, however, policymakers should be mindful that not every number within a range of estimates offered by a conscientious forecaster is believed by the author to have an equal probability of occurring. The extremes in the range offered by Schwartz, Sloan, and Mendelson clearly are believed to be improbable by these authors, even though they cannot be completely ruled out a priori. The authors' "best estimate"—one they believe to have the highest probability of occurring—*is* the projected shortage by the year 2000 of some 7,000 physicians.

Ernest P. Schloss (1988), in a companion piece published in the same issue of the *New England Journal of Medicine*, comes to a similar conclusion, although his forecast is much less explicit and detailed. In the light of recent socioeconomic and demographic factors, he argues, the United States is likely to face a physician shortage within the next three decades, and he warns policymakers not to overreact to predictions of an impending physician surplus.

In between these extreme forecasts are a number of others that generally point to a physician surplus. As already noted, after adjusting the GMENAC forecast for a number of factors, including the ever larger presence of women physicians in the overall supply, Jacobsen and Rimm (1987) concluded that the physician surplus by the year 2000 would be more likely in the range of 6,000 to 39,000, depending on the number of foreign medical graduates entering the physician pool. In its *Sixth Report to the President and Congress on the Status of Health Personnel in the United States* (1988a), the U.S. Bureau of Health Professions projects a physician requirement of 637,000 physicians by the year 2000 and a supply of 708,600, pointing to a surplus of 71,600 (table 2-11, p. 2–22). In its critique of the study by Schwartz, Sloan, and Mendelson (1988), the Bureau judges the growth in future demand posited by these authors (variable g in equation [5] above) to be excessively high (U.S. Bureau of Health Professions, 1988b; especially table 3) and also questions the high number of physicians assumed by the authors to be in activities other than patient care.

Finally, after reviewing all of the studies available on this topic, the Council on Graduate Medical Education concluded in its *First Report* on July 1, 1988: "From the data and testimony it has received, the Council has concluded that there is now or soon will be an aggregate oversupply of physicians in the United States. The Council notes, however, that there are significant uncertainties which could change this assessment" (vol. 1, p. xxi). But the Council hastened to add: "There is conflicting evidence as to whether an oversupply of physicians would necessarily lead to socially undesirable consequences" (vol. 1, p. xxi). Finally, the Council recommended, wisely in my view, that "at the present time, the Federal Government should not attempt to influence physician man-power in the aggregate" (vol. 1, p. xxi).

How Harmful is a Physician Surplus?

The Council's caveat and its recommendation raise the question: who actually is harmed by a physician surplus? Alternatively, it may be asked: are the social consequences of a surplus as serious as those of a short-age? Unfortunately, the research community has not reached a consensus on these questions, in spite of many serious efforts to do so.

In its testimony before the Council on Graduate Medical Education, the American Medical Association argued that a physician surplus could "lower the quality and raise the cost of physician services" (Riddick, 1987, pp. 164–165). Quality of care is thought to suffer when physicians performing complicated procedures do not perform them frequently enough to maintain their skill, or when specialists are driven by com-petition to render primary care services for which they are not properly trained. Costs are driven up, according to the AMA testimony, because there appears to be a high correlation between increases in real physi-cian expenditures and increases in the physician-population ratio, although the AMA was quick to add that the added utilization need not be inappropriate. In any event, the AMA left the Council with the remarkable proposition that "market forces cannot be relied upon to adjust the growth rate of the U.S. physician supply, because the U.S. health care system does not operate in a free market" (Riddick, 1987, p. 170) and vaguely hinted at measures to stem the rise in the number of American physicians without actually calling for direct controls on that growth.

Within the research community itself, the frequently observed posi-tive correlation between the physician-population ratio and per capita spending on physician services has engendered one of the most tena-cious, heated, and, so far, futile debates. One school of thought (for example, Evans, 1973, 1974; Reinhardt, 1978, 1985b; Rice, 1984; and, apparently, Sloan, 1983, 1984) sees in that correlation support for the intuitively appealing hypothesis that physicians respond to the economic pressure triggered by higher physician density by inducing in their patients a higher level of demand for physician services than would genuinely be demanded by fully informed patients technically capable of evaluating the medical merits of their care. That excess utilization, according to this school of thought, is not only costly to the rest of society; it can also be harmful to the patient's health. Other researchers (Sloan and Feldman, 1978; Harris, 1986; Rossiter and Wilensky, 1987; Feldman and Sloan, 1988) have argued, however, that a mere correlation of this sort implies nothing about causation and would, in fact, be data-compatible with hypothetical models that explicitly preclude the physician's ability to induce demand for his services at given levels of fees faced by patients. It is hard to argue with that objection, of course, although by itself such theoretical argumentation clearly cannot not settle the matter conclusively.

Econometric studies designed to test these rival hypotheses with appeal to nonexperimental data have so far not been able to settle the matter one way or the other either, and for a very good reason: such analyses have not been able to distinguish properly between physician services merely *accepted* by often frightened and ill-informed patients, and services *actively demanded* by the patient. Although it is plausible to argue that initial patient visits to a physician are purely patient-initiated, that argument does not extend to the many ancillary services that can be packaged by a physician into such a patient-initiated visit. As Mark Pauly has wisely concluded on this point: "For many reasons it is likely that we [economists] will never fully resolve the demand creation/information imperfection question . . . Thus the fee-for-service market will remain a mystery as far as empirical predictions are concerned" (1988, p. 229).

Unwilling to wait for a resolution of this issue by the experts, and possibly quite innocent of this learned debate, policymakers almost everywhere on the globe appear to have let their policies on this matter be guided by their own intuition. That intuition appears to have sustained the thesis that physicians can, indeed, create demand for their services within broad limits, and that they will usually do so to counteract downward pressure on their incomes. Upon that thesis, for example, has rested the demand by the White House and by the Congress, in 1989, that the introduction of the Resource-Based Relative Value Scale (RBRVS) be accompanied by a global cap on Medicare's expenditures on physician services. That cap is meant to control what is euphemistically called the "volume problem," which however is clearly understood by all to refer to the likelihood that surgeons and other proceduralists will react to the impending reduction in their fees through increases in the recommended use of their services.[14] Thus, policymakers tread boldly beyond the point on the road at which health services researchers remain locked in erudite disputation.

Is Health Manpower Forecasting Worth the Trouble?

It has been the purpose of this chapter to describe to the noninitiated the task of health manpower forecasting, in theory and in practice, and to assess the role of that research effort in the formulation of the nation's health policy. The second section of the chapter was intended to convey to the reader the sheer complexity of this research enterprise. In effect, the forecaster who seeks to project the size of the physician surplus or shortage in some future target year attempts nothing less than projecting for the user of that information the conditional mean (or modal value) of a fairly wide probability distribution of possible values for the variable "projected supply of physicians minus projected physician requirements in future year t." The shape and position of that probability distribution are conditional upon a whole host of influences that must, first, be quantified and, second, projected into the future as well. In short, the task is daunting.

It is no more daunting, however, and no more unsuccessful in practice, than the labor market forecasts regularly issued by the U.S. Bureau of Labor or the macro-economic forecasts regularly issued by the Office of Management and Budget and the Congressional Budget Office. Indeed, the task is no more daunting, nor any less successful in practice, than the annual financial accounting reports and the financial forecasts upon which modern business firms base their strategies and upon which pension and mutual funds place their billion-dollar bets.

Time after time, when health manpower forecasters in the past have submitted precise point estimates of the future health manpower situation, they have found themselves to be widely off the mark, *ex post*. On the other hand, when forecasters have sought to cover their flanks, *ex ante*, by hedging their point estimates with entire ranges of possible, alternative scenarios, these ranges have been sufficiently wide to frustrate policymakers. It may therefore fairly be asked whether the benefits from health manpower forecasting warrant its cost at all.

In exploring that question, one will soon discover that the *cost* of the enterprise has actually been rather modest by comparison with other efforts to structure information for decision makers. The highly elaborate GMENAC exercise, for example, probably cost no more than $3 million or so, a number that pales in comparison with the vast sums spent annually by the typical American corporation to produce its financial reports. As I have argued elsewhere, these corporate reports are much cruder and certainly no more reliable than even the crudest health manpower forecasts produced by health services researchers (Reinhardt, 1981, pp. 1155–56).

In the *New York Times* of March 22, 1990, for example, it was reported that "the Shawmut National Corporation [a bank] said yesterday that after examination by Federal banking regulators it had revised its 1989 earnings to show a loss of $128.9 million. In January, it had reported a profit of $201.7 million" (p. D1). Not in the entire history of health manpower forecasting in the United States have researchers ever been so widely off the mark with their numbers—even for twenty-year forecasts—than were this bank's highly paid accountants and auditors. Yet major revisions of this sort are not at all uncommon among the people who structure financial information for the business world, information upon which powerful decisions may be based. To make this point even more forcefully, one may ask whether there is in the history of health manpower forecasting anything as egregiously wanting as the work of the high-priced accountants who produced, and the high-priced auditors who judged as "fair and accurate," the financial reports of, say, the Lincoln Savings and Loan Association—reports that seduced the present Chairman of the Federal Reserve and former economic consultant Alan Greenspan to pronounce that institution safe, sound, and beyond the need for government regulation, all at an eventual cost to the American taxpayer of some $2 billion or so? Or, are health manpower forecasts usually any wider off the mark than are the longer-range macroeconomic forecasts of the U.S. Treasury Department or the President's Council of Economic Advisors?

In placing health manpower forecasting into this wider perspective, the issue of its *cost* quickly loses significance. There remains the question, however, whether the enterprise yields any benefits at all, or whether it possibly might do more harm than good. To think about this question, one might open for health manpower forecasting an imaginary T-account and credit to it the good thought to flow from that research, while debiting to the account the potential pitfalls of the effort. Upon completion of that exercise, one may conclude that the negative side of health manpower forecasting lies not so much in the production of the forecasts themselves, but in the use to which such forecasts have been put at the level of policy.

The first credit one would enter for health manpower forecasting is the routine baseline inventorying of the already available health manpower that the exercise forces upon the researcher. These inventories by themselves should be useful information bases for policymakers. Next, there is surely merit in having available even simple, computer-based models that permit one to explore "what if" questions through simulation exercises. Coupled with good human judgment on what scenarios are more probable than others, such exercises can identify future pressure points that can be eliminated through judicious policy action. Third, the exacting requirements of health manpower forecasting serve as a perennial incentive to the health services research community to produce empirical information on the many behavioral links illustrated earlier with the aid of Figure 9-5. Information on these behavioral links is important in many policy initiatives other than forecasting per se.

Finally, health manpower forecasting could become potentially more useful if it shifted its focus away from the traditional, narrow preoccupation strictly with numbers of physicians to what Jeffrey Harris (1986) has called "intermediate targets"—time series on physician incomes and the rate of return to medical education, on wait-times to appointments and other measures of access, on the bookings of physician-recruitment firms, on rates of incidence of surgical procedures, and so on. In other words, Harris really calls for the metamorphosis of health manpower forecasting per se into a better coordinated discipline of health manpower *analysis*.

Health manpower forecasting can be less than helpful if the forecasts are carelessly rendered or communicated to the users—for example, if simple point estimates are proffered as gospel truth, without the necessary caveats, or if the projections are deliberately biased to trigger a desired policy action. And even carefully rendered forecasts can do harm if policymakers place undue reliance on numbers and fail to temper these numbers with other information, experience, and good judgment. The history of health manpower forecasting during the 1950s and 1960s suggests that the forecasts produced then may have been too simplistic and too alarmist, possibly seducing policymakers into an excessively expansionist health manpower policy (although, as noted, there were other powerful forces pushing in that direction).

One may describe health services research as an attempt to enhance the accuracy of the folklore upon which policymakers base their decisions. Properly structured, conveyed, and used, health manpower forecasting is one bit of the vast information needed to improve that folklore, but it will never be the *one* sufficient bit of information, and it will never replace that mysterious ingredient fundamental to all good policymaking: judgment. As Eli Ginzberg (1989) has sagely observed on this point: "In a pluralistic society such as the United States, which does not have a national system of health care, it may be futile to pose the question whether the nation will have too many, too few, or just the right number of physicians a decade or two in the future. All we can hope to do is to address selected facets of the supply problem as they force themselves onto the nation's agenda. To do more is likely to lead to frustration; to do less is to stockpile problems for the future." Well said!

10

Maintaining Quality of Care

Robert H. Brook and Elizabeth A. McGlynn

In this chapter we discuss the role that the public should play in maintaining and improving the quality of U.S. health care. The principal goal of the U.S. health care system should be to maximize the health of the population; the goal is not to save money, though a cursory reading of the current literature might suggest that to be the case. We define quality of care in terms of the relationship of medical care to health: high quality care has a positive impact on health whereas poor quality care has a negative impact. In order to identify high quality care, researchers must examine the link between the process of delivering medical services and the resulting changes in health status, both positive and negative. Put simply, health services research should distinguish between processes that produce health improvements and those that either produce no improvements or produce health decrements. Such information will assist policymakers in designing delivery and reimbursement systems capable of maximizing health. Improved systems would eliminate or prohibit reimbursement for poor quality care.

The optimal public role in maintaining or improving the quality of care requires answers to the following questions: (1) What is health? (2) How is health measured? (3) How is quality assessed? (4) Is there evidence that a problem with quality exists? (5) What is the public's role in improving the quality of care? These questions provide the framework for this chapter. In order to agree on what we are trying to maximize, we must define health. Once health is defined, we can discuss methods for measuring it and the populations to which the measurements should be applied. The next step is to determine how high quality care contributes to maximizing health and how an attuned delivery system might produce better health. We next turn to a discussion of whether a problem with quality exists. We conclude with a discussion of the public's role in maintaining and improving the quality of care.

A Conceptual Definition of Health

To build an understanding of the goal of the health delivery system and the methods by which we might achieve that goal, a conceptual and operational definition of health is necessary. Health has been conceptualized both negatively and positively. In one conceptualization, health is the absence of disease (Kostrzewski, 1979). This definition focuses on the effective biological functioning of the various organ systems and defines health as the state in which all organ systems are functioning within "normal" levels. In general, "normal" is defined relative to the average for the population. For example, most people have a body temperature that is close to 98.6 degrees; temperatures one and a half or more degrees higher than the average point to the existence of a health problem. This focus on the absence of disease as the definition of health is typical of the way in which many health professionals view health and has implications for measuring progress toward maximizing health. For instance, most trials that evaluate new cancer drugs assess whether they shrink the tumor rather than whether the patient feels better or is able to work.

An alternate approach is to define health as a state in which multiple dimensions of health are maximized. For example, the World Health Organization has defined health in terms of mental, physical, and social dimensions and has indicated that health is achieved when a person is maximally performing along these dimensions (World Health Organization, 1948). Most of us know intuitively what it means to have good mental or physical health and would readily agree that these areas should be included in defining a person's health status. In particular, nearly everyone would consider as relevant dimensions of health whether one is depressed, anxious, or in good spirits; whether one can take care of one's daily activities such as feeding, dressing, and bathing oneself; whether one can walk, run, and climb steps. Less clear is whether social participation, defined as having friends, belonging to organizations, and participating in activities, is an aspect of health or whether it represents a different dimension involving the quality of life.

Over the last 20 years, substantial interdisciplinary research has addressed questions about the dimensions to be included in a definition of health; whether health differs from quality of life; and whether one can develop an integrated measure of health. Although the health services research literature treats health as multidimensional, there is no agreement on the dimensions to be included nor on a summary measure of health. The dimensions of health depend in part on whose perspective is considered: that of patients, family members, doctors, or the community.

For the patient, health is a multidimensional concept that emphasizes the impact of disease on functioning in everyday life and on the individual's perceptions of personal health (Ware et al., 1978a, 1978b; Lohr and Ware, 1987). The patient is most concerned with those aspects of health that have a direct effect on the perceived or actual capacity to carry out normal life activities.

Similarly, the family is likely to be most concerned with those dimensions of health that have an impact on family functioning. While mild hypertension may have a negative effect on a patient's perceptions of his health, it may not directly affect the family because over long time periods it produces few external symptoms. In contrast, even minor symptoms related to poor mental health may have substantial effects on the functioning of the family.

From the physician's perspective, the key dimensions of health have traditionally been clinical or biological. These are the ways in which the physician thinks about health and acts with respect to treatment. For example, the physician aims to lower the patient's blood pressure or blood sugar through the use of medications.

From the perspective of society, health can be defined either broadly or narrowly depending upon the community's values regarding its social responsibility for providing solutions to health problems. With a narrow definition of health, society may accept responsibility for treating only catastrophic incidents, such as trauma, or life-threatening illnesses. With a more broad definition, society may take responsibility for assisting individuals to perform their social roles. For example, public funds may be used to provide elderly people who have difficulty using the public transportation system with taxi tokens so that they can visit their physicians or improve their social health by going to a movie or senior center.

The multiple dimensions of health are probably interrelated. A person with a chronic physical illness is at higher risk of having a lower mental health status, and the presence of a mental disorder can produce physical limitations as well (Stewart et al., 1989; Wells et al., 1989). Thus, even in a cost-containment atmosphere, it would be short-sighted to consider only a narrow definition of health. If the public is to play a larger role in assuming responsibility for measuring progress toward the goal of maximizing health, agreeing on a definition of health is essential.

An Operational Definition of Health

A minimum acceptable definition of health should include maximizing biological and clinical indicators of organ functions as well as physical, mental, and role functioning in everyday life. With this conceptual definition of health at hand, the next challenge is to make the definition operational. We posit two considerations: how do we measure this broad concept of health, and to whom should the measurements be applied?

Measuring Health

Most biological or clinical markers of health are measurable (for example, blood pressure, blood sugar). Furthermore, in most instances where medical technology is available, we know the dosage of medication required to produce the desired outcome (for instance, blood pressure control).

Physicians have developed instruments that allow them to assess how patients are doing clinically even where no biological measurement exists. For instance, the *Diagnostic and Statistical Manual (DSM)* provides standardized guidelines for diagnosing mental disorders (American Psychiatric Association, 1987). Similarly, instruments such as the Rose Questionnaire provide a standardized patient history approach to diagnosing the presence of angina (Friedman et al., 1985; Wilcosky, Harris, and Weissfeld, 1987). Many other tools have been used by researchers as well as clinicians to measure health.

For broader measures of health, such as functional status and general health perceptions, instruments have also been developed. Measures of functioning provide a common metric for assessing the impact of disease on health. General health perceptions provide information on how the patient is experiencing his clinical health status (Ware et al., 1978a; Bergner et al., 1981; Bergner, 1985; Bush, Kaplan, and Bush, 1982). This allows the individual to assess his health based on the relative weighting of different dimensions.

An example of these measures is shown in Table 10–1. We can assess the impact of disease in terms of deviations from the functional level of individuals without disease. Thus, "impact" is the decrement in each measure that is uniquely attributable to having a particular disease. The

Table 10-1. Comparison of scores for multiple dimensions of health between a general population and patients with and without chronic diseases

Group	Predicted scores			
	Physical function	Role function	Mental health	Health perceptions
General population	91**	92**	78	75**
Patients with no chronic conditions	86	87	78	73
Patients with chronic conditions				
Hypertension	86	88	77	69*
Diabetes	78*	78*	78	60*
Congestive heart failure	63*	59*	73*	59*
Myocardial infarction	60*	54*	75*	63*
Arthritis	77*	77*	75*	65*
Chronic lung problems	73*	74*	73*	60*
Gastrointestinal disorders	79*	73*	70*	59*
Back problems	76*	79*	77	68*
Angina	70*	72*	74*	59*

Source: Stewart et al., 1989.

Note: All scales scored 0–100, with a higher score indicating better health. Scores control for age, sex, education, income, presence of other chronic conditions and serious medical problems.

*Score is significantly lower than average for general patient population.

**General population score significantly higher than that for the general patient population.

a. Not statistically significant, probably due to small sample size and resulting high standard error.

table shows, for example, that individuals who have recently had a myocardial infarction experience a significant impact on their physical and role functioning and on health perceptions, but no substantial difference in terms of mental health. Even hypertension, which does not have, for most individuals, associated physical manifestations, affects how people perceive their health, as shown in the health perceptions measure.

The following general conclusions appear reasonable. First, the broader measures of health are now sufficiently robust to justify their inclusion in any scientific study that is undertaken to establish the effectiveness of any treatment modality (Stewart et al., 1989; Wells et al., 1989). Both physicians and patients desire information about the impact of different treatment modalities on health and functioning. To obtain such information, health measures must be used in clinical trials.

Second, although we know how to measure a patient's health at a given point in time, we are less clear about the role that current medical care can play in changing a person's functional status. We have observed that there is a great deal of variation in how patients function at specified levels of impairment of an organ system (Stewart et al., 1989; Rubenstein et al., 1989). For instance, two people whose hearts have lost equal amounts of muscle and who have had comparable problems in pumping blood through their systems can be affected quite differently in terms of their mental status or their physical capacity. We have surprisingly little knowledge about why this occurs and less knowledge about whether interventions could be designed for any given level of impairment to help patients function maximally.

Third, despite the lack of information on the relationship between medical care practices and patient health and functioning, we can be confident about our ability to define and measure health and to take the next logical step. We believe that quality of care can be defined in terms of health. High quality care is that which produces positive changes, or slows the decline, in health; low quality care fails to prevent or actually accelerates a decline in a person's health.

Whose Health Should be Maximized?

The next step after developing meaningful measures of health is to consider to whom such measurements should be applied and who should bear responsibility for the health of the group. Quality has been assessed at the level of the individual patient, the facility, and among various groups in the population. We believe that the quality of care assessment must occur at a more global level than that defined by a single encounter, episode of care, or facility in which care has been rendered. A public quality assessment system, particularly one conceptualized at a national level, should rely upon population-based approaches (see Mushlin and Appel, 1980). The challenge arises in defining the population for whom a group of providers will take responsibility. In an ideal world, each patient would have a primary care physician who was principally responsible for managing all necessary care. Thus, the population for whom the physician was held accountable would be all patients designating that physician as their primary care doctor. However, because the health care system in the United States is not organized in this manner, assigning responsibility for care is somewhat more difficult.

In organizations that have an enrolled population, such as prepaid health plans, one could stipulate that the organization is responsible for maximizing the health status of its enrollees. Preferred provider organizations could similarly require policyholders to designate a principal care physician. In solo, fee-for-service practice, all those not previously designated by one of the above methods could be assigned on the basis of counties, zip codes, or other areas defined by geographic proximity. Quality could be measured at a level of aggregation greater than the individual physician. There are probably other approaches to defining a matched group of patients and physicians that would be worth exploring as well. This is a crucial step in designing an operational system for quality assessment and improvement.

Dimensions of Quality Assessment

We can now consider the processes by which the health and functioning of the U.S. population might be maximized, that is, how we can assess the quality of care. In judging the quality of care, health services researchers have tended to define two major dimensions of the delivery process: technical process and art of care. Technical process refers to whether a physician, given the preferences of the patient, is using the most appropriate intervention available; art of care refers to the manner in which the physician interacts with the patient. In the definition of quality, both dimensions are important, although reasonable people might disagree about the relative importance of the two.

Technical Process

Technical process of care refers to the amount, type, and manner of resource utilization. Good technical care requires making the correct diagnosis, deciding on the proper course of treatment, successfully implementing that course, adequately monitoring the patient's progress, and discontinuing or modifying treatment as required. The measures of technical process are appropriateness (was the right procedure used for the right reason?) and outcomes (how well did the patient do? was the procedure performed competently?). Further, we should consider how appropriateness and outcomes are related, as shown in Figure 10–1. If there is a direct correlation, we might observe the conditional probabilities shown in the figure. The world is unlikely to be this orderly, but what we are striving for is appropriate uses of procedures that are performed in a competent manner so that positive health outcomes result.

For many conditions, the medical literature, particularly randomized clinical trials, offers the best information available on the efficacy of certain treatments. However, in many instances the ways in which treatment modalities are used have changed over time, and even if they were properly evaluated when first introduced (which is unlikely), they may not have been properly reevaluated. Therefore, judgments from the practicing physician community and academic physicians must be obtained and synthesized in order to identify the elements of technical process that should be used for patients with different conditions. In addition, most of the literature and information from physicians relate to biological or clinical outcomes of care rather than the functional out-

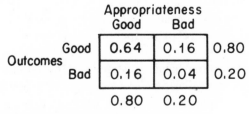

Figure 10-1. Appropriateness-outcome relationship.

comes. More research is required to establish whether there is a linkage between technical processes of care and functional outcomes.

Art of Care

Technical tasks affect the patient's health status, but the art of practice also affects quality. The art of care generally refers to the interpersonal interaction between physician and patient. The measure of art of care most commonly used is patient satisfaction. This is an "outcome" measure that is different from health. If the physician perceives anxiety, reassures the patient, and understands how to make the patient feel comfortable, this may help to elicit better information from the patient. For instance, a physician who practices high art of care may have a patient who is more likely to be compliant in taking prescribed drugs or holding still for an examination.

Content of Public Information

What information does the public need about technical competence and the art of care? The trade-offs between information about clinical, functional, and satisfaction outcomes will vary depending on the circumstances under which the patient is receiving care from a given physician. The choices reflect the relative importance of technical skills versus the art of care.

Let us consider, for example, a situation where a patient has a broken leg. Let us stipulate that one surgeon with poor interpersonal skills is likely to achieve a 99.9 percent probability of a favorable result in setting the fracture. Another orthopedic surgeon might have excellent interpersonal skills, but would achieve only a 97 percent probability of a fully successful outcome. Which physician should the patient select? Most people would choose the physician likely to produce the best technical result, recognizing that because their contacts would be limited they could tolerate a lower level of interpersonal relations in order to achieve the best outcome.

Consider, on the other hand, a patient with diabetes who needed to see the physician on a regular basis. One physician might have excellent technical but poor interpersonal skills, whereas a second might have average technical skills and an excellent interpersonal manner. Which physician would the patient go to? The trade-off in this case would be more complex because of the patient's continuing need for a relationship. The choice made by the patient might change over time as the disease became more severe and technical skill became more critical to achieving positive outcomes.

While most people would probably desire information about both technical and art of care dimensions, we believe that the public should focus first on improved information about the technical aspects of care. There are several reasons for this. First, "art" may be in the eye of the beholder. A satisfactory doctor-patient encounter to one person may be unsatisfactory to another. Some patients prefer a physician who is authoritarian and who does not involve them in the decision-making process; others want to know their options and participate in the decision process. For this reason, information about the art of care may best be secured by the individual seeking care. On the other hand, most people are not competent to judge the technical quality of care. Even a highly trained neurosurgeon may be unclear about the quality of prenatal care that his wife is receiving. Further, it may be possible to set multiple standards for the technical dimensions of care which will provide patients with choices among a set of technically equivalent treatments that may or may not have different side effects.

Problems with the U.S. Health Care System

Before discussing how we might design and implement a public quality assessment system, it is worth considering whether there is any evidence of a current problem with quality. We will not endeavor to list all of the ills facing the U.S. health care delivery system. We have chosen a few examples to illustrate the challenges facing those concerned about the quality of care; these include the cost-quality trade-off, access to care, appropriateness of care, and variations in the use of procedures.

The Cost-Quality Trade-off

As illustrated in Figure 10–2, the real issue facing most countries is the cost-quality trade-off: many people are asking whether the health outcomes achieved justify the expenditures. This trade-off has been represented as a curve that increases for a time during which more resources enhance quality, eventually becomes vertical (more resources

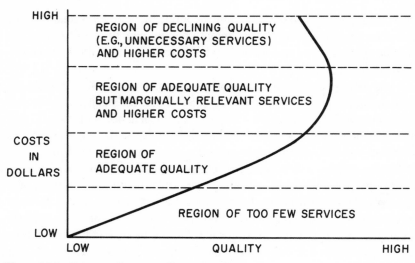

Figure 10-2. Conceptual cost-quality trade-off curve.

achieve the same level of quality), and may ultimately bend back (increased expenditures associated with lower outcomes). Whether the relationship between cost and quality eventually becomes negative remains uncertain; but beyond some point, additional resources spent on care will not enhance health status.

There are vast differences in expenditures on medical care across the Western world, yet those differences, according to available measures, do not result in significant differences in health status (Fuchs, 1974; Cochrane et al., 1978; World Health Organization, 1981; Mizrahi et al., 1983; Newhouse, 1987). In the United States we have evidence for both the upward-sloping and the downward-sloping portions of the curve of cost-quality relationships. Some evidence is provided from looking at the effect of differential access to care on patient outcomes.

Access and Outcomes

If one severely restricts the amount of expenditures on medical care, quality and outcomes suffer. Several years ago the State of California terminated Medi-Cal (California's Medicaid program) coverage for medically indigent adults (McGlynn and Newhouse, 1985). Prior to that action, a group of about 270,000 medically indigent adults were eligible for care under Medi-Cal. California transferred this responsibility to the counties along with a budget amount considerably lower than had earlier been spent on this group. The transfer resulted in greatly restricted access to care for these individuals and forced them to seek care in the already overburdened county system. A group of about 186 such patients had been treated at UCLA.

We followed this group of 186 patients who had earlier been patients at UCLA for a year and discovered the following results (Lurie et al., 1986). Before termination of their insurance benefits, 92 percent could identify a regular physician; after termination, only 50 percent were able to do so. Prior to termination, 3 percent of the patients had a diastolic blood pressure greater than 100 (indicating uncontrolled hypertension); 19 percent had a diastolic greater than 100 following termination. General health status, measured on a 0–100 self-report scale, fell from an average value of 47 to 36 (indicating poorer health status). The percentage of people who indicated they were satisfied with care declined from 97 to 40 percent. Most disturbing, in a one-year period seven deaths occurred among the 186 patients. These seven deaths were preventable; they could be attributed largely to a failure of the patients to obtain needed medication to treat hypertension or diabetes. In the control group there were no changes among the variables discussed above and no deaths.

Thus, a change in health policy reflecting a reduction in the dollars spent on medical care resulted in decreased health status and increased deaths. Extrapolating from these data, this change in health policy may have resulted, among this 1 percent of the population, in about 7,000 excess deaths. This is approximately equal to the total number of deaths that occur annually in California from breast cancer. Inadequate medical care services can result in severe negative outcomes, such as death, and other reductions in health status, such as progressive and inadequately treated chronic disease. Alternatively, this study suggests that increased expenditures on health care can improve health status.

Other data suggest, however, that the existence of too many services may impair health status, providing some evidence for the backward-bending portion of the curve illustrated in Figure 10–2. For instance, in the RAND Health Insurance Experiment, people in six communities were randomly assigned to different health insurance plans (Newhouse, 1974). These plans differed in the amount of cost sharing for which the patient was responsible; the copayment amounts were zero (free care),

25, 50, and 95 percent. Patients were also subject to a deductible (an amount they had to pay before the cost-sharing arrangement went into effect) and were protected by a ceiling on expenditures (an amount above which they did not have to pay).

One of the interesting findings from the HIE was that people who received free care in the fee-for-service system used more drugs than did people who had to cost-share. For instance, a 50 percent increase in the use of minor tranquilizers occurred among people with free care compared to those who cost-shared; narcotic use was 90 percent higher and penicillin prescriptions were 70 percent higher among the former (Lohr et al., 1986). These increases occurred in the absence of any evidence that pain was lessened or that the impact of infectious disease on health was reduced; however, increased numbers of skin rashes, a potential side effect of the drugs studied, did occur among those enrolled in the free plan.

The challenge is to ensure that expenditures are used only on the upward-sloping portion of the curve and to identify utilization that does not improve health status. Two bodies of literature providing such evidence are summarized in the following sections: variations in utilization and appropriateness of care.

Variations in Utilization

There is substantial variation in the United States in the use of procedures. Not only does insurance status predict variations in the use of resources, but a person's geographic location also affects the probability of receiving certain services or procedures. These variations in the use of services have occurred in areas as small as towns and as large as regions. Tables 10–2 and 10–3 show some of these variations. In Table 10–2, figures from the National Center for Health Statistics show variations by region; in Table 10–3, variations are shown for smaller geographic areas. For instance, one study compared the probability of having an organ removed by a given age by the hospital area in which one lived in New England (Wennberg and Gittlesohn, 1973; Wennberg, Gittlesohn, and Shapiro, 1975). After adjusting for differences in the size and characteristics of the populations in the areas, the authors found that: (1) by the age of 20, the likelihood of having tonsils removed varied from 6 percent in the low-service area to 68 percent in the high area; (2) the variation in the removal of a uterus by the age of 70 ranged from

Table 10-2. Geographic variations in rates of procedure use per
100,000 persons, 1983

Procedure	All regions	Northeast	North central	South	West
Hysterectomy	218	197	213	253	187
Cesarean section	348	322	327	389	332
Tonsillectomy	73	58	100	70	61
Cholecystectomy	210	182	243	226	169
Cardiac catheterization	219	134	265	246	204
Lens extraction	271	237	335	226	304
Prostatectomy	154	166	179	135	139

Source: NCHS, Surgical and Nonsurgical Procedures in Short-Stay Hospitals, United States, 1983.

Table 10-3. Geographic variations in the use of surgical procedures by county of
residence, rate per 10,000 persons

Procedure	Vermont (1969)			Maine (1973)		
	High	Average	Low	High	Average	Low
Tonsillectomy	151	43	13	122	62	23
Appendectomy	32	18	10	22	17	11
Hemorrhoidectomy	10	6	2	19	7	3
Herniorrhaphy	48	41	29	60	45	35
Prostatectomy	38	20	11	40	25	18
Hysterectomy	60	30	20	93	59	39
Cholecystectomy	57	27	17	55	35	27

Sources: Wennberg and Gittelsohn, 1973; Wennberg and Gittelsohn, 1975; as reported in Leape, 1989.

20 to 75 percent; (3) prostate removal by the age of 80 varied from 20 to 60 percent.

Another study examined the variations in the annual rates of selected procedures among people over 65 years of age living in different geographic areas (Chassin et al., 1986a). The average Medicare population in each area was 340,000 people. This study did not focus on differences caused by one or more deviant physicians or hospitals, but rather looked at the degree to which care rendered in the United States today is homogeneous. The use of the selected procedures varied greatly. For example, the likelihood that a person would undergo coronary artery bypass surgery varied from 7 per 10,000 persons to 23 per 10,000. The rate of variation for carotid endarterectomy ranged from 6 to 232 per 10,000 population, and for coronary angiography from 22 to 51 per 10,000.

There is no doubt that deviant or outlier physicians and hospitals exist. Variations in utilization across geographic and hospital service areas, while worrisome, might not result in a call for immediate action, but rather in a call for research to understand what produces these variations and to explore which rates can result in optimal health status.

Appropriateness of Care

The problem with data about variations is that we do not necessarily know that high use is bad and low use is good (or vice versa); we are unclear about the clinical implications of the variations. What is needed is an additional body of research that examines the extent to which procedures are used for appropriate reasons.

We define medical care as appropriate when the benefits of providing a particular service to a class of patients exceed the risks associated with such care. Inappropriate care occurs when the risks exceed the benefits. Benefits and risks are defined broadly in health status terms and do not include economic considerations. The outcomes of medical care are consequences (benefits and risks) associated with various procedures. Outcomes are measured in a variety of ways, including clinical or physiologic measures (for example, blood pressure) and functional status (for example, ability to walk a set distance).

Table 10–4 summarizes some of the relevant literature on appropriateness of care, which shows a considerable amount of inappropriate use of procedures, hospital use, office visits, and medications (Brook et al., 1989). The methods used to arrive at the conclusions vary, but what is consistent is the finding of substantial amounts of inappropriate care. The focus for procedures and hospital use has traditionally been on overuse; however, one study of underuse of hip arthroplasty revealed an equally important failure. The literature on medications looked at all aspects of inappropriate use, and problems were reported for each area.

Appropriateness ratings among institutions also demonstrate considerable variation (Table 10–5). The studies of appropriateness consis-

Table 10-4. Appropriateness of medical care for elderly: Summary of literature

Type of service	Overuse	Misuse	Underuse	Reference
Procedures				
Coronary artery bypass surgery	14%	—	—	Winslow, 1988
Coronary angiography	17%	—	—	Chassin, 1987
Carotid endarterectomy	32%	—	—	Winslow, 1988
Carotid endarterectomy	13%	—	—	Merrick, 1986
Upper GI endoscope	17%	—	—	Chassin, 1987
Hip arthroplasty	—	—	40%	Melton, 1982
Preoperative lab screening	60%	—	—	Kaplan, 1985
Cardiac pacemaker	20%	—	—	Greenspan, 1988
Cardiac pacemaker	30–75%	—	—	Phibbs, 1985
Hospital use				
Admission and days of care	10–35%	—	—	Siu, 1986
Admissions	12–28%	—	—	Restuccia, 1984
Days of care	7%	—	—	Studnicki, 1984
Days of care	27–33%	—	—	Siu, 1988
Breast cancer hosp. care	—	4–17%	4–17%	Greenfield, 1987
Office visits for 5 common conditions	—	—	26–80%	Heller, 1984
Medications				
All types				
Hosp.-admission	—	5.3%	—	Gosney, 1984
Hosp.-discharge	—	2.9%	—	Gosney, 1984
Outpatient	33%	18%	—	Mas, 1983
Outpatient	—	50%	—	Helling, 1982
Outpatient	37%	—	—	Laporte, 1983
Psychoactives (outpatient)	7%	44%	—	Wells, 1988
Anti-infectives				
Nursing home	—	—	67%	Satia, 1985
Theoretical	—	—	65–80%	Sisk, 1986
Emergency room	22%	—	—	Bernstein, 1982
Hospital	—	69%	—	Crossley, 1984
Hospital	—	74%	—	Shapiro, 1979
Emergency room	17%	—	6%	Brand, 1983
Outpatient	—	44%	—	Mullooly, 1984
Hospital	—	60–90%	—	Avorn, 1988
Hospital	17%	37%	—	Jewesson, 1983
Gastrointestinal	35%	31%	—	Ulaszek, 1984
(outpatient)	25%	71%	—	Stander, 1988

Source: Brook et al., 1989.

tently find differences at the level of the individual site, although there appears to be no relationship between rates of use of a procedure and resulting variations in appropriateness (Chassin et al., 1987b).

Considerable work has been done to demonstrate that something is amiss in the health care system. There are people who die or suffer poor health status because they do not have access to care or receive a poor quality of care. There are other people who appear to be exposed to too much care, some of whom suffer iatrogenic outcomes.

The Public's Role in Assessing Quality

What role should the public take in acquiring information, monitoring progress, providing information, and improving the quality of care? The answer is not simple. There are two competing schools of thought on

Table 10-5. Variations in appropriateness of procedure use

Procedure	Site	Appropriateness rating		
		Inappropriate (%)	Equivocal (%)	Appropriate (%)
Coronary	1	18	10	72
angiography	2	17	7	77
	3	15	4	81
Carotid	1	30	34	37
endarterectomy*	4	40	30	30
	2	29	29	42
Upper GI tract	5	18	11	71
endoscopy*	2	19	8	73
	1	15	14	72
Coronary artery	1	12	29	59
bypass surgery**	2	6	17	78
	3	23	40	37
Carotid	A	0	35	65
endarterectomy**	B	20	13	67
	C	23	27	50
	D	9	36	55
	E	9	41	50

Sources: Chassin et al., 1987b; Winslow et al., 1988; Merrick, 1986.
*Sites were geographic areas.
**Sites were hospitals.

the optimal approach to ensuring high quality care. The first is an external monitoring system that examines quality and makes the results generally available. The second is an internal system, called continuous improvement, that assumes that every professional is trying to produce the highest quality product possible and will seek to identify and correct problems without pressure from outside bodies.

Assessing and making public the quality of performance of a professional is likely to produce a negative emotional reaction. For example, if teachers' promotions were to depend upon students' evaluations or performance, there would be considerable anxiety among the members of the teaching profession. Such a response would be characteristic of all types of workers, from blue-collar laborers to physicians and judges.

But the quality of the output of most workers is in fact known. Let us consider the auto industry. The public does not know the performance records of individual workers, nor that of individual plants, but independent assessments as well as consumer ratings are available for both the technical and design features of different makes of cars. This information is used by some consumers when they are deciding which car to purchase. Factors relating to technical quality, such as safety records, repair records, and resale values, and design characteristics, such as style, are combined with cost considerations when the buyer is making his selection. Generally, adequate information is available for consumers to assess quality. The information is provided through a combination of public and private sources. It is unlikely that, if left to its own devices, the industry itself would provide such information.

Continuous improvement requires entering into cooperative arrangements with suppliers, developing internal systems of control, and utilizing statistical techniques by which to improve the reward system so that the entire work force is encouraged to pursue quality improvement at all times (Deming, 1986). However, tensions can develop between the goal of constant improvement and releasing information to the public about the quality of one's product. Those who advocate continuous improvement argue that enhancements cannot continue to be made in a fishbowl environment; this will sooner or later produce ill will on the part of those whose work is being evaluated. The advocates of external monitoring suggest that internal systems become co-opted over time by other organizational objectives and eventually fail to ensure continuing quality improvement.

We take the position that both internal and external approaches are required, and that one will not work without the other. In the absence of external information about quality, constant improvement in medical care will not occur at an optimal rate. On the other hand, if too much information about quality is publicly released, the environment necessary to support continuous innovation might not be sustainable.

Up to the present, the resolution of this tension has been to release virtually no information about quality of health care to the public. When an individual selects a health plan from among the choices offered by the employer, the choice is likely to be based almost entirely on cost considerations. Some individuals may incorporate other considerations, such as freedom of provider choice, accessibility of the provider, and word-of-mouth reputation of the provider. Similar levels of information are available when individuals are making decisions regarding the selection of a surgeon and where to have an elective operation.

Since the turn of the century, and even before, informed observers have pointed to the desirability of providing the public with more details about quality. For instance, Florence Nightingale, more than a century ago, studied survival rates of the injured in the Crimean War. She observed vastly different survival rates among the hospitals in which the patients were operated on, and she found that large hospitals had higher death rates than small hospitals. When studying leg amputations, she adjusted her data for the severity of injuries by stratifying on the basis of whether the amputation occurred below or above the knee. She prepared tables setting out her findings and submitted them to the Queen of England in an effort to make such information available so the public could respond (Nightingale, 1858, 1862, 1863).

Ernest Groves, a surgeon in the United Kingdom in the early 1900s, collected data reflecting the death rate following simple operations such as appendectomies and prostatectomies. He developed methods to collect such standardized data by hospital and recommended that they be made available to the public (Groves, 1908).

Edward Codman, a surgeon at the Massachusetts General Hospital in Boston, considered it the responsibility of every hospital to inform its patients of its outcomes. He suggested that every patient be recalled one year after his or her operation to assess whether the procedure was indicated and whether the patient had improved or suffered an iatrogenic complication. Making use of a primitive set of punch cards, he presented his data to the public in tabular form (Codman, 1914).

Seventy years later, the issue of health providers making quality of care measures available to the public remains moot. The medical profession, although interested and involved in developing better measures to police itself internally, has been reluctant to make its findings generally available to the public. In turn, the public's lack of access to such information has slowed the progress of quality improvement. Since the profession's internal efforts have failed to inform the public, a systematic, national effort to address the information gap in quality and to understand how high quality care is produced will be required.

The reason we argue for a systematic national approach is that we seek greater standardization of the health care product. This suggests the adoption of at least minimal acceptable standards of practice that are endorsed by practitioners and policymakers alike. In order to accomplish this goal, the public must play a role. Providing the public with information about the quality of care would represent a revolution in contemporary medicine. Most people think of revolutions in medicine in terms of new technologies or new drugs that are effective in treating disease or injuries, but in the last 40 years or so, during which most of this new technology has become available, the real medical revolution has been the way in which physicians have exchanged information with patients. Physicians first began to tell patients that they had a terminal illness only about 20 years ago. Up to that point, physicians would inform the patient's family that the patient had a terminal illness, but the physician did not discuss the matter with the patient for fear that if the latter learned the truth he would give up all desire to live, the disease would spread more rapidly, and death would come sooner.

The same arguments are being advanced today as one prepares for the new revolution that would inform patients about the quality of the care they receive from their physician or their hospital. If this revolution comes to pass, it will shift the balance of power between patients and physicians, which in turn will affect the way in which medical care is sought and provided. The issue for patients will be whether such changes will result in better or worse medical care (or better or worse outcomes). The issue for physicians will be how the new environment will influence the quality of medical care they deliver. It may also affect a person's decision whether or not to study medicine, as well as the practice norms of those currently active in the profession.

Designing a Public Quality Information System

If one puts together these observations from health services research and the earlier remarks about definitions affecting the quality of care, one has the foundation for a system that would provide the public with information about quality of care focusing on both appropriateness and outcomes of care.

Example 1: Appropriateness

Providing the public with valid information about appropriateness of care requires a method for measuring it. How does one judge whether a diagnostic test, such as an electrocardiogram, was appropriate for the condition and appropriately used? How does one determine whether a therapeutic procedure, such as a hysterectomy, was undertaken for appropriate reasons? Such determinations require prior agreement about an operational definition of health benefit and health risk.

To develop such operational definitions, one could rely on a review of the scientific literature. For instance, one could review the entire literature on the risks and benefits of having a hysterectomy. When we undertook such a comprehensive literature review for six procedures—coronary artery bypass surgery, coronary angiography, cholecystectomy, colonoscopy, endoscopy, and carotid endarterectomy—we found that the available information on which to make an appropriateness decision was very limited (see Table 10–6). Few experiments had made use of a randomized design to assess whether the procedure should be undertaken and to determine whether the patient benefited from it. We also found that clinical indications or circumstances for performing the procedure had seldom been carefully appraised. We concluded that it would be impossible to assess appropriateness solely on the basis of a literature review (Fink et al., 1987). A technique for combining expert opinion with such a literature review was required to judge appropriateness.

Previously, judgments about appropriateness were made in terms of sweeping generalizations. Few specific indicators had been developed to assess the use of a procedure. Moreover, the measurements were often ambiguous. We developed a method for measuring appropriateness that had the following characteristics. First, a thorough review of the literature was undertaken. Next, based on the literature review and conversations with experts, a detailed set of indications for all the possible uses of a procedure was developed. The indications were sufficiently detailed so that clinicians could agree on whether or not the patient should have the procedure. The indications contained five or six clinical parameters (see Table 10–7), and the list of indications included all possible reasons

Table 10-6. Content of publications on six procedures

Procedure	Article content				
	Indications	Use rate	Efficacy	Complications	Costs
Coronary angiography	31	6	77	33	7
Coronary artery bypass surgery	29	7	116	73	6
Carotid endarterectomy	56	0	50	43	0
Upper GI tract endoscopy	53	0	52	38	9
Colonoscopy	50	0	22	54	4
Cholecystectomy	57	32	19	39	5
Total (Percent)	276 (34)	45 (6)	336 (42)	280 (35)	31 (4)

Source: Fink et al., in press; based on a review of 803 articles.

Table 10-7. Sample indications for coronary angiography

APPROPRIATE

In patients with stable angina (Class III or IV), who have received less than maximal medical therapy but who have a positive or very positive treadmill test result.

EQUIVOCAL

In patients with no angina (asymptomatic, post-MI, or previous stable angina); positive treadmill test result; negative or absent thallium scan test result.

INAPPROPRIATE

In patients with no angina, no exercise tests performed, post-MI, post-CABS, following unstable angina, or previous stable angina.

Source: Chassin et al., 1987a.

for undertaking the procedure (Chassin et al., 1986b, 1986c; Kahn et al., 1986a, 1986b; Solomon et al., 1986).

After developing this preliminary list of indications, we convened an expert panel that had access to the detailed literature review as well as to the list of preliminary indications. The panel was asked to address two tasks: first, to consider the list of indications and, if necessary, to modify it by making some of them either more or less specific; second, to rate the indications on a 9-point scale of appropriateness. The panel consisted of generalists and specialists, representatives from all regions of the country drawn from both the academic and practice communities. Such a panel prevented any single specialty from dominating the decision about the use of a procedure in its own domain (Park et al., 1986; Merrick et al., 1987; Kahn et al., 1988).

If the panel did not disagree about the use of the procedure and placed it within 1 to 3 on a 9-point scale, we concluded that it was inappropriate to use the procedure. We defined as equivocal a situation where the panel rated the use of the indication between 4 and 6 on the same 9-point scale or disagreed about the use of the procedure. An appropriate indication was one in which the median rating was 7 to 9 and there was no disagreement about the use of the procedure.

We used the structure of these indications to design a medical records form to abstract relevant information (Kosecoff et al., 1987a). The purpose of the form was to collect relevant data about the reasons for performing the procedure, in particular the clinical status of the patient and the earlier therapies that had been used. Based on the information on the forms, we were able to classify the proportion of patients whose procedures were judged to be appropriate, equivocal, or inappropriate (Kosecoff et al., 1987b). These results, shown for three procedures in Table 10–8, suggest that there is a considerable amount of inappropriate use (Chassin et al., 1987b).

Example 2: Patient Outcomes

Appropriateness is only one dimension; the second relates to outcomes of care. In the last few years there has been significantly increased activ-

Table 10-8. Appropriateness of procedure use in Medicare population

Procedure	Appropriate (%)	Equivocal (%)	Inappropriate (%)
Coronary angiography	74	8	17
Carotid endarterectomy	35	32	32
Upper GI endoscopy	72	11	17

Source: Chassin et al., 1987b.

Table 10-9. Sample Medicare hospital mortality information, 1986

Diagnostic category	Hospital				
	1	2	3	4	5
Overall					
No. of patients	729	1,820	1,208	2,271	1,344
Actual mortality rate	8	14	9	16	19
Range of predicted mortality	8–16	10–16	8–15	9–16	11–18
Cancer					
No. of patients	63	99	118	162	72
Actual mortality rate	13	17	14	30	24
Range of predicted mortality	11–35	13–33	13–32	18–35	14–36
Stroke					
No. of patients	35	80	49	77	60
Actual mortality rate	29	33	22	38	37
Range of predicted mortality	13–43	18–39	16–42	18–39	18–41
Severe acute heart disease					
No. of patients	11	75	39	74	51
Actual mortality rate	45	45	33	42	53
Range of predicted mortality	16–69	27–51	25–55	27–51	28–56
Pulmonary disease					
No. of patients	62	190	87	262	216
Actual mortality rate	11	26	25	29	34
Range of predicted mortality	11–33	14–27	14–33	14–26	15–29
Severe trauma					
No. of patients	24	62	46	87	47
Actual mortality rate	4	8	4	7	9
Range of predicted mortality	3–30	5–22	3–21	4–18	3–21
Urology					
No. of patients	50	59	47	130	72
Actual mortality rate	2	5	4	7	10
Range of predicted mortality	1–17	2–17	1–18	2–12	3–17
Gynecology					
No. of patients	22	12	11	14	11
Actual mortality rate	0	0	0	0	0
Range of predicted mortality	0–98	0–98	0–99	0–94	0–99
Low-risk heart disease					
No. of patients	34	195	72	152	101
Actual mortality rate	0	3	1	7	7
Range of predicted mortality	1–19	2–9	2–13	2–10	2–11

Source: U.S. Department of Health and Human Services, HCFA, Medicare Hospital Mortality Information, 1986, vol. 1.

ity in this arena. Outcome data are used even in newspaper advertise-
ments. A few years ago, an advertisement appeared in the *Los Angeles
Times* which claimed that a department store's raincoat collection demonstrated "quality down to the last detail." On the opposite page, the
Eisenhower Medical Center stated: "If you are considering heart surgery, read this. Eisenhower Medical Center had the lowest mortality in
the country." What was the basis for this medical center's advertisement?

In 1986 and 1987, the Health Care Financing Administration (HCFA)
published data that described, after adjustment for the variables contained in the data base, the likelihood of a person over the age of 65
dying in a given hospital (U.S. DHHS, 1987, 1989). The HCFA data base
for hospitalized patients contains the following information: demographic
data, the patient's diagnosis, and the procedures performed during the
patient's hospitalization. This data file can be linked to another data file
that permits one to determine whether the patient was alive or dead at
certain periods following hospitalization. With these data files as a basis,
a multivariate analysis can be undertaken of selected diagnostic groups
that describes the expected number of deaths that a hospital will experience for a given procedure or within a specific diagnostic category. It
also enables one to report the number of deaths that actually occurred
and compare the two statistically (Jencks et al., 1988b). A sample of the
information produced by HCFA is shown in Table 10–9.

The major weakness of HCFA's statistical system is that it does not
contain sufficient clinical data to allow for adjustments for differences in
severity of illness among patient populations in different hospitals
(Greenfield et al., 1988; Jencks et al., 1988a).[1] But the data do contain
information that relates to severity, such as the patient's age. These
data were the basis for Eisenhower Medical Center's advertisement in
the *Los Angeles Times*.

There have been more clinically detailed studies, however, that have
examined the question of outcomes across hospitals. One of the best of
these focused on the efficacy of coronary artery bypass surgery in 15
academic teaching hospitals. That study collected data about men who
had stable angina but who underwent coronary artery bypass surgery.
After adjusting for almost every conceivable clinical difference between
the patient populations in these hospitals, this study found the following
(Kennedy et al., 1980): the observed mortality rates varied twenty-fold,
from 0.3 to 6.6 percent; the ratio of observed to expected mortality also

varied twenty-fold from 0.08 to 2.52 percent. A good hospital is one in which the ratio of observed mortality to expected mortality is low; a poor hospital is one in which the observed to expected ratio is high. Hospitals that did well on the observed mortality also did well on the observed to expected mortality ratio.

If such information were available, could future patients make constructive use of it? Let us say that the reader of this chapter is going to have coronary artery bypass surgery but does not know that the hospital down the street from his home has a 0.03 percent mortality rate, whereas the hospital to which he is scheduled to be admitted, despite a prestigious reputation, has a 6.6 percent mortality rate, a twenty-fold higher mortality rate for the procedure. The patient would be able to make a more fully informed choice of hospitals if he had access to such data.

Although these data about surgical patients are interesting and important, most people die from medical conditions. In particular, diseases such as heart failure, pneumonia, stroke, and heart attack are the causes for most deaths in hospitals. We know that there are large differences among hospitals in mortality for these medical conditions. For instance, mortality from heart attacks varies from 12 percent in the lowest tenth percentile of hospitals to 32 percent in the highest percentile of hospitals (Chassin et al., 1989). What patients really want to know is whether any of those deaths could have been prevented or whether the observed variation merely reflects case-mix differences. To answer that question, we examined data from one large chain of about 100 hospitals. We determined for three conditions—stroke, heart attack, and pneumonia—that one could identify hospitals whose death rate was better or worse than expected. In making this determination we adjusted for some differences in the case mix of patients, using such variables as the percentage of patients admitted from a nursing home or through an emergency department and the patient age distribution (Dubois et al., 1987a).

We then asked the question, how many patients in hospitals with better or worse than expected outcomes experienced a preventable death? We determined preventable deaths by having three physicians, who were blinded as to the hospitals involved, independently read the medical records of patients who had died as a result of one of these conditions. We found that the potential preventable death rate varied from 18 percent for people with strokes to 37 percent for people with heart attacks, while pneumonia had a 24 percent rate (Dubois et al., 1987b).

When we analyzed the data, we found that about 6 percent of all patients admitted to high outlier hospitals (whether they died or not) and 3 percent in low outlier hospitals experienced potentially preventable deaths (Dubois et al., 1988).

How does one interpret this information? There are substantial differences in outcomes depending on the physician or the hospital where the procedure is performed. For procedures with medium risks, such as bypass surgery, or hospitalization for pneumonia, stroke, or heart attack, the mortality differences among physicians and hospitals labeled as good or less good appear to be of the order of 2 to 3 percentage points per hundred patients who are admitted or treated for these specific diagnoses. Are these differences so minor that they should be overlooked? If they are too large to be ignored, what should be done about them?

Where Do We Go from Here?

We have sought to demonstrate that the methods for assessing appropriateness and outcomes of medical care exist and, in several areas, have been successfully applied. Further, the evidence to date suggests that a considerable amount of inappropriate care is currently being delivered. We have also demonstrated that poor patient outcomes can be identified for some conditions. What should become of this information? Currently such information is published in peer-reviewed medical journals, with subsequent haphazard efforts to pass such information in comprehensible language along to the public. There are steps that could be taken immediately and additional steps that should be considered for future action; we consider each in turn.

Action to Be Taken Now

Appropriateness methods have been applied to only a few conditions, and in many instances advances in medical knowledge and technique require updating of these standards. Undertaking a systematic assessment of appropriateness would require developing criteria for, let us say, the top 50 procedures. For initial development, this would cost about $500,000 to $1 million per procedure, which would cover analyzing the literature, constructing criteria, convening expert panels, developing a tool for abstracting data from medical records, and pilot testing the instrument.

At the same time as we develop criteria for the major procedures, we need to advance the state of the art in measurement. The methodology used in the RAND studies described earlier is at best a Model-T approach to measuring appropriateness. The methodology needs to be improved, and the sciences of decision analysis, meta-analysis, and clinical epidemiology need to be drawn upon to strengthen the study of appropriateness. Developing new standards will provide a good opportunity for more sophisticated work. David Eddy in particular has pointed to directions for developing improved and new standards (Eddy et al., 1987; Eddy and Billings, 1988). To date, most studies have focused on retrospective reviews of practice. We believe that prospective methods must be tried. Such an approach seeks to intervene before a procedure is undertaken and can contribute to improving practice by eliminating problems before they occur.

The appropriateness methodology also needs to be expanded to measure underuse. It is much easier to determine whether a procedure that was undertaken was appropriate than to assess whether a procedure that should have been used was not provided. The issue of underuse of appropriate procedures becomes that much more important as the incentives in the health care system change from encouraging overuse to encouraging underuse, that is, as fee-for-service is replaced by capitated or prepaid plans. Very little work has been done to establish the amount of underuse of beneficial procedures.

Assuming that we are successful in expanding the number of procedures for which practice standards are established, the next step would be to publish appropriateness criteria in a form that patients could use for guidance. In the case of an elective diagnostic or therapeutic procedure, a patient could take the guidelines to his physician and explore the indications for their use. Such discussions could lead to a reduction in inappropriate procedures or an increase in the use of appropriate ones and would also modify the physician-patient relationship in a favorable direction.

Further, such information could be incorporated into background material that prospective subscribers could review before enrolling in a health care plan. If one believes that our pluralistic health care system will continue into the foreseeable future, it would be helpful if in addition to information about premium cost and the location of facilities, information were presented about the use of key procedures. If appropriateness varied substantially among plans, people could choose on the basis of characteristics that went beyond cost and accessibility. Data about plans that were presented by relatively small geographic areas, such as counties or cities, would be more useful to prospective enrollees.

Steps for the Future

In the long term, one could aim at developing a system such as that described above that would be maintained on a national basis. Some of the required information for people over 65 is available through HCFA. Suppose a Medicare enrollee could call an 800 number and initiate the following interchange. First the enrollee would be asked to enter her name and social security number. The voice, having identified the patient, would then inquire into the operation that the patient was considering. After a response was elicited, the inquiree would be asked to enter the names or the identification numbers of the hospitals that she was considering. The computer would whirl and, after adjusting for possible differences in case mix among hospitals and physicians, would report the expected and observed mortalities for the operation at the identified hospitals. The message could end at that point, or it could go further and issue some warnings. Based on this interchange, the patient might reconsider whether or not she should undergo the procedure at a specific institution. Similar data could also be made available by plan or hospital for appropriateness and thus help the patient decide how to choose when she is selecting a health insurance plan.

For the non-elderly, a consumer reports system could be developed. Such a system would monitor on a regular basis several dimensions of the quality of care delivered by various health care systems, including solo practitioners. These dimensions should cover care for the conditions most relevant to different age and gender groups in the population. An annual report could be published that would rate the performance of different systems on each of the critical dimensions. Because no such system currently exists, we do not know how much variation is likely to occur within as compared to between systems. For example, one hypothesis is that an organization that delivers high quality care does so across most conditions and procedures. Alternatively, some organizations might be better at providing health care to children and young adults and would do less well with the elderly, whereas another might provide excellent services for the elderly and do less well with younger persons.

Summary

In this chapter we have discussed how quality of care can be defined and measured and given some examples of what the public's role could be in improving the quality of acute hospital care. A comparable analysis could be undertaken with respect to ambulatory and nursing home care. In the ambulatory arena, measures of mortality would need to be expanded by including more comprehensive outcome measures such as measures of functioning. With respect to nursing home care, much more consideration would need to be given to the circumstances surrounding and the timing of death. In all areas, some attention would have to be paid to the art of care and patient satisfaction, but it must be emphasized that the goal of the health care system is not to produce satisfied patients in the absence of contributing to their improved health and functioning.

We have called attention to only a few of the thousands of studies carried out over the last two decades on the quality of care. One consistent finding from this extensive literature is the existence of substantial deficiencies in quality regardless of the measurements and analytic procedures used. This points to the need to accelerate progress toward introducing more systematic efforts to assess and improve quality. The tremendous resource investment that the American people are making in their health care system—about $620 billion in 1989—underscores this urgency. We must launch a systematic national effort to assess, monitor, and improve the quality of care delivered. If we undertake such a task, it is possible that with the same outlay of resources we could meet the basic health needs of all Americans.

We believe that the quality of health care in the United States is not sufficiently high, and that the variation in quality of care is sufficiently great to require a greater involvement of the public. We likewise believe that without a strong public commitment to improving quality of care, major progress will not occur. We have sought to provide some examples of what needs to be done. It is regrettable that we were unable to set forth a more scientific epidemiology of variations in quality of care, but the information base to do so does not exist. The generation of new information should be one of the first goals that the public pursues as it expands its role in improving the quality of care delivered in the United States.

11

The Challenges Ahead

Eli Ginzberg

Those who have read the preceding chapters with care will recognize the substantial contributions that health services research has made in enlarging the knowledge pool about how the U.S. health care system operates and in pointing out how the system might be modified in order to improve its efficiency and effectiveness. In this concluding chapter, the progress that health services research has made, the challenges that it faces today, and some of the actions that might be taken to enable it to increase its productivity in the future will be reviewed anew. The following disclaimer should be made: the analysis and recommendations that follow are the editor's best judgments. They do not reflect prior agreement with either the contributors or the sponsoring organizations—the Commonwealth Fund and the Foundation for Health Services Research. An additional reminder: as is true of all research and book writing, what is gained in depth is paid for in coverage, and vice versa. The contributors to this volume are drawn heavily from among members of the economics branch of health services research. Clearly such a concentration has led to an underrepresentation of members of other branches, in particular the sociocultural and the political.

There is no possible way to extract all or even most of the constructive contributions that the authors have made in the preceding chapters to enlarging and deepening the field of health services research without making this chapter unduly long. Rather, I will select one critical point from each of the chapters to demonstrate the considerable progress that has characterized health services research in the quarter-century since 1965, noting in passing that the roots of health services research go back much further.

The model that Lawrence Brown sets out in Chapter 2 distinguishes among three basic tasks of health services research—documentation, analysis, and prescription. Brown demonstrates how the first two functions have contributed greatly to widening the knowledge pool. However, he emphasizes the much greater difficulty that health services research faces when it comes to prescription. Identifying what health services research can do well and pointing out where it faces major hurdles are important contributions to clarifying goals, a critical step in the progress of any research endeavor.

Stuart Altman and Ellen Ostby's account in Chapter 3 of the problems that faced the federal government in finding a substitute for cost reimbursement to hospitals treating Medicare patients and in adjusting the prospective payment system (PPS), once it was in place, reveals the critical role that health services research played in the design of the new system. Had it not been for the imaginative work carried out by the researchers at Yale in the 1970s, Congress would not have had a ready substitute for cost reimbursement. Although the authors are cautious not to claim too much for the new system, they suggest that it has probably contributed substantially to restraining cost increases for inpatient care and otherwise moving hospitals in the direction of more efficient and effective use of their resources—in short, no small victory for health services research and the new PPS system.

Paul Ginsburg and Philip Lee in Chapter 4 deal with a new system of physician payments that is much closer to the present. They point out that the increase in physician payments in the 1980s under Medicare Part B has been so steep (roughly threefold between 1980 and 1988) that the administration and the Congress had to explore all reasonable alternatives in order to slow the rise in expenditures, to introduce more rationality into the relative earnings of different groups of physicians, and to offer Medicare beneficiaries better protection from excessive balance billing. The story they relate about William Hsiao's imaginative research to develop a resource-based relative value scale, the many steps that the Physician Payment Review Commission (PPRC) took to review and tighten Hsiao's proposal, and the final modifications introduced by the Congress is an outstanding example of the full range of the model of health services research—from documentation through analysis to prescription. As good scholars, Ginsburg and Lee make no promises about the long-term ability of the new payment system to restrain physician expenditures, but they are hopeful that it will contribute to this goal.

In many respects, Joseph Newhouse's account in Chapter 7 of the design, execution, and policy implementations of the Health Insurance Experiment (HIE) is the key insider's review of the single most ambitious health services research effort ever launched in this or any other country. Newhouse shows how this long-term, costly, controlled experiment to explore the interrelations among individuals paying varying out-of-pocket amounts for care, the amount of services that they sought, and the effects of the services that they obtained on their health status and satisfaction yielded a large amount of new knowledge and understanding and led to policy changes. As a cautious scholar, he does not claim that everything that the investigatory team planned and carried out was optimal, but he concludes that any health services research program needs to find financing for such ambitious long-term investigations.

In reviewing in considerable depth in Chapter 5 the transformation of the Medicaid legislation since 1965, Karen Davis and Diane Rowland call attention to the constructive point-counterpoint between health services research and the legislators and administrators who have the ongoing responsibility to find accommodations between raising tax revenues and financing essential health care services for the poor and the near-poor. They note how health services research, by calling attention to the differentially high infant mortality of the United States relative to other advanced economies and to the favorable cost/benefit ratio of investing more money in prenatal care, spurred Congress to revise its restrictive Medicaid policies after 1984 and to mandate and encourage the states to increase their Medicaid outlays so that more health benefits would be available for pregnant women and young children. On a related front, they demonstrate how health services research also encouraged Congress to improve coverage for the elderly and the disabled and even to rescue a small part of the entitlements that were voted in 1988 in the catastrophic care amendments to Medicare and then rescinded in 1989.

Diane Rowland's Chapter 6 on financing health care for the elderly is rich in details about the continuing interaction between health services research and the growing accumulation of knowledge about the met and unmet needs of the elderly for different types of health care services. She reviews systematically the major health status, health financing, and related studies that were carried out by the federal government in the 1970s and 1980s and shows how the results enlarged our understanding of the unmet health needs of the elderly. Hers is another demonstration of the role of documentation and analysis as critical preludes to setting the stage for policy changes.

In Chapter 8 on alternative delivery systems (ADS), Harold Luft and Ellen Morrison demonstrate the critical importance of documentation and analysis in clarifying the options facing policymakers as they struggle with a highly dynamic but very costly health care system. Unless health services research is able to take into account and study the consequences of the major changes that are occurring on each of several fronts—the characteristics of the population seeking medical care, the changing structures that condition how services are provided, and the many changes among the principal payors for care—policymakers and the public at large will be at sea. Improved public policy with respect to the structuring and operation of our complex health care system depends in the first instance on the contributions of health services research to develop appropriate criteria for measuring the effectiveness and economy of the system and, second, on applying the criteria in a balanced fashion.

The subject of physician supply, the central issue of Uwe Reinhardt's analysis in Chapter 9, provides a case study of the use of economic theory to model the supply issue, with recourse to history and case material to evaluate and test various parts of the model; in the concluding section, Reinhardt investigates the inherent limitations of health services research in providing definitive answers to alternative public policies. This chapter helps the reader to confront both the potential and the limits of health services research when it deals with such an inherently complex issue as the appropriate number of physicians that a society should educate. But if the growth of knowledge is needed for improved policy, then Reinhardt's contribution in clarifying the confusions surrounding the various approaches to the issue represents a significant advance, even if he is forced to stop short of providing a definitive answer to the question: how many physicians are enough?

The concluding chapter by Robert Brook and Elizabeth McGlynn on maintaining quality of care opens up one of the most exciting current approaches of health services research, which is directed toward moving analysis from measuring access and the cost of health care to the quality of care, a major step ahead. The authors describe the necessity for studying the quality of care and point out that much of the health care that patients currently receive is ineffective if not downright harmful, while at the same time, many other patients do not receive services from which they could benefit. Brook and McGlynn carry their analysis a step further by pointing out the need for the public to play a critical role in pressing for the systematic study of quality and the release of the new knowledge both to the profession and to the consumer so that each can profit by making better choices about future treatment modalities. Health services research has taken the first steps to move the critical role of quality in the provision of health care out of the definitional stage to data collection, analysis, and protocol writing.

By way of recapitulation, one can identify the following three major lines of advance of health services research during the last quarter-century, as detailed in the chapters of this book. The first important line of progress grew out of efforts directed toward improving the operations of the new legislation of 1965—Medicare and Medicaid—particularly to expand access for the eligible groups and to control costs. The chapters on hospital reimbursement, physician payment, Medicaid, and the elderly all deal with these complexities. Although effective cost containment remains a major challenge, a reading of these four chapters demonstrates how much progress we have made as a result of health services research's contribution to enlarging our understanding of the issues involved in expenditure controls and in putting initial controls in place.

Three of the contributions, those of Brown, Luft and Morrison, and Reinhardt, can be grouped as advances in model building and analysis, the foundations for continuing advances in health services research. The fashioning of new tools of analysis and the systematic assessment of the strengths and weaknesses of the existing body of knowledge are the sine qua non for continuing progress in any research endeavor, and health services research is no exception.

The last group of contributions, by Newhouse and Brook and McGlynn, are the most closely tied to public policy: the HIE, through a controlled, randomized trial, was able to garner critical new knowledge about the ways in which money outlays by consumers, access, and health status are linked. And Brook and McGlynn have sketched out an approach that, if followed and supported by additional resources and collaborative efforts, holds promise of contributing significantly to the effectiveness of the health care system.

One unequivocal conclusion emerges from this summary review: health services research has demonstrated its capacity to make important and continuing contributions to the improved understanding of how our health care system operates and how it can be made to perform more effectively and efficiently for the benefit of the American people. But it would be an error to end the assessment at this point. We need to go two steps further to focus on some of the major challenges that confront health services research and explore at least briefly some of the possible responses to these challenges.

The major problem areas confronting health services research at the present time can be categorized as follows: informational, intellectual, financing, and policy planning. In the concluding pages of this chapter I point to some of the responses to these problem areas that health services research needs to follow.

Informational. The availability of quantitative data and improvements in their scale and quality are key requirements for the continuing progress of health services research as in most other scientific arenas, natural or social. While model building is possible in the absence of data, model testing is not. Moreover, in the absence of adequate data, investigators are likely to remain in the dark about important facets of their problem, unless they are fortunate enough to have an intuitive understanding of the relationship among factors that hold the key to understanding and action.

There is broad agreement within the health services research community that the development of data bases, particularly from the treatment of Medicare patients, has been an important spur to deepening analysis of inpatient care, treatments, and, to a lesser degree, cures. Moreover, the growing accumulation of information about the 6.5 million Medicare patients admitted to hospitals every year is a major resource for studying various aspects of health care administration from variations in admissions to variations in treatment; soon, it is hoped, this information will lead to a much greater understanding of variations in outcomes. The Medicare discharge data also provide a basis for looking at variations in lengths of stay among different groups of patients in different hospitals in various locations. But the informational base needs strengthening. We have relatively little information based on longitudinal experience. How much do we know about the health status and treatments of selected groups of patients before they were admitted to a hospital, and similarly, how much do we know about what happened to them after discharge, taking account of the different treatment modalities that they underwent while in the hospital?

Slow but steady progress is being made in splicing together routine data sets containing information about the short-term and longer-term outcomes of various medical and surgical interventions. But significant advances lie ahead once an adequate planning mechanism is put in place that stipulates the types of data that need to be collected and an agreed-to system for the collecting. A much improved data base will enable physicians and others to gain new insights into the changing health status of patients in response to changing modalities of treatment.

One can go further and state that on a great many different fronts involving questions of access, cost, quality, and outcomes, the existing data bases are in an early stage of construction or for the most part do not currently exist. The design and implementation of the mechanisms for collecting data, organizing it for use, and making it readily accessible to the health services research community still lie in the future. Improving the data bases is an essential task if health services research is to realize more of its potential.

Intellectual. It may be helpful to recall the central theme of Robert Blendon's address at the organizing meeting of the Association for Health Services Research (AHSR) in 1984 when, searching for an analogy for the newly emerging field, he noted that health services research faced the same problems as "area studies." In drawing this analogy, Blendon noted that health services research was not a recognized academic discipline, nor was it likely to become one in the conventional meaning of the term *discipline,* but was most likely to continue to be a field of research that would draw its intellectual strengths and its methodologies from an array of different disciplines, as in fact it has—from medicine, public health, economics, sociology, psychology, and many more. Blendon could also have drawn an analogy between health services research and urban studies, and, if he had wanted to stretch the point a bit, he could have compared the new field to the emerging centers on various campuses focused on the exploration of gender or race issues, fields that are also multidisciplinary and draw on a wide range of conventional disciplines for their personnel and methodologies.

But having noted that health services research has some intellectual company on campus and off, it would be a mistake to underestimate the special problems that all emerging interdisciplinary fields, including health services research, encounter in the dominant academic environment in which they are rooted. There is no point in arguing whether the life of academe would be strengthened if the fields of inquiry were less discipline-centered. The fact is that they have been for most of this century and are likely, as far as one can see ahead, to remain discipline-oriented. That means that most young people looking forward to doctoral work are likely to select one or another of the classic disciplines to major in; and later most, if not all of them, will aim to advance their careers by contributing articles and occasionally books that fall within the mainstream of their chosen area. In selecting the subjects to explore and write about they will follow the established folkways, seeking to make some improvement or some new application in the currently fashionable theories in their field. That is the conventional way for a young scholar to get ahead—and it matters not whether the field is economics, political science, sociology, psychology, or any of the related disciplines. Only a very small percentage (about 3.5 percent) of all the members of AHSR report that they have received a doctorate within health services research, a fact that reflects its recent establishment as a discipline in its own right as well as its continuing dependence on attracting and retaining investigators from other disciplines.

Even though there is an ongoing need for individuals with interdisciplinary training and skills to study the rapidly changing health care industry, health services research does not fit easily into the academic establishment. Health services research programs may be located in medical schools, schools of public health, or in policy centers, as well as in departments of economics, business, sociology, or political science, and in still other academic subdivisions. But it is no secret that many programs in health services research have encountered difficulties in seeking an appropriate niche within the discipline-bound academic environment.

Financing. The preceding references to the problems that health services research is encountering on both the informational and intellectual fronts are closely linked to questions of financing. Federal and state legislators have been resistant to the appropriation of substantial sums for the collection of more and better data. Hence the present and prospective gaps in strengthening the informational resources available to health services research are likely to continue, though they will, it is hoped, moderate as Congress perceives more clearly the critical importance of improved data bases.

In terms of training grants and research funding, financing issues dominate. The pursuit of a doctorate in any of the cognate disciplines involves about five years of graduate study, which if paid for out of pocket at a leading private university carries a price tag of more than $125,000 plus earnings forgone, and amounts to a sizable sum even in state-supported institutions. Currently there are a limited number of training programs financed by the Department of Health and Human Services (HHS) including dissertational grant support from the former National Center for Health Services Research and Health Care Technology, which recently was renamed the Agency for Health Care Policy and Research, and from the National Institute of Mental Health, the National Institute on Aging, and still other subdivisions of HHS, as well as some training funds in the Department of Defense and the Veterans Administration. But the 1980s have seen the federal government cut back significantly on its total funding for training grants. The 1990s might see, as part of new legislation discussed below, a more expansionary posture at least as far as health services research is concerned.

Training grants or alternative ways of financing the costs of educating doctoral and particularly postdoctoral students are a necessary but not a sufficient condition to assure a field the trained personnel that it needs. Talented individuals will make the sizable investment of time and effort only if they see the prospects for an attractive career ahead of them, and for those attracted to research such prospects depend in no small measure on the availability of research funding. The 1980s have not dealt kindly with health services research, but once again the trend appears to be pointing upward.

Policy Planning. One of the most difficult challenges facing health services research is the sizable gap that exists between its analytical activities and its policy prescriptions. There are tools and techniques available that enable health services research to analyze various facets of the changing health care sector and in the process to illuminate hitherto unrecognized or misunderstood relationships and to put forward improved formulations. But when it comes to the policy arena, scholarship and analytical work take one only as far as the threshold, where an array of interest blocs, competing politicians, the media, and still other potent groups are likely to be engaged participants. Some illustrations can help to illuminate the nature of the difficulties that the health services research community encounters when it enters the policy arena, or, conversely, when it attempts to steer clear of the policy arena. Let us look briefly at Medicare, Medicaid, and long-term care (LTC), three problem areas that have commanded the attention of health services research during the last quarter-century.

Medicare was passed by Congress under the promptings and persuasion of President Johnson with the aim of relieving the elderly, once they had retired and were no longer covered by employer-based health insurance, of the large costs of medical care, particularly hospital care. Although Medicare accomplished much of its objective, it early became clear, and with time even clearer, that protection against high-cost, acute care was not synonymous with protection against catastrophic expenditures. Even in the arena of acute care, an unlucky few faced multiple long-stay hospital admissions or were forced to remain on costly drugs for long periods of time. There were relatively few contributions from the health services community that addressed this shortfall in catastrophic coverage for acute care, probably because the commercial insurance companies succeeded in offering MediGap policies to cover most, if not all, of the uncovered acute care risks of Medicare, and these policies were bought by most of the exposed population.

The catastrophic amendments upheaval of 1988–1989 reflected in the first instance serious political miscalculations by members of the Congress. In addition, the health services research community did not focus adequate attention on the elderly's exposure to higher taxes versus expanded benefits. Although there is sufficient embarrassment from the 1989 repeal of these amendments to spread among all of the parties, in particular the American Association for Retired Persons, which lobbied for the amendments; congressional leadership, which pushed for passage of the amendments; the administration, which acquiesced to their acceptance; and the National Committee to Save Social Security and Medicare, which lobbied successfully for their repeal, the role of health services research was peripheral rather than central.

When Medicaid was passed in 1965 with little deliberation and less debate, the optimists believed that the United States had taken a major step forward to a one-class system of medical care that would sooner rather than later cover the entire population. And by the mid-1970s about two-thirds of all persons living in poverty were in fact covered by Medicaid. But that was the high point. Over the next decade, the country retrogressed to a point where only about 45 percent of the poverty population continued to be covered.

During this period Medicaid did not engage much of the attention of the health services research community, with a few notable exceptions including Karen Davis, Robert Blendon, and Thomas Moloney. The backsliding noted above occurred with little public knowledge, much less indignation or calls for remedial action. But as Davis and Rowland note in their chapter on Medicaid, health services research played an increasingly important role in getting the attention of Congress in the mid-1980s and keeping it in the following years, with the result that many new beneficiaries, particularly pregnant women and young children, were added to the Medicaid rolls.

It would not be fair to overlook the critical fact that since Medicaid is a federal-state program and the fifty states differ greatly in their criteria of eligibility, range of services, and administrative mechanisms, the health services research community confronts a horrendous task in staying abreast of such a large, diversified system of health care financing and delivery. But this reminder of the size and complexity of the United States—roughly four times more populated than the largest of the western European nations—is yet one more challenge across the board that health services research continues to confront.

As for long-term care, responses to the problem, with relatively minor exceptions, have proved elusive. The principal exception was congressional action in the early 1970s that made all victims of kidney disease requiring renal dialysis, as well as all persons between 55 and 65 years of age defined as permanently disabled after a wait of two years, eligible for Medicare.

Although the elderly have become increasingly vocal about the shortcomings of a government-financed system for health care that ignores their needs for nursing home and home health care benefits, both the Congress and state legislators have been skirting the issue because of the complexity and the costs. They continue to take refuge in the availability of Medicaid to pay the costs of nursing home care for those elderly persons who require prolonged institutionalization.

Health services research has played a role in the design and evaluation of demonstrations currently under way to admit Medicare beneficiaries to nursing homes as well as efforts to use home care and community-based services as alternatives to institutionalization. The resources of health services research were also used in the in-depth analysis carried out in the recent study by Alice Rivlin and Joshua Wiener of the potentialities of a social insurance system for LTC. But by their actions and non-actions, it is clear that both federal and state legislators are leery about placing LTC on their calendars for debate and are even less eager for early action. They sense that with the debacle of the catastrophic care amendments with their self-financing feature, the potential costs of LTC are far above what their respective budgets can readily absorb, not only in their present constrained condition but even in less pressured circumstances.

No matter how enthusiastic one is about the potential of health services research to illuminate how our present very large and costly system of health care could be made more effective and how it could be modified and changed to provide more and better services to the population, there is nothing in health services research per se that should lead one to look to it for definitive answers, if the underlying problem is a gross discrepancy between public needs and desires and available or prospective tax revenues. The only reasonable demand on health services research under these conditions would be that it alert both the public and the politicians to the nature, scale, and scope of the revenue deficiencies and possibly point the way to initial steps that might be taken even in the face of a fiscally constrained environment.

Some might read the foregoing as a criticism of health services research. Others, more accurately, will conclude that a major contribution of health services research is to recognize and illuminate unpleasant realities. The truth, even if it is unpleasant, is the ally rather than enemy of progress.

The remainder of this chapter deals with possible selected responses to the problems identified above. I will take note of some of the more important developments that are currently under way, leaving for final comments some additional responses that might be pursued to increase the potential of health services research. Under the leadership of Representatives Gradison, Stark, and Waxman, and with much encouragement from the health services research activists, Congress in the closing days of its 1989 session legislated the termination of the National Center for Health Services Research (NCHSR) and the creation of a successor institution, the Agency for Health Care Policy and Research within the Public Health Service of the Department of Health and Human Services, with multiple sources of funding including in particular general revenues and contributions from the Medicare Trust Fund. In contrast to the recent level of funding for the NCHSR and related research support that it replaces, which had been in the mid-$30 million level in 1987 and 1988, the new legislation provides for steady and substantial increases in authorizations over the next four years. In FY 1992, half of the total.

authorization of $220 million is allocated to outcomes research alone. By FY 1994, the authorization for outcomes research is scheduled to rise to $185 million. Clearly the mood of the Congress has begun to shift from that of suspicion about the potential of health services research to contribute significantly to improving the performance of the U.S. health care system, to one of approbation, if one looks at the proposed authorizations. The prior lack of congressional enthusiasm for health services research was related, aside from administrative infighting, to the remorseless increase in total national expenditures for health care, from $280 billion in 1980 to $600 billion at the decade's end. What lies behind this recent change, as reflected in the upward trend in authorizations? The single simplest answer is the new governmental interest in outcomes research with practice guidelines that hold promise of both saving large sums and at the same time improving the quality of care that patients receive. The sources for the new enthusiasm come from RAND (see Brook and McGlynn's chapter); from Dr. William Roper, the former head of HCFA and recently designated head of the Centers for Disease Control; and from such advocates as Paul Elwood, whose 1988 Shattuck Lecture was directed to outcomes research, and John Wennberg, a pioneer in small area analysis of medical practice variations.

New approaches touted as the cure for cost inflation have led to disappointment in the past, and the most recent approach focused on outcomes research may repeat the cycle. But there are several reasons for Congress, the medical profession, and other interested parties to look favorably on outcomes research and practice guidelines, cost saving aside. The prospect of improving medical and surgical care for the American people is basis enough for the new enthusiasm.

To see the funding future in its entirety, one must look not only to the new Agency for Health Care Policy and Research but also to the sizable funds at the disposal of HCFA for the support of both research and demonstrations and evaluations, and to the federal funding that comes via grants and contracts through various institutes of the National Institutes of Health and the Alcohol, Drug Abuse, and Mental Health Administration (ADAMHA), often under nomenclature that conceals or at least does not call attention to the fact that they are to be used for health services research. And one must also recall the point made earlier that departments other than HHS are involved in health services research, including Defense and the Veterans Aministration. Further, much of the General Accounting Office's increasingly broad program of evaluations is not readily distinguishable from health services research. And the same holds for the detailed analyses undertaken by the Office of Technology Assessment (OTA) for its congressional constituency. Another major agency is the Congressional Budget Office, which has demonstrated considerable skill in assessing the costs of alternative health care policy initiatives.

But the fact worth stressing is that until the recent turnaround, the health services research leadership had good reasons to be concerned, if not distressed, because of the congressional unwillingness to increase funding for health services research. As of the beginning of the 1990s the outlook has taken a turn for the better, but the supporters of health services research will emphasize that although the projected budget for FY 1994 is a move in the right direction, one must place it in context. According to HCFA, national expenditures for health care in 1994 are projected to total $917 billion, resulting in a relative outlay for federal support for health services research under the most optimistic assumptions of a very small fraction of one percent.

But to see the picture whole, not just the critical role played by the federal government, one must call attention to the fact that a few of the state governments provide modest support for health services research, and that some of the principal parties of interest in the health sector, including the AMA, the AHA, the AAMC, other professional and political associations such as AARP, large business enterprises, hospitals, HMOs, and still other organizations, have been appropriating more money and building larger and more competent staffs to improve their informational base and their analytical capabilities in order to sharpen and reinforce their policy positions. We are long past the day when recourse to an advertising campaign based on opposition to "socialized medicine" was the principal response by the AMA to the threat of Medicare legislation.

There are other interested parties that play a role in the funding of health services research directly or as a by-product of their operational functions. The Robert Wood Johnson Foundation and Pew Charitable Trusts have for the last decade or two been among the leading supporters of health services research, particularly in regard to the training of future researchers. And there are a number of smaller health foundations including the Henry J. Kaiser Family Foundation, the John A. Hartford Foundation, the Commonwealth Fund, the Milbank Memorial Fund, and several others that have been allocating a significant share of their philanthropic dollars to health services research. Further, passing reference must be made to the data collection and analysis of changing aspects of the health insurance coverage of the American people by, among others, Kaiser Permanente, RAND, and the Health Insurance Association of America (HIAA).

As emphasized earlier, funding is the necessary, though not the sole, factor in assuring the viability and growth of health services research. There are at least two additional factors of critical importance that bear on the rate at which the future potential of health services research can be developed and utilized. The first relates to the distribution of effort between operational research and larger system-wide inquiries directed to cross-cutting issues such as possible responses to the challenge of the uninterrupted upward trend in health care costs; the substantial and growing numbers of uninsured persons; the excess number of acute care hospitals and hospital beds, with national occupancy reported in the middle 60 percent range; the implications of radical declines in the number of applicants to medical and nursing schools, and many more critical areas that call for early and comprehensive analyses and recommendations for policy changes.

Many of these issues are not being researched and are not likely to be studied, not because they are unimportant or would fail to attract the interest of the health services research community but rather because there are no patrons (that is, funders) who are particularly interested in these issues. Without a constant flow of external funds, the academically based health services research community cannot become engaged, and those who hold positions in administrative agencies, even in special research units, are overloaded by an avalanche of operational questions to which early answers are required.

If this analysis is more or less on target, then it follows that one of the agenda items that the federal government as well as nongovernmental funders need to consider and resolve is how some small part of what is likely to become a considerably increased stream of funding for health services research can be directed to the general and specific support of a number of strong research groups, preferably located in different regions of the country so that their specialized knowledge of regional, state, and local conditions can be tapped. Health services research needs the perspective and the depth that can result from some longer-term strategies that address important questions, the answers to which are needed both for better understanding and for better policy formulation. Some enthusiasts have sought for years to develop a model for health services research similar to that used to fund biomedical research, but for various reasons they have failed to date to make much progress. In one respect they are surely right: health services research needs a number of centers with levels of funding that permit the staff to pursue questions that are not necessarily of immediate interest and concern to harassed administrators and besieged politicians. A modest amount of long-term funding for long-term research is a challenge that a sophisticated society that spends currently one out of every nine dollars of its GNP on health care should be able to meet.

The other open issue shows more promise of early resolution—at least one can see evidence that various constructive actions are under way and that many more are likely to be introduced before long. There is little or no point in the nation's investing heavily in outcomes research if the federal government is to assume the task of determining practice guidelines as well as the responsibility for enforcing them. Such a system would be doomed to failure from the start, since the improvement of medical care depends primarily on altering the knowledge base and the practice modes of physicians. To accomplish this, the physician community must be actively and continuously involved at every stage of the process. It is encouraging therefore to note that the AMA, the RAND Corporation, and a group of academic health centers may soon enter into a cooperative venture aimed at developing useful new knowledge based on outcomes research that will provide the basis for practice guidelines that should improve the quality of medical care received by the American people.

In a multi–interest group society such as ours, there is clearly an ongoing role for state and federal governments to play in shaping and reshaping the nation's health care system, the more so since together they are the largest single funders, accounting for roughly 40 percent of all health expenditures. But it is also critically important that other interested and concerned groups be actively involved. Hence the prospective AMA/RAND/academic health centers (AHCs) cooperative venture is encouraging not only for the specific effort it is making, important as that is, but also for the model that it offers for future cooperative undertakings. Health services research has long confronted a serious challenge in moving from research to policy. As other groups become alert to the value of research, they can help provide the bridge. And with more bridges in place, health services research will be in a strengthened position to develop its full potential.

One final observation both about the accomplishments of health services research since the mid-1960s, the focus of this book, as well as about the potential of health services research, the concern of this concluding assessment: the United States has begun to learn the hard way that ideology and party preferences are not trustworthy bases for the structuring, operation, and change of a health care system that has grown to a point where it exceeds one-ninth of the total economy and is likely before the end of the present decade to exceed one-eighth. Aside from scale, the U.S. health care sector is characterized by great scope and diversity in terms of the numbers of parties involved in the financing, provision, and control of health care services.

The Congress, state legislatures, and employers as well as other concerned parties have no alternative but to look to health services research for the analysis and evaluation of how the health care sector is performing in meeting the priority needs of the American public, and further to seek leads and directions from health services research concerning how the health care system might be modified to make more efficient and effective use of its resources, which are great but not unlimited. Health services research faces a challenge in fulfilling its potential, but its accomplishments to date emphasize that it is the only game in town that holds the promise of making the health care provided to the American people more effective and less costly.

Notes

2. Knowledge and Power

1. Reactions and skirmishes through 1978 are discussed in Abernathy and Pearson (1979), pp. 95–181.
2. On November 15, 1979, the House rejected Carter's proposed cost controls by a vote of 234–166, with 99 Democrats voting against the president's position (see Congressional Quarterly Weekly Report, 1979).
3. For a lively dissent, see Glaser, 1989a; for some rebuttals and a response, see Glaser, 1989b.
4. Reviewing his interviews on agenda-setting in Washington in the late 1970s, Kingdon observed that "one reason that medical care costs dominated the health interviews was that the numbers simply spoke to these people." His interviews also showed how the documentary concerns of politicians and bureaucrats generate demand for analytical and prescriptive responses by researchers: "Much of the time the agenda is set by forces and actors outside the researcher-analyst community. Then politicians turn to that community for proposals that would be relevant to their concerns and that might constitute solutions to their problems." (See Kingdon, 1984, pp. 96, 59.)
5. Not always, however. In the move to deregulate airlines, trucking, and telecommunications, the economic image of free market forces had a powerful influence on policy. (See Derthick and Quirk, 1985, especially pp. 237–258.) But these reforms mainly entailed dismantling or curtailing the existing regulatory apparatus and then allowing allegedly natural market dynamics to assert themselves. In the health field, few who advocate market-based solutions contend that they would work well without a sophisticated regulatory framework that would at once preserve and encourage competition and inhibit and correct for its undesirable consequences.

4. Physician Payment

1. Balance bills are the difference between what the physician charges and what the third-party payor approves for payment.
2. For Blue Shield plans, physicians are also a potent constituency. Indeed, the history of Blue Shield includes many instances of physician majorities on boards of directors. For a summary of the economic literature on physician control of Blue Shield plans, see Arnould and DeBrock, 1985.
3. Although some Blue Shield plans had pioneered the mechanism, it was in limited use before its adoption by Medicare.
4. For researchers interested in this work, our suggested reference is the October 28, 1988, issue of the *Journal of the American Medical Association,* which includes nine articles by Hsiao and his colleagues. A brief description was published in the *New England Journal of Medicine* (Hsiao et al., 1988a). The contract report to the Health Care Financing Administration (Hsiao et al., 1988b) is not very accessible to those with a casual interest in the study because of its bulk and resultant high cost.
5. The methodology employed in the Hsiao study is discussed in the second part of this chapter in the section on developing a fee schedule for Medicare.
6. For example, if relative payments were distorted among broad categories of services but were not distorted for individual services within a category, R-squared could be high and prediction error less than two standard deviations. See Hammons (in press) for a discussion of other methodological issues pertaining to this study.
7. Assuming that physician practice decisions are influenced more by supply than by demand considerations (since patients have extensive health insurance that pays all or a high proportion of the bill), classical models would suggest that decreased fees would lead to a reduction in the amount of the service provided, but target income models would suggest that physicians would increase services to maintain a target income. See the section on overall fee levels for additional discussion of models of physician behavior.
8. The equity issue for beneficiaries is complex. Higher payment would mean lower balance bills but higher coinsurance amounts. As long as changes in balance billing offset more than 20 percent of the changes in fee levels, beneficiaries in rural areas would seem to be better off as a result of a geographic realignment of payment. The presence of private supplemental insurance (Medigap) makes the change even more favorable to rural beneficiaries as long as premium rating areas are broader.
9. Roughly 80 percent of Medicare beneficiaries have supplemental insurance that pays the coinsurance. For unassigned claims, the demand response will generally parallel the supply response. When price is reduced, the net price to the patient—the balance bill—will tend to increase.
10. For a recent exchange on the issue, see Feldman and Sloan (1988) and Rice and Labelle (1989).
11. When analyzing the effects of changes in relative values, CBO applies these asymmetric assumptions at the level of a physician. Thus, the net change in

overall fee levels is computed for each physician and then the asymmetric behavioral assumptions are applied.

12. Disaggregation of Part B into physician services and other components is not available as far back as 1980.

13. The study defined surgery to include operations and invasive procedures.

14. The bill reported by the House Energy and Commerce Committee envisioned an immediate revision of the prevailing charges for about 400 procedures for which relative values were available from PPRC. Although this approach was not reflected in the final legislation, the related budget reduction provisions used the same information to identify procedures that were overvalued by at least 10 percent. For the 245 procedures that met this criterion, the legislation prescribed a reduction in prevailing charge screens of the lesser of one-third of the difference between the current level and that projected under the fee schedule and 15 percent.

15. See note 14.

7. Controlled Experimentation as Research Policy

1. Newhouse (1974) and Brook et al. (1979) provide fuller descriptions of the design. Newhouse et al. (1979) discuss the measurement issues for the second generation of social experiments, to which the HIE belongs. Ware et al. (1980a, 1980b) discuss many aspects of data collection and measurement for health status.

2. For a skeptical voice about whether cost sharing reduced use, see Fein, 1971.

3. There was one other randomized experiment conducted at an HMO (Perkoff, Kahn, and Haas, 1976). Perhaps the fact that it was newly established accounts for the anomalous result (relative to the vast nonexperimental literature) that although the HMO did reduce hospital use, outpatient use was sufficiently higher to more than offset the saving.

4. There was a higher refusal rate among the HMO experimentals than among the fee-for-service experimentals, but any bias from this higher refusal seems minimal. See the discussion in Newhouse, Manning, et al., 1987, especially the discussion of Tables 5, 6, and 7.

5. For example, the Xerox Corporation in 1983 announced an increase in its deductible from $100 per person per year or $200 per family to 1 percent of family earnings. It raised coinsurance on hospital and surgical services from 0 to 20 percent. In addition, it lowered its cap on out-of-pocket expenditures (analogous to the MDE) from 6 percent of earnings to 4 percent of earnings. In a brochure distributed to its employees it said: "According to a study by the RAND Corporation, when consumers are required to increase their share of medical costs, there is a significant decrease in the total amount spent for these services. Furthermore, this study—and other similar studies—does not indicate that the health of the employees was adversely affected by the decrease in costs."

6. The Individual Deductible plan also had free inpatient care.

7. Admissions in community hospitals rose from 31 million in 1970 to 36 million in 1982, but had fallen back to 32 million by 1986 (American Hospital Association, 1987). During this time nominal total expenses rose from $25 billion to $141 billion. Using the GNP personal consumption deflator, this represents an increase of 2.26 in real terms. In other words, if one decomposes the change in costs into the change in admissions and the change in cost per admission, virtually all the increase is in the latter component.

8. Unless the cost sharing became larger than that employed in the Health Insurance Experiment; specifically, unless it was large enough so that most hospitalized individuals at the margin would be paying out of pocket for their care. Both common sense and HIE data suggest that individuals and families do not want to incur the risk that such large amounts of cost sharing would impose. Even at a 30 percent loading fee, 75 percent of the participants said they would have reduced their Maximum Dollar Expenditure if given an opportunity to do so (though only a third would have reduced it to zero) (Marquis and Phelps, 1985).

9. The number of group HMO plans, to which the experimental results apply, grew from 139 as of June 30, 1980, to 195 in December 1984 and 250 as of June 30, 1986. Enrollment grew from 7.4 million in 1980 to 13.1 million and 15.2 million in 1984 and 1986, respectively (U.S. Bureau of the Census, 1988).

10. Medicare eligibles were not included in the HIE for three reasons. (1) As noted earlier, at the time the Experiment began, Medicare was viewed as a successful government program, one not to be tampered with. As a result of this perceived success, the federal government did not want to include Medicare beneficiaries. (2) A case could be made that the response to cost sharing might well differ among the elderly—in particular, the prevalence of chronic conditions is much greater—and in any event the variance of expenditure is greater among the elderly. Hence, at a minimum, if one were to include the elderly, one would probably oversample them. This, in turn, would have resulted in either substantially reduced precision among the under-65 group or a substantially increased budget. (3) When the HIE began, there was doubt about whether it was feasible, even among the non-elderly. It was clear, however, that an experiment with the elderly would pose greater logistical problems. Informed consent might be more difficult to obtain in some cases; it might be difficult for some elderly to get to a screening examination center; and it would be difficult for some elderly to give lengthy personal interviews.

11. Note that inappropriate hospitalization was at approximately the same rate on the Individual Deductible plan as on the free plan, implying that physicians did not inappropriately hospitalize participants to avoid the cost sharing.

12. The HIE can also be contrasted with the National Medical Care Expenditure Survey (NMCES), another prospective observational study which was approximately contemporaneous with the HIE. The NMCES gathered data on utilization, insurance coverage, and some measures of health status during 1977. In principle, the NMCES could be seen as a control group for the HIE, although it has not been used in that fashion. Instead, the main use of the NMCES in the policy debate has been to study the uninsured, though the data from it have

been used more to quantify the number and describe the characteristics of the uninsured (or underinsured) than to estimate the consequences for use or health status of being uninsured. As noted in the text, the HIE by definition cannot say anything about the consequences of being uninsured because no one was uninsured in the HIE.

9. Health Manpower Forecasting

1. In principle, it is possible to identify empirically a truly *efficient* production function through linear programming techniques (see, for example, Farrell, 1957). Unfortunately, that approach is extremely sensitive to measurement error in the underlying observations (see Reinhardt, 1973).
2. The slope of these lines is determined by the relative prices of the two inputs.
3. For an early attempt to construct such a model, see Yett, Drabek, Intriligator, and Kimbal (1971).
4. Most econometric models for sectors of the economy or for the economy as a whole tend to have very short forecast horizons. Furthermore, most of them are subject to considerable forecasting error.
5. This section draws heavily on Ginzberg (1987) and Reinhardt (1975, chaps. 2 and 3).
6. In 1971–72 alone, some 13,000 FMGs entered the United States.
7. Dickinson was then Director of Medical Economic Research of the American Medical Association, which at that time vigorously opposed federal intrusion into medical education. As Ginzberg remarks in "The Politics of the U.S. Physician Supply" (1987, p. 19), Dickinson's identification with the AMA probably gave his quite sensible idea less currency than it deserved.
8. In these estimates, physician productivity was typically measured not in terms of visits per week but by annual gross revenue per physician, deflated by a medical care price index.
9. For an extended assessment of the merits and demerits of that approach, see Reinhardt (1973, pp. 212–223).
10. For a contrast of the two methods, see Reinhardt (1973).
11. For a well-written, concise description of the GMENAC's methodology, see McNutt (1981). For a relatively kind and gentle critique of that methodology, see Reinhardt (1981).
12. That etiquette has been clearly demonstrated, once again, in the stakeholders' reaction to the Resource-Based Relative Value Scale (RBRVS) recently developed by researchers at Harvard University. Spokespersons for medical specialties whose members would lose income under the RBRVS (for example, surgical specialists) have found much fault with the scientific merits of the underlying study. Medical specialties who stand to gain from the RBRVS (family practitioners and internists), on the other hand, have praised the scientific virtue of that same methodology. Income has never been mentioned in these discussions. Even so, an economist could easily have predicted these reactions to scientific

inquiry strictly on the basis of economic theory and merely by knowing the likely impact of the RBRVS on the critics' own income.

13. If d denotes the continuously compounded annual growth rate in per capita demand and q the continuously compounded positive or negative annual growth rate in physician productivity, then we may express the projected, required physician-population ratio as

$$(D_t/Q_t) = (D_0/Q_0) \, e^{(d - q)t},$$

where subscript zero denotes a base year. Note: $\{d - q\} = g$.

14. The policy does not rest on the thesis that volume will increase because the patient's 20 percent coinsurance is lowered with the lowered fees. If that had been the thesis, Congress would simply have raised the coinsurance rate.

10. Maintaining Quality of Care

1. HCFA has developed a medical records abstraction system that can be used by hospitals to interpret mortality statistics by using information about the clinical condition of the patient on admission. The system, known as the Medicare Mortality Predictor System (MMPS), applies only to patients who are admitted with stroke, pneumonia, myocardial infarction, or congestive heart failure. These conditions account for about 12.5 percent of admissions and 33 percent of mortality for the Medicare population. HCFA developed the system to assist hospitals to respond to the published mortality reports but does not intend to implement the system itself on a routine basis (Daley et al., 1988).

References

2. Knowledge and Power

Abernathy, David S., and David A. Pearson. 1979. *Regulating Hospital Costs: The Development of Public Policy.* Washington, D.C., and Ann Arbor, Mich.: AUPHA Press.

Bell, Daniel. 1969. The idea of a social report. *The Public Interest* no. 15 (Spring):72–97.

Biles, Brian, et al. 1980. Hospital cost inflation under state rate-setting programs. *New England Journal of Medicine* 303 (September 18):664–668.

Brown, Lawrence D. 1983a. *Politics and Health Care Organization: HMOs as Federal Policy.* Washington, D.C.: Brookings Institution.

——— 1983b. *New Policies, New Politics: Government's Response to Government's Growth.* Staff paper. Washington, D.C.: Brookings Institution.

——— 1988. Afterword. In Warren Greenberg, ed., *Competition in the Health Care Sector: Ten Years Later.* Durham, N.C.: Duke University Press, pp. 139–141.

Brown, Lawrence D., and Catherine McLaughlin. 1988. "May the third force be with you": community programs for affordable health care. In Richard M. Scheffler and Louis F. Rossiter, eds., *Advances in Health Economics and Health Services Research.* Greenwich, Conn.: JAI Press, pp. 187–271.

Coelan, Craig, and Daniel Sullivan. 1981. An analysis of the effects of prospective reimbursement programs on hospital expenditures. *Health Care Financing Review* 2 (Winter):1–40.

Coleman, James S., et al. 1966. *Equality of Educational Opportunity.* Washington, D.C.: U.S. Government Printing Office.

Congressional Quarterly Weekly Report. 1979. Vol. 37 (November 17):2575.

Derthick, Martha, and Paul J. Quirk. 1985. *The Politics of Deregulation.* Washington, D.C.: Brookings Institution.

Eby, Charles L., and Donald R. Cohodes. 1985. What do we know about rate-setting? *Journal of Health Politics, Policy, and Law* 10 (Summer):299–327.

Enthoven, Alain C. 1980a. *Health Plan.* Reading, Mass.: Addison-Wesley.

——— 1980b. How interested groups have responded to a proposal for economic competition in health services. *American Economic Review,* Papers and Proceedings 70 (May):142–148.

Enthoven, Alain, and Richard Kronick. 1989. A consumer choice health plan for the 1990s: universal health insurance in a system designed to promote quality and economy. Two parts. *New England Journal of Medicine* 320 (January 5):29–37 and (January 12):94–101.

Feldman, Roger, and Frank Sloan. 1988. Competition among physicians, revisited. *Journal of Health Politics, Policy, and Law* 13 (Summer):239–261.

———— 1989. Reply. *Journal of Health Politics, Policy, and Law* 14 (Fall):587–625.

Glaser, William A. 1970. *Paying the Doctor.* Baltimore: Johns Hopkins University Press.

———— 1978. *Health Insurance Bargaining: Foreign Lessons for Americans.* New York: Gardner Press.

———— 1987. *Paying the Hospital.* San Francisco: Jossey-Bass.

———— 1989a. The politics of paying physicians. *Health Affairs* 8 (Fall):129–146.

———— 1989b. *Health Affairs* 8 (Winter):67–96.

Harvard Educational Review. 1969. *Equal Educational Opportunity.* Cambridge, Mass.: Harvard University Press.

Hiatt, Howard H. 1987. *America's Health in the Balance: Choice or Chance?* New York: Harper and Row.

Hsiao, William C., et al. 1988. Results and policy implications of the resource-based relative-value study. *New England Journal of Medicine* 319 (September 29): 835–841.

Kingdon, John W. 1984. *Agendas, Alternatives, and Public Policies.* Boston: Little, Brown.

Majone, Giandomenico. 1989. *Evidence, Argument and Persuasion in the Policy Process.* New Haven, Conn.: Yale University Press.

Marmor, Theodore R. 1973. *The Politics of Medicare.* Chicago: Aldine.

McIlrath, Sharon. 1989. New era of Medicare payment to be accompanied by MVPs. *American Medical News,* December 8, pp. 1, 40, 42–43.

Menges, Joel. 1986. From health services research to federal law: the case of DRGs. In Marion Ein Lewin, ed., *From Research into Policy: Improving the Link for Health Services.* Washington, D.C.: American Enterprise Institute for Public Policy Research, pp. 20–33.

Moynihan, Daniel P. 1970. *Maximum Feasible Misunderstanding* (paperback ed.). New York: Free Press.

Nelson, Barbara J. 1984. *Making an Issue of Child Abuse: Political Agenda Setting for Social Problems.* Chicago: University of Chicago Press.

Olson, Mancur, Jr. 1969. The purpose and plan of a social report. *The Public Interest* no. 15 (Spring):72–97.

Paul-Shaheen, Pamela, et al. 1987. Small area analysis: a review and analysis of the North American literature. *Journal of Health Politics, Policy, and Law* 12 (Winter):741–809.

Rice, Thomas H., and Roberta J. Labelle. 1989. Do physicians induce demand for medical services? *Journal of Health Politics, Policy, and Law* 14 (Fall):587–625.

Roemer, Milton I., and Max Shain. 1959. *Hospital Utilization under Insurance*. Chicago: American Hospital Association.
Tierney, John. 1987. Organized interests in health politics and policymaking. *Medical Care Review* 44 (Spring):89–118.
U.S. Bureau of the Census. 1989. *Statistical Abstract of the United States, 1989*. 109th ed., table 144, table 162. Washington, D.C.
U.S. Department of Health, Education, and Welfare. 1989. *Toward a Social Report*. Washington, D.C.: U.S. Government Printing Office.
Wedig, Gerard, et al. 1989. Can price controls induce optimal physician behavior? *Journal of Health Politics, Policy, and Law* 14 (Fall):587–625.
Weiss, Carol H. 1977. Research for policy's sake: the enlightenment function of social research. *Policy Analysis* 3 (Fall):531–547.
Winsten, Jay A. 1976. The Utah professional review organization as a prototype for PSRO's. In Richard Green, ed., *Assessing Quality in Medical Care: The State of the Art*. Cambridge, Mass.: Ballinger, pp. 213–239.

3. Paying for Hospital Care

Altman, Stuart, and Joseph Eichenholz. 1976. Inflation in the health industry: causes and cures. In Michael Zubkoff, ed., *Health: A Victim or Cause of Inflation?*, pp. 7–30. New York: Prodist–Milbank Memorial Fund.
Anderson, Odin, and Duncan Neuhauser. 1969. Rising costs are inherent in modern health care systems. *Hospitals* 43 (February 16):50–52.
Anderson, Ronald, and John Hull. 1969. Hospital utilization and cost trends. *Health Services Research* 4 (Fall):198–221.
Biles, Brian, Carl Schramm, and Graham Atkinson. 1980. Hospital cost inflation under state rate-setting programs. *New England Journal of Medicine* 303 (September 18):664–668.
Carr, W. John, and Paul Feldstein. 1967. The relationship of cost to hospital size. *Inquiry* 4 (June):45–65.
Davis, Karen. 1981. Recent trends in hospital costs: failure of the voluntary effort. Testimony before the U.S. House of Representatives, Committee on Energy and Commerce, December 15. Washington, D.C.: U.S. Government Printing Office.
Dowling, William. 1976. Prospective rate setting, concept and practice. *Topics in Health Care Financing* 3 (Winter):7–37.
Editorial. 1978. Voluntary effort: a new spirit of cooperation. *Hospitals* 52 (July 1): 55–59.
Feder, Judith, and Bruce Spitz. 1980. The politics of hospital payment. In Judith Feder, John Holahan, and Theodore Marmor, eds., *National Health Insurance: Conflicting Goals and Policy Choices*, pp. 301–347. Washington, D.C.: The Urban Institute.
Fetter, Robert, Youngshoo Shin, Jean Freeman, Richard Averill, and John Thomp-

son. 1980. Case mix definition by diagnosis-related groups. *Medical Care Supplement* 18 (February):1–53.

Gaus, Clifton, and Fred Hellinger. 1976. Results of prospective reimbursement. *Topics in Health Care Financing* 3 (Winter):83–96.

Gibson, Robert. 1980. National health expenditures, 1979. *Health Care Financing Review* 2 (Summer):1–36.

Ginsburg, Paul. 1976. Inflation and the economic stabilization program. In Michael Zubkoff, ed., *Health: A Victim or Cause of Inflation?*, pp. 31–51. New York: Prodist–Milbank Memorial Fund.

Hellinger, Fred. 1979. Hospital rate-regulation programs and proposals: a survey and analysis. *Topics in Health Care Financing* 6 (Fall):5–14.

Horn, Susan, Bette Chachich, and Cathy Clopton. 1983. Measuring severity of illness: a reliability study. *Medical Care* 21 (July):705–714.

Klarman, Herbert. 1969. Approaches to moderating the increases in medical care costs. *Medical Care* (May-June):174–190.

Lave, Judith, Lester Lave, and Lester Silverman. 1973. A proposal for incentive reimbursement for hospitals. *Medical Care* 11 (March–April):79–90.

Letsch, Suzanne, Katharine Levit, and Daniel Waldo. 1988. National health expenditures, 1987. *Health Care Financing Review* 10 (Winter):109–129.

Lipscomb, Joseph, Ira Raskin, and Joseph Eichenholz. 1978. The use of marginal cost estimates in hospital cost-containment policy. In Michael Zubkoff, Ira Raskin, and Ruth Hanft, eds., *Hospital Cost Containment: Selected Notes for Future Policy*, pp. 514–537. New York: Prodist–Milbank Memorial Fund.

Mills, Ronald, Robert Fetter, Donald Riedel, and Richard Averill. 1976. AUTOGRP: an interactive computer system for the analysis of health care data. *Medical Care* 14 (July):603–615.

Morrisey, Michael, Frank Sloan, and Joseph Valvona. 1988. Shifting Medicare patients out of the hospital. *Health Affairs* 7 (Winter):52–64.

Newhouse, Joseph. 1976. Inflation and health insurance. In Michael Zubkoff, ed., *Health: Victim or Cause of Inflation?*, pp. 210–224. New York: Prodist–Milbank Memorial Fund.

Newman, John, William Elliott, James Gibbs, and Helen Gift. 1979. Attempts to control health care costs: the United States experience. *Social Science and Medicine* 13A (August):529–540.

Pauly, Mark, and David Drake. 1970. Effect of third-party methods of reimbursement on hospital performance. In Herbert Klarman, ed., *Empirical Studies in Health Economics*, pp. 297–314. Baltimore: Johns Hopkins University Press.

Pearson, David, and David Abernethy. 1980. A qualitative assessment of previous efforts to contain hospital costs. *Journal of Health Politics, Policy, and Law* 5 (Spring):120–141.

Prospective Payment Assessment Commission. 1989. *Medicare Prospective Payment and The American Health Care System: Report to the Congress*. Washington, D.C.: ProPAC, June.

Roemer, Milton, and Max Shain. 1959. *Hospitalization Utilization under Insurance*. Chicago: American Hospital Association.

Russell, Louise, and Carrie Manning. 1989. The effect of prospective payment on

Medicare expenditures. *New England Journal of Medicine* 320 (February 16):439–444.

Salkever, David, and Thomas Bice. 1978. Certificate of need legislation and hospital costs. In Michael Zubkoff, Ira Raskin, and Ruth Hanft, eds., *Hospital Cost Containment: Selected Notes for Future Policy,* pp. 429–460. New York: Prodist–Milbank Memorial Fund.

Sloan, Frank, and Bruce Steinwald. 1980. Effects of regulation on hospital costs and input use. *Journal of Law and Economics* 23 (April):81–109.

Steinwald, Bruce, and Laura Dummit. 1989. Hospital case-mix change: sicker patients or DRG creep? *Health Affairs* 8 (Summer):35–47.

U.S. Congress, House of Representatives. 1971. *Social Security Amendments of 1971.* Report of the Committee on Ways and Means, 92nd Congress, 1st Session.

U.S. Department of Health and Human Services. 1987. Health Care Financing Administration, Office of Research and Demonstrations. *Report to Congress: Impact of the Medicare Hospital Prospective Payment System.* HCFA Publication no. 03251, August.

Wallack, Stanley, and Henya Handler. 1983. *Report on the Impact of the Medicare Hospital Prospective Payment System (PPS).* Report to the Health Care Financing Administration. Waltham, Mass.: Bigel Institute for Health Policy, Heller Graduate School, Brandeis University.

4. Physician Payment

Arnould, R. J., and L. M. DeBrock. 1985. The effect of provider control of Blue Shield plans on health care markets. *Economic Inquiry* 23 (3):449–476.

Burney, I., G. Schieber, et al. 1978. Geographic variation in physicians' fees. *Journal of the American Medical Association* 240 (3):1368–71.

Burstein, P. L., and J. Cromwell. 1985. Relative incomes and rates of return for U.S. physicians. *Journal of Health Economics* 4 (March):63–78.

Christensen, S. 1989. Volume responses to exogenous changes in Medicare's payment policies. Technical Memorandum, U.S. Congressional Budget Office, August.

Christensen, S., and S. Harrison. 1989. Comparison of current congressional proposals for changing Medicare's system for paying physicians. Technical Memorandum, U.S. Congressional Budget Office, September.

Colby, D., and D. Juba. In press. The effect of a Medicare fee schedule on beneficiary out-of-pocket costs and physicians' payments. In H. E. Frech, ed., *Regulating Doctors' Fees: Costs, Competition, and Controls under Medicare.* Washington, D.C.: American Enterprise Institute.

Cromwell, J., J. B. Mitchell, M. L. Rosenbach, W. B. Stason, and S. Hurdle. 1989. Using physician time and complexity to identify mispriced procedures. *Inquiry* 26 (1):7–23.

Feldman, R., and F. Sloan. 1988. Competition among physicians, revisited. *Journal of Health Economics, Policy, and Law* 13 (2):239–261.

Frech, H. E. III, and P. B. Ginsburg. 1978. *Public Insurance in Private Medical Markets.* Washington, D.C.: American Enterprise Institute.

Ginsburg, P. B., J. Newhouse, et al. 1986. Planning a demonstration of per-case reimbursement for inpatient physician services under Medicare. RAND Pub. no. R-3378-HCFA. Santa Monica, Calif.: The RAND Corporation, April.

Gold, M., and I. Reeves. 1987. Preliminary results of the GHAA–BC/BS survey of physician incentives in health maintenance organizations. Research Brief no. 1. Washington, D.C.: Group Health Association of America, November.

Greenberg, G. 1988. Project officer's overview. In P. McMenamin, H. West, and L. Marcus, eds., Changes in Medicare Part B physician charges: final report. Springfield, Va.: Mandex Inc., October.

Hammons, G. T. In press. Commentary. In H. E. Frech, ed., *Regulating Doctors' Fees: Costs, Competition, and Controls under Medicare.* Washington, D.C.: American Enterprise Institute.

Health Care Financing Administration. 1989. Reports to Congress: Medicare physician payment. October.

Hillman, A. L. 1987. Special report: financial incentives for physicians in HMOs. *New England Journal of Medicine* 317 (27):1743–48.

Hsiao, W. C., and W. B. Stason. 1979. Toward developing a relative value scale for medical and surgical services. *Health Care Financing Review* 1 (2):23–28.

Hsiao, W. C., et al. 1988a. Results and policy implications of the resource-based relative value study. *New England Journal of Medicine* 319(13):881–88.

———— 1988b. A national study of resource-based relative values for physician services: final report. Health Care Financing Administration contract no. 17-C-98795-03, September 27.

Labelle, R., J. Hurley, and T. Rice. 1989. Financial incentives and medical practice: evidence from Ontario on the effect of changes in physician fees on medical care utilization. Background Paper 89-3, December. Washington, D.C.: Physician Payment Review Commission.

Lasker, R. D., et al. 1989. Variation in Medicare global service policies: relationship to current payment and implications for a fee schedule. Physician Payment Review Commission, Background Paper 89-2, November.

McMenamin, P., H. West, and L. Marcus. 1988. Changes in Medicare Part B physician charges: final report. Springfield, Va.: Mandex Inc., October.

Mitchell, J. B., K. A. Calore, J. Cromwell, et al. 1984. Creating DRG-based physician reimbursement schemes: a conceptual and empirical analysis. Year I report prepared for the Health Care Financing Administration, U.S. Department of Health and Human Services, Baltimore, Md., October.

Mitchell, J. B., and J. Cromwell. 1982. Physician behavior under the Medicare assignment option. *Journal of Health Economics* 1:245–64.

Mitchell, J. B., G. Wedig, and J. Cromwell. 1989. The Medicare physician fee freeze. *Health Affairs* 8 (1):21–33.

National Rural Health Care Association. 1988. Letter to the Physician Payment Review Commission, November 2. Washington, D.C.

Nelson, L., A. Ciemnecki, N. Carlton, and K. Langwell. 1989. Assignment and the participating physician program: an analysis of beneficiary awareness, understanding, and experience. Physician Payment Review Commission. Background Paper no. 89-1, September.

Paringer, L. 1980. Medicare assignment rates of physicians: their responses to changes in reimbursement policy. *Health Care Financing Review* 1 (3):75–89.

Physician Payment Review Commission. 1988. *Annual Report to Congress,* March.

——— 1989. *Annual Report to Congress,* April.

Rice, T. 1984. Determinants of physician assignment rates by type of service. 1984. *Health Care Financing Review* 5 (4):33–42.

——— 1988. Statement to Physician Payment Review Commission, December.

Rice, T., and N. McCall. 1982. Changes in Medicare reimbursement in Colorado: impact on physicians' economic behavior. *Health Care Financing Review* 3 (4):67–85.

——— 1983. Factors influencing physician assignment decisions under Medicare. *Inquiry* 20 (1):45–56.

Rice, T., and R. J. Labelle. 1989. Do physicians induce demand for medical services? *Journal of Health Policy and Law* 14 (3):459–75.

Rodgers, J. F., and R. A. Musacchio. 1983. Physician acceptance of Medicare patients on assignment. *Journal of Health Economics* 2 (March):55–73.

Rodwin, V., H. Grable, and G. Thiel. In press. Updating the fee schedule for physician reimbursement: comparative analysis of selected experience abroad and of policy options for the United States. *Quality Assurance and Utilization Review.*

Schieber, G. J., and J-P. Poullier. 1989. International health care expenditure trends: 1987. *Health Affairs* 8 (3):169–177.

Sunshine, J., and J. Swartzman. 1989. Medicare's share in U.S. physicians' revenues. Washington, D.C.: Physician Payment Review Commission.

Welch, W. P. 1989. Prospective payment to medical staffs: a proposal. *Health Affairs* 8 (1):34–49.

Welch, W. P., S. Zuckerman, and G. Pope. 1989. The geographic Medicare economic index: alternative approaches. Urban Institute Working Paper 3839-01-01, June.

Welch, W.P., S. Zuckerman, G. Pope, and M. G. Henderson. 1989. Cost of practice and geographic variation in fees. *Health Affairs* 8 (3):117–128.

Zuckerman, S., W. P. Welch, and G. C. Pope. 1987. The development of an interim geographic Medicare economic index. Urban Institute Working Paper, December.

5. Financing Health Care for the Poor

Aday, Lu Ann, and Ronald Andersen. 1984. The national profile of access to medical care. *American Journal of Public Health* 74:1331–38.

Aday, Lu Ann, Ronald Andersen, and Gretchen V. Fleming. 1980. *Health Care in the U.S.: Equitable for Whom?* Beverly Hills, Calif.: Sage Publications.

Alan Guttmacher Institute. 1987. *Blessed Events and the Bottom Line.* New York.

American Academy of Pediatrics. 1982. *Medicaid and Children: A Policy Analysis.* November. Evanston, Ill.: AAP Division of Pediatric Practice.

Anderson, Maren D., and Peter D. Fox. 1987. Lessons learned from Medicaid managed care approaches. *Health Affairs* 6(1):71–86.

Axnick, N. W., S. M. Shavell, and J. J. Witte. 1969. Benefits due to immunization against measles. *Public Health Reports* 84:673–680.

Bachman, Sara S., Stuart H. Altman, and Dennis F. Beatrice. 1988. What influences a state's approach to Medicaid reform? *Inquiry* 24 (Summer):243–250.

——— 1987. Implementing change: lessons for Medicaid reformers. *Journal of Health Politics, Policy, and Law* 12(2):237–251.

Berwick, D. M., and A. L. Komaroff. 1982. Cost effectiveness of lead screening. *New England Journal of Medicine* 306:1392–98.

Blendon, Robert J., and Thomas W. Moloney. 1982. Perspectives on the Medicaid crisis. In Robert J. Blendon and Thomas W. Moloney, eds., *New Approaches to the Medicaid Crisis.* New York: F&S Press, Frost and Sullivan.

Bovbjerg, R. R., and John Holahan. 1982. *Medicaid in the Reagan Era: Federal Policy and State Choices.* Washington, D.C.: Urban Institute Press.

Braveman, Paula, Geraldine Oliva, Marie Grisham Miller, et al. 1989. Adverse outcomes and lack of health insurance among newborns in an eight-county area of California, 1982 to 1986. *New England Journal of Medicine* 321(8):508–513.

Brown, E. R., M. R. Cousineau, and W. T. Price. 1985. Competing for Medi-Cal business: why hospitals did, and did not, get contracts. *Inquiry* 22:237–250.

Burwell, Brian O., and Marilyn P. Rymer. 1987. Trends in Medicaid eligibility: 1975 to 1985. *Health Affairs* 6(4):31–45.

Butler, John A., Peter Budetti, Margaret A. McManus, Suzanne Stenmark, and Paul W. Newacheck. 1985. Health care expenditures for children with chronic illnesses. In Nicholas Hobbs and James M. Perrin, eds., *Issues in the Care of Children with Chronic Illness.* San Francisco: Jossey-Bass.

Butler, John A., Sara Rosenbaum, and Judith S. Palfrey. 1987. Ensuring access to health care for children with disabilities. *New England Journal of Medicine* 317 (July 16):162–164.

Butler, John A., William D. Winter, Judith Singer, and Martha Wenger. 1985. Medical care use and expenditure among children and youth in the United States: analysis of a national probability sample. *Pediatrics* 76(4):495–507.

Children's Defense Fund. 1985. *The Health of America's Children: The Maternal and Child Health Data Book.* Washington, D.C.: Children's Defense Fund.

Christianson, Jon. 1984. Provider participation in competitive bidding for indigent patients. *Inquiry* 21:161–177.

Cohen, Harold. 1982. State price controls. In Robert J. Blendon and Thomas W. Moloney, eds., *New Approaches to the Medicaid Crisis.* New York: F&S Press, Frost and Sullivan.

Commonwealth Fund Commission on Elderly People Living Alone. 1987. *Medicare's Poor: Filling the Gaps in Medical Coverage for Low-Income Elderly Americans.*

Prepared by Diane Rowland and Barbara Lyons. Baltimore, Md.: The Commonwealth Fund Commission on Elderly People Living Alone, November.

Congressional Budget Office. 1979. *A Profile of the Uninsured: The Haves and Have Nots*. Washington, D.C.

——— 1981. *Medicaid: Choices for 1982 and Beyond*. Washington, D.C.: U.S. Government Printing Office.

Congressional Research Service. 1988a. *Health Insurance and the Uninsured: Background Data and Analysis*. A report prepared for the U.S. House of Representatives, Energy and Commerce Committee, Subcommittee on Health and the Environment, Committee Print Serial 100 X. Washington, D.C.: U.S. Government Printing Office.

——— 1988b. *Medicaid Source Book: Background Data and Analysis*. A report prepared for the use of the Subcommittee on Health and the Environment of the Committee on Energy and Commerce, U.S. House of Representatives. Washington, D.C.: U.S. Government Printing Office, November.

Cromwell, J., and S. Hurdle. 1984. *The Evolution of State Medicaid Programs*. Chestnut Hill, Mass.: Center for Health Economics Research.

Cromwell, J., and J. Kanak. 1982. The effects of prospective reimbursement programs on hospital adoption and service sharing. *Health Care Financing Review* 4(2):67–88.

Davidson, Stephen M., Jerry Cromwell, and Rachel Schurman. 1986. Medicaid myths: trends in Medicaid expenditures and the prospects for reform. *Journal of Health Politics, Policy, and Law* 10(4):699–728.

Davis, Karen 1973. Lessons of Medicare and Medicaid for national health insurance. Hearings on National Health Insurance, Subcommittee on Public Health and Environment, Committee on Interstate and Foreign Commerce, U.S. Congress, Washington, D.C., December 12.

——— 1975. *National Health Insurance: Benefits, Costs, and Consequences*. Washington, D.C.: The Brookings Institution.

——— 1976. Achievements and problems of Medicaid. *Public Health Reports* 912(4):309–316.

——— 1979. Child health assurance plan. Testimony before the U.S. Congress, House of Representatives, Interstate and Foreign Commerce Committee, Subcommittee on Health and the Environment, June 7.

——— 1983. Child health assurance. Testimony before the U.S. Congress, House of Representatives, Committee on Energy and Commerce, Subcommittee on Health and the Environment, Washington, D.C., July 15.

——— 1986. Medicaid: Medigap for the poor elderly. Testimony before the U.S. Congress, House of Representatives, Committee on Energy and Commerce, Subcommittee on Health and the Environment, Washington, D.C., March 26.

Davis, Karen, Gerard Anderson, Diane Rowland, and Earl Steinberg. 1990. *Health Care Cost Containment*. Baltimore, Md.: Johns Hopkins University Press.

Davis, Karen, and Roger Reynolds. 1976. The impact of Medicare and Medicaid on access to medical care. In Richard N. Rosett, ed., *The Role of Health Insurance in the Health Services Sector*. Cambridge, Mass.: National Bureau of Economic Research.

Davis, Karen, and Diane Rowland. 1983. Uninsured and underserved: inequities in health care in the United States. *Milbank Memorial Fund Quarterly/Health and Society* 61(2):149–176.

———— 1986. *Medicare Policy: New Directions for Health and Long-Term Care.* Baltimore, Md.: Johns Hopkins University Press.

———— 1990. Old and poor: policy challenges in the 1990s. *Journal of Aging and Social Policy,* forthcoming.

Davis, Karen, and Cathy Schoen. 1978. *Health and the War on Poverty: A Ten Year Appraisal.* Washington, D.C.: The Brookings Institution.

Feder, Judith, and John Holahan. 1985. Medicaid Program Evaluation: A Synthesis of Interim Findings. Report to the Health Care Financing Administration, Washington, D.C., March, unpublished.

Fox, Harriette B., and Ruth Yoshpe. 1987. Medicaid financing for early intervention services. Washington, D.C.: Fox Health Policy Consultants, June.

Freeman, Howard E., Robert Blendon, Linda Aiken, Seymour Sudman, Connie Mullinix, and Christopher Corey. 1987. Americans report on their access to health care. *Health Affairs* 6(1):6–18.

Freund, Deborah A. 1984. *Medicaid Reform: Four Studies of Case Management.* Washington, D.C.: American Enterprise Institute.

Freund, Deborah A., and Robert F. Hurley. 1987. Managed care in Medicaid: selected issues in program origins, design, and research. *Annual Review of Public Health* 8:137–163.

Freund, Deborah A., and Edward Neuschler. 1986. Overview of Medicaid capitation and case management initiatives. *Health Care Financing Review* 7 (December):21–30.

Gortmaker, Steven L. 1981. Medicaid and the health care of children in poverty and near poverty: some successes and failures. *Medical Care* 19 (6):567–582.

Gortmaker, Steven L., and William Sappenfield. 1984. Chronic childhood disorders: prevalence and impact. *Pediatric Clinics of North America* 31(1):3–18.

Griffith, Jeanne E., and Joseph A. Cislowski. 1986. *Infant Mortality: Are We Making Progress?* Washington, D.C.: Congressional Research Service Review, Library of Congress, January.

Holahan, John. 1978. *Financing Health Care for the Poor: The Medicaid Experience.* Lexington, Mass.: D. C. Heath.

———— 1987. *The Impact of Alternative Medicaid Hospital Payment Systems on Hospital's Medicaid Revenues, Admissions, and Lengths of Stay.* Washington, D.C.: The Urban Institute.

Holahan, John, and Joel Cohen. 1986. *Medicaid: The Cost Containment Access Trade-Off.* Washington, D.C.: The Urban Institute.

Howell, Embry. 1988. Low-income persons' access to health care; NMCUES Medicaid data. *Public Health Reports* 103(5):507–514.

Iglehart, John K. 1983. Medicaid turns to prepaid managed care. *New England Journal of Medicine* 308(16):976–980.

———— 1985. Medical care of the poor: a growing problem. *New England Journal of Medicine* 313(1):59–63.

Institute of Medicine. 1985. Committee to Study the Prevention of Low Birth-weight. *Preventing Low Birthweight.* Washington, D.C.: National Academy Press.

Iryes, Henry T. 1981. Health care for chronically disabled children and their families. In *Better Health for Our Children: A National Strategy. The Report of the Select Panel for the Promotion of Child Health to the United States Congress and the Secretary of Health and Human Services,* vol. 4, Background papers. Washington, D.C.: U.S. Government Printing Office.

Johns, L., M. D. Anderson, and R. A. Derzon. 1985. Selective contracting in California: experience in the second year. *Inquiry* 22:335–347.

Kasper, Judith D. 1986a. Children at risk: the uninsured and the inadequately insured. Paper presented at the annual meeting of the American Public Health Association, Maternal and Child Health Section, Las Vegas, Nevada, September.

——— 1986b. Health status and utilization: differences by Medicaid coverage and income. *Health Care Financing Review* 7(4):1–17.

Kidder, D., and D. Sullivan. 1982. Hospital payroll costs, productivity, and employment under prospective reimbursement. *Health Care Financing Review* 4(2):89–100.

Kleinman, Joel C., Marsha Gold, and Diane Makuc. 1981. Use of ambulatory medical care by the poor: another look at equity. *Medical Care* 19(10):1011–36.

Lewin, Lawrence S., and Marion Ein Lewin. 1987. Financing charity care in an era of competition. *Health Affairs* 6(1):47–60.

Lurie, Nicole, Nancy B. Ward, Martin F. Shapiro, and Robert H. Brook. 1984. Termination from Medi-Cal: does it affect health? *New England Journal of Medicine* 311(7):480–484.

Martin, J., D. Dolkart, and D. Freko. 1984. *Reasons for the Downturn in Under-65 Admissions.* Policy Brief no. 52, Office of Public Policy Analysis. Chicago: American Hospital Association, September 21.

Mitchell, Janet, and Gerald Cromwell. 1980. Medicaid mills: fact or fiction? *Health Care Financing Review* 2(3):37–49.

Moloney, Thomas W. 1982. *What's Being Done about Medicaid?* A Commonwealth Fund Paper. New York: The Commonwealth Fund.

Muse, Donald N. 1987. *Medicaid Trends: Past, Present, and Future.* Presentation to the National Health Policy Forum, Washington, D.C., January.

Neuschler, E. 1985. *Prepaid Managed Care under Medicaid: Overview of Current Initiatives.* Washington, D.C.: National Governors' Association.

Newacheck, Paul W. 1987. The costs of caring for chronically ill children. *Business and Health* 4(3):18–24.

——— 1988. Access to ambulatory care for poor persons. *Health Services Research* 12(3):401–419.

Newacheck, Paul W., and Margaret A. McManus. 1988. Financing health care for disabled children. *Pediatrics* 81(3):385–394.

Oberg, Charles N., and Cynthia Longseth Policy. 1988. Medicaid: entering the third decade. *Health Affairs* 7(4):83–96.

Office of Technology Assessment. 1987. *Technology-Dependent Children: Hospital v. Home Care: A Technical Memorandum.* Washington, D.C.: U.S. Government Printing Office, May.

—— 1988. *Healthy Children: Investing in the Future.* OTA-H-345. Washington, D.C.: U.S. Government Printing Office.

Olinger, L. 1986. Medicaid program evaluation: interim findings—inpatient hospital reimbursement. Unpublished report. Cambridge, Mass.: Abt Associates.

Omenn, Gilbert S. 1987. Lessons from a fourteen-state study of Medicaid. *Health Affairs* 6(1):118–122.

Orr, Suezanne T., and C. A. Miller. 1981. Utilization of health services by poor children since advent of Medicaid. *Medical Care* 19(6):583–590.

Perrin, James M. 1985. Introduction. In Nicholas Hobbs and James M. Perrin, eds., *Issues in the Care of Children with Chronic Illness.* San Francisco: Jossey-Bass.

President's Commission for the Study of Ethical Problems in Medicine and Biomedical and Behavioral Research. 1983. *Securing Access to Health Care.* Washington, D.C.: U.S. Government Printing Office.

Rabin, D. L., and E. Schach. 1975. Medicaid, morbidity, and physician use. *Medical Care* 13:68–78.

Reinhardt, Uwe. 1985. Comments on 20 years of Medicaid and Medicare. *Health Care Financing Review* (supplement):105–111. Baltimore: U.S. Department of Health and Human Services.

Rogers, D. E., and R. J. Blendon. 1977. The changing American health scene: sometimes things get better. *Journal of the American Medical Association* 237:1710–14.

Rogers, D. E., R. J. Blendon, and T.W. Moloney. 1982. Who needs Medicaid? *New England Journal of Medicine* 307:13–18.

Rosenbach, Margo L. 1985. *Insurance Coverage and Ambulatory Medical Care of Low-Income Children, United States, 1980.* National Medical Care Utilization and Expenditure Survey, Series C, Analytical Report no. 1, DHHS pub. no. 85-20401, National Center for Health Statistics, Public Health Service. Washington, D.C.: U.S. Government Printing Office, September.

Rosenbaum, Sara, Dana C. Hughes, and Kay Johnson. 1988. Maternal and child health services for medically indigent children and pregnant women. *Medical Care* 26(4):315–332.

Rosenbaum, Sara, Dana Hughes, Elizabeth Butler, and Deborah Howard. 1988. Incantations in the dark: Medicaid, managed care, and maternity care. *Milbank Quarterly* 66(4):661–693.

Rosenbaum, Sara, and Kay Johnson. 1986. Providing health care for low-income children: reconciling child health goals with child health financing realities. *Milbank Quarterly* 64(3):442–478.

Rowland, Diane. 1989. Financing of care: a critical component. In Ruth E. K. Stein, ed., *Caring for Children with Chronic Illness.* New York: Springer.

Rowland, Diane, and Clifton R. Gaus. 1982. Reducing eligibility and benefits: current policies and alternatives. In Robert J. Blendon and Thomas W. Moloney, eds., *New Approaches to the Medicaid Crisis.* New York: F&S Press, Frost and Sullivan.

Rowland, Diane, and Barbara Lyons. 1987. Medicaid in Milwaukee: mandatory HMO care for the poor. *Health Affairs* 6(1):87–100.

—— 1989a. Triple jeopardy: rural, poor, and uninsured. *Health Services Research* 23(6):975–1004.

—— 1989b. The utilization of acute care health services by frail elderly people. The Public Policy Institute, American Association of Retired Persons. Washington, D.C.

Rowland, Diane, Barbara Lyons, and Jennifer Edwards. 1988. Medicaid: health care for the poor in the Reagan era. *Annual Review of Public Health* 9:427–450.

Rymer, Marilyn P., and Gerald S. Adler. 1987. Children and Medicaid: the experience in four states. *Health Care Financing Review* 9(1):1–20.

Schoen, Cathy. 1984. Medicaid and the poor: Medicaid myths and reality and the impact of recent legislative changes. *Bulletin of the New York Academy of Medicine* 60(1):54–65.

Short, Pamela Farley, Joel C. Cantor, and Alan C. Monheit. 1988. The dynamics of Medicaid enrollment. *Inquiry* 25:504–516.

Southern Governors' Association. 1985. *Infant Mortality: Final Report.* Washington, D.C.

Spiegel, Alan D. 1979. *The Medicaid Experience.* Germantown, Md.: Aspen Systems.

Spitz, Bruce. 1982. Contracting with health maintenance organizations. In Robert J. Blendon and Thomas W. Moloney, eds., *New Approaches to the Medicaid Crisis.* New York: F&S Press, Frost and Sullivan.

—— 1987. A national survey of Medicaid case-management programs. *Health Affairs* 6(1):61–70.

Starfield, Barbara. 1985a. *The Effectiveness of Medical Care: Validating Clinical Wisdom.* Baltimore, Md.: Johns Hopkins University Press.

—— 1985b. Motherhood and apple pie: the effectiveness of medical care for children. *Milbank Memorial Fund Quarterly* 63(3):523–546.

Stevens, Robert, and Rosemary Stevens. 1974. *Welfare Medicine in America: A Case Study of Medicaid.* New York: Free Press, MacMillan.

Swartz, Katherine. 1988. How the overlap between the poverty and Medicaid populations changed between 1979 and 1983, or lessons for the next recession. *Journal of Human Resources* 24(2):319–330.

Thorpe, Kenneth E., Joanne E. Siegel, and Theresa Dailey. 1989. Including the poor: the fiscal impacts of Medicaid expansion. *Journal of the American Medical Association* 261(7):1003–7.

Torres, Aida, and Asta M. Kenney. 1989. Expanding Medicaid coverage for pregnant women: estimates of the impact and cost. *Family Planning Perspectives* 21(1):19–24.

U.S. Congress. Committee on Energy and Commerce, U.S. House of Representatives. 1986. Statement to the committee on the budget regarding the administration's FY87 budget. Washington, D.C.: U.S. Government Printing Office, March.

U.S. Congress. Committee on Interstate and Foreign Commerce, U.S. House of

Representatives. 1979. Child health assurance act of 1979. Washington, D.C.: U.S. Government Printing Office.

U.S. Congress. Committee on Ways and Means, U.S. House of Representatives. 1985. *Children in Poverty.* Washington, D.C.

—— 1989. *Background Material and Data on Programs within the Jurisdiction of the Committee on Ways and Means.* Washington, D.C.: U.S. Government Printing Office, March 15.

U.S. Congress. Select Committee on Children, U.S. House of Representatives. 1985. *Opportunities for Success.* Washington, D.C.

U.S. Department of Health and Human Services, Health Care Financing Administration. 1982. *Medicare and Medicaid Data Book, 1981.* Baltimore, Md.

—— 1986. *Medicare and Medicaid Data Book 1984.* Baltimore, Md.

—— 1987. *Analysis of State Medicaid Program Characteristics, 1986.* Baltimore, Md.: Office of Research and Demonstrations.

U.S. Department of Health, Education, and Welfare. 1977. *The Revised FY 1978 Budget of the U.S. Department of Health, Education and Welfare, February.* Washington, D.C.

U.S. General Accounting Office. 1987. *Prenatal Care: Medicaid Recipients and Uninsured Women Obtain Insufficient Care.* GAP/HRD 87-137. Washington, D.C.

Vladeck, Bruce. 1982. Paying hospitals. In Robert J. Blendon and Thomas W. Moloney, eds., *New Approaches to the Medicaid Crisis.* New York: F&S Press, Frost and Sullivan.

Vogel, Ron. 1984. An analysis of structural incentives in the Arizona HCCCS. *Health Care Financing Review* 5:13–22.

Walden, D., G. Wilensky, and J. Kasper. 1985. Changes in health insurance status: full-year and part-year coverage. NMCES, Data Preview no. 21. NCHSR, DHHS. Washington, D.C.: U.S. Government Printing Office.

Wilensky, Gail R., and Marc L. Berk. 1982. Health care, the poor, and the role of Medicaid. *Health Affairs* 1(4):93–100.

Zuckerman, Stephen, and John Holahan. 1988. PPS waivers: implications for Medicare, Medicaid, and commercial insurers. *Journal of Health Politics, Policy, and Law* 13(4):663–681.

6. Financing Health Care for Elderly Americans

Aday, Lu Ann, Ronald Anderson, and Gretchen Fleming. 1980. *Health Care in the U.S.: Equitable for Whom?* Beverly Hills, Calif.: Sage Publications.

Advisory Council on Social Security. 1983. *Medicare Benefits and Financing.* Washington, D.C.: U.S. Government Printing Office.

Applebaum, Robert, Frederick Seidl, and Carol Austin. 1980. The Wisconsin community care organization: preliminary findings from the Milwaukee experiment. *Gerontologist* 20 (June):350–355.

Avorn, Jerry. 1983. Drug policy in the aging society. *Health Affairs* 2(3):23–32.

Birnbaum, Howard, and David Kidder. 1984. What does hospice cost? *American Journal of Public Health* 74(7):689–697.

Blumenthal, David, Mark Schlesinger, and Pamela Brown Drumheller. 1988. *Medicare: Renewing the Promise*. New York: Oxford University Press.

Blumenthal, David, Mark Schlesinger, Pamela Brown Drumheller, and the Harvard Medicare Project. 1986. The future of Medicare. *New England Journal of Medicine* 314(11):722–728.

Bowen, Otis, and Thomas Burke. 1985. Cost neutral catastrophic care proposed for Medicare recipients. *Federation of American Hospitals Review* (November/December):42–45.

Breslow, Lester, and Anne Somers. 1977. The lifetime health monitoring program: a practical approach to preventive Medicare. *New England Journal of Medicine* 296 (March 17):601–608.

Brooks, C. H., and K. Smyth-Staruch. 1984. Hospice home care cost savings to third-party insurers. *Medical Care* 8:691–703.

Bulkin, Wilma, and Herbert Lukashok. 1988. Rx for dying: the case for hospice. *New England Journal of Medicine* 318 (6):376–378.

Cafferata, Gail. 1984a. Private health insurance coverage of the Medicare population. *National Health Care Expenditures Study Data Preview 18*. Washington, D.C.: U.S. Government Printing Office, September.

—— 1984b. Knowledge of their Medicare coverage by the elderly. *Medical Care* 22:835–847.

—— 1985a. Private health insurance of the Medicare population and the Baucus legislation. *Medical Care* 23:1086–96.

—— 1985b. The elderly's private insurance of nursing home care. *American Journal of Public Health* 75(6):655–656.

Caldwell, Janice, and Marshall Kapp. 1981. The rights of nursing home patients: possibilities and limitations of federal regulation. *Journal of Health Politics, Policy, and Law* 6(1):40–48.

Callahan, James. J., and Stanley S. Wallack. 1981. *Reforming the Long-Term Care System*. Boston: Lexington Books.

Callahan, James J., Lawrence D. Diamond, Janet Z. Giele, and Robert Morris. 1980. Responsibility of families for their severely disabled elders. *Health Care Financing Review* 1(3):29–48.

Christensen, Sandra, and Richard Kasten. 1988. Covering catastrophic expenses under Medicare. *Health Affairs* 7(1):80–93.

Christensen, Sandra, Stephen Long, and Jack Rodgers. 1987. Acute health care costs for the aged Medicare population: overview and policy options. *The Milbank Quarterly* 65(3):397–425.

Christianson, Jon. 1986. *Channeling Effects on Informal Care*. Report prepared for DHHS. Princeton, N.J.: Mathematica Policy Research.

Cohen, Donna, and Margaret Hastings. 1989. Mental health and the elderly. In Carl Eisdorfer, David Kessler, and Abby Spector, eds., *Caring for the Elderly: Reshaping Health Policy*. Baltimore, Md.: Johns Hopkins University Press.

Cohen, M., Eileen Tell, and Stanley Wallack. 1986. Client related risk factors of nursing home entry among elderly adults. *Journal of Gerontology* 20(6):785–792.

Commonwealth Fund Commission on Elderly People Living Alone. 1987. *Medicare's Poor: Filling the Gaps in Medical Coverage for Low-Income Elderly People.* Report prepared by Diane Rowland and Barbara Lyons. Baltimore, Md.

—— 1989. *Help at Home: Long-Term Care Assistance for Impaired Elderly People.* Report prepared by Diane Rowland. Baltimore, Md.

Consumers Union. 1984. Medicare supplement insurance. *Consumer Reports* (June):347–355.

—— 1989. Beyond Medicare. *Consumer Reports* (June):375–391.

Corder, Larry, and Steven Garfinkel. 1985. Supplemental health insurance coverage among aged Medicare beneficiaries. NMCUES Series B, Descriptive Report no. 5, DHHS pub. no. 85-20205 ORD HCFA.

Coward, Raymond T., and Stephen J. Cutler. 1989. Informal and formal health care systems for the rural elderly. *Health Services Research* 23(6):785–806.

Davis, Feather Ann. 1988. Medicare hospice benefit: early program experience. *Health Care Financing Review* 9(4):99–111.

Davis, Karen. 1973. Lessons of Medicare and Medicaid for national health insurance. Hearings before the Subcommittee on Public Health and the Environment, Committee on Interstate and Foreign Commerce, U.S. House of Representatives, December 12.

—— 1975. Equal treatment and unequal benefits: the Medicare program. *Milbank Memorial Fund Quarterly/Health and Society* 53 (Fall):449–488.

—— 1986. Medicaid: Medigap for the poor elderly. Testimony before the U.S. House of Representatives Committee on Energy and Commerce, Subcommittee on Health and the Environment, Hearing on Economic Status and Financial Burden for Health Care of the Elderly, Washington, D.C., March 26.

Davis, Karen, and Roger Reynolds. 1976. The impact of Medicare and Medicaid on access to medical care. In Richard Rosett, ed., *The Role of Health Insurance in the Health Services Sector.* New York: National Bureau of Economic Research, pp. 391–423.

Davis, Karen, and Diane Rowland. 1986. *Medicare Policy: New Directions for Health and Long Term Care.* Baltimore, Md.: Johns Hopkins University Press.

Davis, Karen, and Cathy Schoen. 1978. *Health and the War on Poverty.* Washington, D.C.: Brookings Institution.

DeNovo, A., and Gail Shearer. 1978. *Private Health Insurance to Supplement Medicare.* Washington, D.C.: Office of Policy Planning, Federal Trade Commission.

Doty, Pamela. 1986. Family care of the elderly: the role of public policy. *Milbank Quarterly* 64:34–75.

Doty, Pamela, Korbin Liu, and Joshua Wiener. 1985. Overview of long-term care. *Health Care Financing Review* 6(3):69–78.

Dunlop, Burton. 1980. Expanded home-based care for the elderly: solution or pipe dream. *American Journal of Public Health* 70(4):514–518.

—— 1983. The Medicare hospice benefit: unanticipated cost and access impacts? *Health Affairs* 2(3):127–131.

Ecosometrics, Inc. 1981. *Review of Reported Differences between Urban and Rural Elderly: Needs, Services, and Service Costs.* Administration on Aging Contract no. 105-80-065. Washington, D.C.: Ecosometrics, Inc.

Eggert, Gerald, Joyce Bowlyow, and Carol Nichols. 1980. Gaining control of the long term care system: first returns from the ACCESS experiment. *Gerontologist* 20 (June):356–363.

Employee Benefit Research Institute. 1985. *Medicare Reform: The Private Sector Impact.* Washington, D.C.: EBRI.

Feder, Judith. 1989. Financing home care for the elderly: roles and limits of public programs. Background paper prepared for the Commonwealth Fund Commission on Elderly People Living Alone. Background Series no. 15. Baltimore, Md.: Commonwealth Fund Commission on Elderly People Living Alone.

Feder, Judith, Marilyn Moon, and William Scanlon. 1987. Medicare reform: nibbling at catastrophic costs. *Health Affairs* 6(4):5–19.

Fox, Peter D., and Steven B. Clauser. 1980. Trends in nursing home expenditures: implications for aging policy. *Health Care Financing Review* 2(2):65–70.

Garfinkel, Steven, Arthur Bonito, and Kenneth McLeroy. 1987. Socio-economic factors in Medicare supplemental health insurance. *Health Care Financing Review* 9(1):21–30.

Gaumer, Gary, et al. 1986. Impact of the New York long-term home health care program. *Medical Care* 24 (July):647.

Ginzberg, Eli. 1984. Comment on Medicare benefits: a reassessment. *Milbank Memorial Fund Quarterly* 62(2):230–236.

Gornick, Marion. 1976. Ten years of Medicare: impact on the covered population. *Social Security Bulletin* 39:7–9.

Gornick, Marion, James Beebe, and Ronald Prihoda. 1983. Options for change under Medicare: impact of a cap on catastrophic illness expense. *Health Care Financing Review* 5(1):33–43.

Gornick, Marion, Jay Greenberg, Paul Eggers, and Allen Dobson. 1985. Twenty years of Medicare and Medicaid: covered populations, use of benefits, and program expenditures. *Health Care Financing Review* (Annual Supplement):13–59.

Greenberg, Jay, Walter Leutz, and R. Abrahams. 1985. The national social health maintenance organization demonstration. *Journal of Ambulatory Care Management* 8(November):32–61.

Greenberg, Jay, Walter Leutz, Merwyn Greenlick, Joelyn Malone, Sam Ervin, and Dennis Kodner. 1988. The social HMO demonstration: early experience. *Health Affairs* 7(3):66–79.

Greenfield, Margaret. 1968. *Medicare and Medicaid: The 1965 and 1967 Social Security Amendments.* Berkeley, Calif.: University of California, Institute of Government Studies, September.

Greer, D., Vincent Mor, J. Morris, et al. 1986. An alternative in terminal care: results of the national hospice study. *Journal of Chronic Diseases* 39:9–26.

Hamm, Linda, Thomas Kickham, and Dorothy Cutler. 1982. Research, demonstrations and evaluations. In Ronald Vogel and Hans Palmer, eds., *Long-Term Care*

Perspectives from Research and Demonstrations. Health Care Financing Administration. Washington, D.C.: U.S. Government Printing Office.

Harrington, Charlene, ed. 1985. *Long Term Care of the Elderly: Public Policy Issues.* Beverly Hills, Calif.: Sage Publications.

Harvard Medicare Project. 1986. *Medicare: Coming of Age. A Proposal for Reform.* Harvard University. Boston, Massachusetts. March.

Haskins, Brenda et al. 1985. *Evaluation of Coordinated Community-Oriented Long-Term Care Demonstration Projects.* Report prepared for HCFA. Berkeley, Calif.: Berkeley Planning Associates.

Hedrick, Susan, and Thomas Inui. 1986. The effect and cost of home care: an information synthesis. *Health Services Research* 20(6):851–880.

Hing, Esther. 1981. Characteristics of nursing home residents, health status and care received: national nursing home survey, United States, May–December 1977. *Vital and Health Statistics.* Series 13, no. 51. DHHS Pub. no. (PHS) 80-1712. Hyattsville, Md.: Public Health Service, National Center For Health Statistics.

——— 1987. Use of nursing homes by the elderly. Preliminary data from the 1985 national nursing home survey. *Advance Data from Vital and Health Statistics.* No. 135. DHHS Pub. no. (PHS) 87-1250. Hyattsville, Md.: Public Health Service, National Center For Health Statististics.

Hsiao, William. 1984. Medicare benefits: a reassessment. *Milbank Memorial Fund Quarterly Health and Society* 62(2):207.

Hughes, Susan, David Cordray, and V. Alan Spiker. 1984. Evaluation of a long-term home care program. *Medical Care* 22:469.

Institute of Medicine. 1977. *A Policy Statement: The Elderly and Functional Dependency.* Washington, D.C.: National Academy of Science.

——— 1981. Racial differences in the use of nursing homes. In *Health Care in a Context of Civil Rights.* Washington, D.C.: National Academy Press.

——— 1986. *Improving the Quality of Care in Nursing Homes.* Washington, D.C.: National Academy Press.

Kane, Robert L. 1988. Post-acute care: packages, bows, and strings. In Mark Pauly and William Kissick, eds., *Lessons from the First Twenty Years of Medicare: Research Implications for Public and Private Sector Policy.* Philadelphia: University of Pennsylvania Press.

Kane, Robert, Rosalie Kane, and Sharon Arnold. 1985. Prevention and the elderly: risk factors. *Health Services Research* 19(6)(part 2):945–1006.

Kane, Robert, R. Matthias, and S. Sampson. 1983. The risk of placement in a nursing home after acute hospitalization. *Medical Care* 21(11):1055–61.

Kane, Robert, J. Wales, L. Bernstein, et al. 1984. A randomized controlled trial of hospice care. *Lancet* 1:890–894.

Kasper, Judith. 1990. Cognitive impairment among functionally limited elderly people in the community: future considerations for long-term care policy. *Milbank Memorial Quarterly* 68(1), forthcoming.

Katz, S., T. Downs, M. Cash, and R. Grotz. 1970. Progress in the development of the index of ADL. *The Gerontologist* 10:20–30.

Katz, Sidney, Amasa Ford, Roland Moskowitz, Beverly Jackson, and Marjorie Jaffe. 1963. Studies in illness in the aged: the index of ADL: a standardized measure of biological and psychosocial function. *Journal of the American Medical Association* 185(12):914–919.

Kemper, Peter, et al. 1986. *The Evaluation of the National Long Term Care Demonstration: Final Report.* Prepared for DHHS. Princeton, N.J.: Mathematica Policy Research.

Kemper, Peter, Robert Applebaum, and Margaret Harrigan. 1987. Community care demonstrations: what have we learned? *Health Care Financing Review* 8(4): 87–100.

Kovar, Mary Grace. 1986. Expenditures for the medical care of elderly people living in the community. *Milbank Quarterly* 64(1):100–132.

Lave, Judith. 1985. Cost containment policies in long-term care. *Inquiry* 22(1):7–23.

———— 1988. The structure of the Medicare benefits package: evolution and options for change. In Mark Pauly and William Kissick, eds., *Lessons from the First Twenty Years of Medicare: Research Implications for Public and Private Sector Policy.* Philadelphia: University of Pennsylvania Press.

Lave, Judith, Allen Dobson, and Randall Walton. 1983. The potential use of the Health Care Financing Administration data bases on health services research. *Health Care Financing Review* 5(1):93–98.

Lavor, Judith, and Marie Callender. 1976. Home health cost effectiveness: what are we measuring? *Medical Care* 14(10):866–872.

Lawton, M., and E. Brody. 1969. Assessment of older people: self-maintaining and instrumental activities of daily living. *Gerontologist* 9:179–186.

Leader, Shelah. 1986. *Home Health Benefits under Medicare.* Report prepared for the Public Policy Institute of the American Association of Retired Persons. No. 8601. Washington, D.C.: American Association of Retired Persons.

Leaf, P. J., M. M. Livingston, G. L. Tischler, et al. 1985. Contact with health professionals for the treatment of psychiatric and emotional problems. *Medical Care* 23(12):1322–37.

Leutz, Walter, R. Abrahams, M. R. Greenlick, et al. 1988. Targeting expanded care to the aged: early SHMO experience. *Gerontologist* 28 (February):4–17.

Lingle, E., K. Kirk, and W. Kelly. 1987. The impact of outpatient drug benefits on the use and costs of health care services for the elderly. *Inquiry* 24:203–211.

Link, Charles, Stephen Long, and Russell Settle. 1980. Cost-sharing, supplementary insurance, and health services utilization among the Medicare elderly. *Health Care Financing Review* 2(2):25–31.

Liu, Korbin, and Elizabeth Cornelius. 1989. ADLs and eligibility for long-term care services. Report prepared for the Commonwealth Fund Commission on Elderly People Living Alone. Background Paper Series no. 14. Baltimore, Md.: Commonwealth Fund Commission on Elderly People Living Alone.

Liu, Korbin, Kenneth Manton, and Barbara Liu. 1985. Home care expenses for disabled elderly. *Health Care Financing Review* 7(2):51–58.

Loeser, William, Emil Dickerstein, and Leonard Schiavone. 1981. Medicare coverage in nursing homes: a broken promise. *New England Journal of Medicine* 304:353–354.

Long, Stephen, and Russell Settle. 1982. Equity and the utilization of health care by the Medicare elderly. *Journal of Human Resources* 17(2):195–212.

———— 1984. Medicare and the disadvantaged elderly. *Milbank Memorial Fund Quarterly Health and Society* 62(4):609–656.

Long, Stephen, Russell Settle, and Charles Link. 1982. Who bears the burden of Medicare cost-sharing? *Inquiry* 19 (Fall):222–234.

Lubitz, James, and R. Deacon. 1982. The rise in the incidence of hospitalizations for the aged, 1968–1979. *Health Care Financing Review* 3(3):21.

Lubitz, James, and Ronald Prihoda. 1984. Use and costs of Medicare services in the last 2 years of life. *Health Care Financing Review* 5(3):117–132.

Macken, Candace. 1986. A profile of functionally impaired elderly persons living in the community. *Health Care Financing Review* 7(2):51–58.

McCall, Nelda. 1984. Utilization and costs of Medicare services by beneficiaries in their last year of life. *Medical Care* 22(4):329–42.

McCall, Nelda, Thomas Rice, and Arden Hall. 1983. *Medigap-Study of Comparative Effectiveness of Various State Regulations.* Menlo Park, Calif.: SRI International.

———— 1987. Medigap: study of comparative effectiveness of various state regulations. *Journal of Health Politics Policy and Law* 12(1):56–76.

McCall, Nelda, Thomas Rice, and Judith Sangl. 1986. Consumer knowledge of Medicare and supplemental health insurance benefits. *Health Services Research* 20(6):633–658.

McMillan, Alma, and Marion Gornick. 1984. The dually-entitled elderly Medicare and Medicaid population living in the community. *Health Care Financing Review* 6(4):73–86.

McMillan, Alma, Penelope L. Pine, Marion Gornick, and Ronald Prihoda. 1983. A study of the cross-over population: aged persons entitled to both Medicare and Medicaid. *Health Care Financing Review* 4(4):19–46.

Meiners, Mark. 1983. The case for long-term care insurance. *Health Affairs* 2(2):55–79.

Meiners, Mark, and R. Coffey. 1985. Hospital DRGs and the need for long-term care services: an empirical analysis. *Health Services Research* 20(3):359–384.

Meiners, Mark, and Gordon Trapnell. 1983. Long term care insurance: premium estimates for prototype policies. NCHSR Working Paper. Baltimore, Md.: National Center for Health Services Research.

Meltzer, Judith, Frank Farrow, and Harold Richmond. 1981. *Policy Options in Long-Term Care.* Chicago: University of Chicago Press.

Merriam, Ida A. 1964. Testimony. Hearing on Blue Cross and other Private Health Insurance for the Elderly. U.S. Congress. Senate Special Committee on Aging. Document 88-2 pt. 1, pp. 3–13. Washington, D.C.: U.S. Government Printing Office.

Mor, Vincent, and Howard Birnbaum. 1983. Medicare legislation for hospice care: implications of national hospice study data. *Health Affairs* 2(2):80–90.

Mor, Vincent, David Greer, and Robert Kastenbaum, eds. 1988. *The Hospice Experiment.* Baltimore, Md.: Johns Hopkins University Press.

Nagi, Saad. 1976. An epidemiology of disability among adults in the U.S. *Milbank Memorial Fund Quarterly* 54(4):439–467.

Neuschler, Edward. 1988. Medicaid eligibility for frail elders. Report prepared for the Commonwealth Fund Commission on Elderly People Living Alone. Background Series no. 10. Baltimore, Md.: Commonwealth Fund Commission on Elderly People Living Alone.

Nocks, Barry, et al. 1986. The effects of a community-based long-term care project on nursing home utilization. *Gerontologist* 26 (April):153.

Pauly, Mark, and William Kissick, eds. 1988. *Lessons from the First Twenty Years of Medicare: Research Implications for Public and Private Sector Policy.* Philadelphia: University of Pennsylvania Press.

Peel, Evelyn, and Jack Scharff. 1973. The impact of cost-sharing on use of ambulatory services under Medicare, current Medicare survey, 1969. *Social Security Bulletin* 36(10):3–24. Washington, D.C.: U.S. Government Printing Office.

Pfeiffer, Elizabeth. 1975. Short portable mental status questionnaire for the assessment of organic brain deficit in elderly patients. *Journal of the American Gerontological Society* 23:433–441.

Piro, A., and T. Lutins. 1973. Utilization and reimbursement under Medicare for persons who died in 1967 and 1968. *Health Insurance Statistics.* DHEW/SSA 74-11702. October. Washington, D.C.: U.S. Government Printing Office.

Rice, Thomas, and Jon Gabel. 1986. Protecting the elderly against high health care costs. *Health Affairs* 5(3):5–21.

Rice, Thomas, and Nelda McCall. 1985. The extent of ownership and characteristics of the Medicare supplemental policies. *Inquiry* 22(2):188–200.

Ricker-Smith, Katherine, and Brahna Trager. 1978. In-home health services in California: some lessons for national health insurance. *Medical Care* 16(3):173–190.

Riley, Gerald, James Lubitz, Ronald Prihoda, and Evelyne Rabey. 1987. The use and cost of Medicare services by cause of death. *Inquiry* 24(3):233–244.

Rivlin, Alice M., and Joshua Wiener. 1988. *Caring for the Disabled Elderly: Who Will Pay?* Washington, D.C.: The Brookings Institution.

Rosenblum, Robert. 1985. Medicare revisited: a look through the past to the future. *Journal of Health Politics, Policy, and Law* 9(4):669–681.

Rovin, Sheldon, and Zoe Boniface. 1988. Health promotion and prevention: a Medicare issue. In Mark Pauly and William Kissick, eds., *Lessons from the First Twenty Years of Medicare: Research Implications for Public and Private Sector Policy.* Philadelphia: University of Pennsylvania Press.

Rowland, Diane. 1989. Measuring the elderly's need for home care. *Health Affairs,* 8(4):39–51.

Rowland, Diane, Barbara Lyons, and Karen Davis. Catastrophic coverage under the Medicare program. In Carl Eisdorfer, ed., *Reshaping Health Care for the Elderly: Recommendations for National Policy.* Baltimore, Md.: Johns Hopkins University Press.

Rowland, Diane, Barbara Lyons, Patricia Neuman, Alina Salganicoff, and Lydia Taghavi. 1988. *Defining the Functionally Impaired Older Population.* Report prepared for the Public Policy Institute of the American Association of Retired Persons. Washington, D.C.: American Association of Retired Persons.

Russell, Louise. 1986. *Is Prevention Better than Cure?* Washington, D.C.: The Brookings Institution.

Ruther, Martin, and Allen Dobson. 1981. Equal treatment and unequal benefit: a reexamination of the use of Medicare services by race, 1967–1976. *Health Care Financing Review* 2(3):55–84.

Ruther, Martin, and Charles Helbing. 1988. Use and cost of Medicare home health agencies. *Health Care Financing Review* 10(1):105–108.

Scallet, Leslie. 1983. Practical approaches for meeting the mental health needs of the elderly. *Health Affairs* 2(2):103–116.

Scanlon, William. 1980. Nursing home utilization patterns: implications for policy. *Journal of Health Politics, Policy, and Law* 4(4):619–641.

Scharff, Jack. 1967. Current Medicare survey: the medical insurance sample. *Social Security Bulletin* 30 (April):4–9. Washington, D.C.: U.S. Government Printing Office.

Schlenger, William, and Larry Corder. 1984. *Access to Health Care among Aged Medicare Beneficiaries*. NMCUES. Series B. DHHS Pub. 84-20203. Washington, D.C.: U.S. Government Printing Office, April.

Schlenger, William, William Wadman, and Larry Corder. 1983. Health status of aged Medicare beneficiaries. NMCUES Report 2. DHHS Pub. 83-20202. HCFA Sept. Washington, D.C.: U.S. Government Printing Office.

Schlesinger, Mark, and Terrie Wetle. 1988. Medicare's coverage of health services. In D. Blumenthal, M. Schlesinger, and P. Drumheller, eds., *Renewing the Promise: Medicare and Its Reform*. New York: Oxford University Press.

Scitovsky, Anne. 1988. Medical care in the last twelve months of life: the relation between age, functional status, and medical care expenditures. *Milbank Quarterly* 66(4):640–660.

Sekscenski, E. 1987. Discharges from nursing homes: preliminary data from the 1985 national nursing home survey. *Advance Data from Vital and Health Statistics*. No. 142. National Center for Health Statistics. DHHS Pub. no. (PHS) 87-1250. Hyattsville, Md.: Public Health Service.

Shapiro, Samuel, Elizabeth Ann Skinner, Morton Kramer, et al. 1985. Measuring the need for mental health services in a general population. *Medical Care* 23(9):1033–43.

Shaughnessy, Peter, Robert Schlenker, and Herbert Silverman. 1988. Evaluation of the national swing-bed program in rural hospitals. *Health Care Financing Review* 10(1):87–94.

Sirrocco, A., and H. Koch. 1977. Nursing homes in the United States: 1973–1974: national nursing home survey. *Vital and Health Statistics*. Series 14, no. 17. National Center for Health Statistics. DHEW Pub. no. (HRA) 78-1812. Washington, D.C.: U.S. Government Printing Office.

Skellie, Albert, Melton Mobly, and Ruth Coan. 1982. Cost-effectiveness of community-based long-term care: current finding of Georgia's alternative health services project. *American Journal of Public Health* 72 (April):356.

Smith, David B. 1981. *Long-Term Care in Transition: The Regulation of Nursing Homes.* Ann Arbor, Mich.: AUPHA Press.

Smits, Helen, Judith Feder, and William Scanlon. 1982. Medicare nursing home benefit variation in interpretation. *New England Journal of Medicine* 307(14):855–862.

Somers, Anne. 1978. The high cost of health care for the elderly: diagnosis, prognosis, and some suggestions for therapy. *Journal of Health Politics, Policy, and Law* 3(2):163–180.

——— 1982. Long-term care for the elderly and disabled: a new health priority. *New England Journal of Medicine* 307(22):221–226.

——— 1984. Why not try preventing illness as a way of controlling Medicare costs? *New England Journal of Medicine* 311(13):853–856.

——— 1987. Insurance for long-term care: some definitions, problems, and guidelines for action. *New England Journal of Medicine* 317(1):23–29.

Spector, William, Sidney Katz, and John Fulton. 1987. The hierarchical relationship between activities of daily living and instrumental activities of daily living. *Journal of Chronic Diseases* 40(6):481–489.

Stassen, Margaret, and Jon Holohan. 1980. *A Comparative Analysis of Long-Term Care Demonstrations and Evaluations.* Draft report prepared for the Administration on Aging. Washington, D.C.: The Urban Institute, pp. 193–194.

Stone, Robyn, Gail L. Cafferata, and Judith Sangl. 1987. Caregivers of the frail elderly: a national survey. *The Gerontologist* 27:616–626.

U.S. Congress. Committee on Finance, U.S. Senate. 1970. *Medicare and Medicaid: Problems, Issues, and Alternatives.* February 9. Washington, D.C.: U.S. Government Printing Office.

U.S. Congress. Committee on Ways and Means, U.S. House of Representatives. 1975. *Selected Issues in Medicare Program Policy.* June 16. Washington, D.C.: U.S. Government Printing Office.

——— 1987. Background materials on health care coverage and expenses of the Medicare population. May 5. Washington, D.C.: U.S. Government Printing Office.

——— 1989. *Background Material and Data on Programs within the Jurisdiction of the Committee on Ways and Means.* WMCP:101-4. (1988 edition, WMCP:100-29; 1987 edition, WMCP:100-4; 1986 edition, WMCP:99-14). Washington, D.C.: U.S. Government Printing Office.

U.S. Congress. Congressional Budget Office. 1976. *Working Papers on Major Budget and Program Issues in Selected Health Programs.* December 10. Washington, D.C.: U.S. Government Printing Office.

——— 1977. *Long-Term Care for the Elderly and Disabled.* CBO Budget Issue Paper. February.

——— 1983. *Changing the Structure of Medicare Benefits: Issues and Options.* March.

——— 1986. Health Care for the elderly. Testimony by Nancy Gordon, Director, before the Energy and Commerce Committee.

———— 1989. *Updated Estimates of Medicare's Catastrophic Drug Insurance Program.* October. Memorandum.

U.S. Congress. Energy and Commerce Committee, U.S. House of Representatives. 1981. Report on experimental efforts in long-term health care for the elderly. Committee Print 97-N. Washington, D.C.: U.S. Government Printing Office.

———— 1986a. Health care for the elderly. Serial no. 99-139. Washington, D.C.: U.S. Government Printing Office.

———— 1986b. Long-term care services for the elderly: background materials on financing and delivery of long-term care services for the elderly. Committee print 99-EE. Washington, D.C.: U.S. Government Printing Office.

———— 1988. *Medicaid Source Book: Background Data and Analysis.* Prepared by the Congressional Research Service. Washington, D.C.: U.S. Government Printing Office.

U.S. Congress. Office of Technology Assessment. 1987a. Prescription drugs and elderly Americans: ambulatory use and approaches to coverage for Medicare. Staff Paper.

———— 1987b. *Losing a Million Minds: Confronting the Tragedy of Alzheimer's Disease and Other Dementias.* April (OTA-BA-324). Washington, D.C.: U.S. Government Printing Office.

———— 1989. The use of preventive services by the elderly. Preventive Health Services under Medicare Series: Paper 2. Washington, D.C.: U.S. Government Printing Office.

U.S. Congress. Select Committee on Aging, U.S. House of Representatives. 1978. Abuses in the sale of health insurance to the elderly in the supplementation of Medicare: a national scandal. Washington, D.C.: U.S. Government Printing Office.

———— 1987. Long-term care and personal impoverishment: seven in ten elderly living alone are at risk. Pub. no. 100-631. Washington, D.C.: U.S. Government Printing Office.

———— 1989. Health care costs for America's elderly, 1977–1988. Comm. Pub. no. 101-712. Washington, D.C.: U.S. Government Printing Office.

U.S. Congress. Special Committee on Aging, U.S. Senate. 1984. Medicare and the health costs of older Americans: the extent and effects of cost sharing. S.Prt. 98-166. Washington, D.C.: U.S. Government Printing Office.

U.S. Department of Health and Human Services. 1986a. *Report to the Secretary on Private Financing of Long-Term Care for the Elderly.* Washington, D.C.

———— 1986b. *Catastrophic Illness Expense: Report to the President.* Washington, D.C.

U.S. Department of Health and Human Services. Health Care Financing Administration. 1977–1989. Demonstrations Summaries. *Health Care Financing Status Report: Research and Demonstrations in Health Care Financing.* Washington, D.C.: U.S. Government Printing Office.

———— 1981. *Long-Term Care: Background and Future Directions.* Baltimore, Md.: Bureau of Data Management and Strategy.

—— 1982–1987. *Annual Medicare Program Statistics: Medicare Enrollment, Reimbursement, and Utilization.* Available for 1981, 1982, 1983, and 1984. Baltimore, Md.: Bureau of Data Management and Strategy.

—— 1982–1989. *Medicare and Medicaid Data Book.* Available for 1981, 1984, 1986, and 1988. Baltimore, Md.: Office of Research and Demonstrations.

—— 1987a. Medicare hospice benefit program evaluation. *Health Care Financing Extramural Report.* Baltimore, Md.: Office of Research and Demonstrations.

—— 1987b. Evaluation of community-oriented long-term care demonstration projects. *Health Care Financing Extramural Report.* USDHHS. HCFA Pub. no. 03242. May. Washington, D.C.: U.S. Government Printing Office.

U.S. Department of Health, Education, Welfare. 1976. *Forward Plan for Health FY 1976–1982.* Public Health Services, August. Washington, D.C.

U.S. General Accounting Office. 1974. *Home Health Care Benefits under Medicare and Medicaid.* B-164031(3). July 9. Washington, D.C.

—— 1977. *Home Health: The Need for a National Policy to Better Provide for the Elderly.* GAO/HRD-78-19. December 30. Washington, D.C.

—— 1979. *Entering a Nursing Home: Costly Implications for Medicaid and the Elderly.* Report to the Congress. Washington, D.C.

—— 1982. *The Elderly Should Benefit from Expanded Home Health Care, but Increasing These Services Will Not Insure Cost Reductions.* GAO/IPE-83-1. December 7. Washington, D.C.

—— 1983. *Medicaid and Nursing Home Care: Cost Increases and the Need for Services are Creating Problems for the States and the Elderly.* Report to the Chairman of the Subcommittee on Health and the Environment, Committee on Energy and Commerce, House of Representatives. Washington, D.C.

—— 1986a. *Medigap Insurance: Law Has Increased protection against Substandard and Overpriced Policies.* Report to the Subcommittee on Health, Committee on Ways and Means, House of Representatives. Washington, D.C.

——1986b. *Medicare: Need to Strengthen Home Health Care Payment Controls and Address Unmet Needs.* GAO/HRD-87-9. December 2. Washington, D.C.

—— 1987. *Medicare: Prescription Drug Issues.* Report to the Chairman, Special Committee on Aging, U.S. Senate. July. Washington, D.C.

Van Nostrand, Joan, A. Sappolo, E. Hing, et al. 1979. The national nursing home survey: 1977 summary for the United States. *Vital and Health Statistics.* Series 13, no. 423. National Center for Health Statistics. DHEW Pub no. (PHS) 79-1794. Public Health Service. Washington, D.C.: U.S. Government Printing Office.

Vertrees, James C., Kenneth G. Manton, and Gerald S. Adler. 1989. Cost-effectiveness of home and community-based care. *Health Care Financing Review* 10(4):65–78.

Vladeck, Bruce. 1980. *Unloving Care: The Nursing Home Tragedy.* New York: Basic Books.

—— 1987. History of the Medicare extended care benefit. In Bruce Vladeck and G. Alfano, eds., *Medicare and Extended Care: Issues, Problems, and Prospects.* Owings Mills, Md.: Rynd Communications.

Vogel, Ronald, and Hans Palmer. 1982. *Long-Term Care Perspectives from Research and Demonstrations*. Health Care Financing Administration. Washington, D.C.: U.S. Government Printing Office.

Waldo, Daniel. 1987. Out-patient prescription drug spending by the Medicare population. *Health Care Financing Review* 9(1):83-90.

Waldo, Daniel, Sally T. Sonnefeld, David R. McKusick, and Ross H. Arnett, III. 1989. Health care expenditures by age group, 1977 and 1987. *Health Care Financing Review* 10(4):111–120.

Weiss, Lawrence, and June Okazawa Monarch. 1983. San Francisco Project OPEN; a long term care health system development and demonstration program for the elderly. *Pride Institute Journal of Long Term Home Health Care* 4 (Winter):13–24.

Weissert, William. 1985. Estimating the long-term care population: prevalence rates and selected characteristics. *Health Care Financing Review* 6(4):83–92.

————— 1986. Hard Choices: targeting long-term care to the "at-risk" aged. *Journal of Health Politics, Policy, and Law* 11(3):463–481.

Weissert, William, et al. 1980. Effects and costs of day care services for the chronically ill: a randomized experiment. *Medical Care* 18 (June):576.

West, Howard. 1971. Five years of Medicare—a statistical review. *Social Security Bulletin* 34(12):17–27. Washington, D.C.: U.S. Government Printing Office.

White House Conference on Aging. 1981. *Final Report of the 1981 White House Conference on Aging*. Washington, D.C.: U.S. Government Printing Office.

Wiener, Joshua. 1987. *Swing Beds: Assessing Flexible Health Care in Rural Communities*. Washington, D.C.: The Brookings Institution.

Wiener, Joshua, and Ray Hanley. 1989. Measuring the activities of daily living among the elderly: a guide to national surveys. Report prepared for the Interagency Forum on Aging-Related Statistics, Committee on Estimates of Activities of Daily Living in National Surveys. October. Washington, D.C.: Interagency Forum on Aging-Related Statistics.

Yordi, Cathleen, and Jacqueline Waldman. 1985. A consolidated model of long-term care: service utilization and cost impacts. *Gerontologist* 25 (August):393.

Zawadski, R. T. 1984. Policy implications of the community-based long-term care demonstrations. *Home Health Care Services Quarterly* 4(3–4):229–247.

Zimmer, James, Annemarie Groth-Juncker, and Jan McCusker. 1985. A randomized controlled study of a home health team. *American Journal of Public Health* 75 (February):134–141.

7. Controlled Experimentation as Research Policy

American Hospital Association. 1987. *Hospital Statistics 1987*. Chicago: The AHA.

Bailit, H. L., J. P. Newhouse, R. H. Brook, et al. 1985. Does more generous dental insurance coverage improve oral health? *Journal of the American Dental Association* 110 (May):701–707.

Ballard, C. L., J. B. Shoven, and J. Whalley. 1985. General equilibrium computations of the marginal welfare costs of taxes in the United States. *American Economic Review* 75 (March):128–138.

Brook, R. H., K. N. Lohr, G. A. Goldberg, et al. 1980 and subsequent. *Conceptualization and Measurement of Physiologic Health for Adults.* R-2262-HHS, vols. 2-1 through 17. Santa Monica, Calif.: The RAND Corporation.

Brook, R. H., J. E. Ware, A. Davies-Avery, et al. 1979. Overview of adult health status measures fielded in RAND's health insurance study. *Medical Care* (Supplement) 17:1–131.

Brook, R. H., J. E. Ware, Jr., W. H. Rogers, et al. 1983. Does free care improve adults' health? Results from a randomized controlled trial. *New England Journal of Medicine* 309 (December 8):1426–34.

Browning, E. 1987. On the marginal welfare cost of taxation. *American Economic Review* 77 (March):11–23.

Chassin, M. R., et al. 1987. Does inappropriate use explain geographic variations in the use of health care services? A study of three procedures. *JAMA* 258(18):2533–37.

Davies, A. R., et al. 1986. Consumer acceptance of prepaid and fee-for-service medical care: results from a randomized trial. *Health Services Research* 21(3):429–452.

Davies, A. R., et al. 1988. *Scoring Manual: Adult Health Status and Patient Satisfaction Measures Used in RAND's Health Insurance Experiment.* N-2190-HHS, April. Santa Monica, Calif.: The RAND Corporation.

Davis, K., and L. B. Russell. 1972. The substitution of hospital outpatient care for inpatient care. *Review of Economics and Statistics* 54 (May):109–120.

Enthoven, A. Management of competition in the FEHBP. *Health Affairs* 8(3):33–50.

Fein, R. 1971. Testimony. *Health Care Crisis in America, 1971.* Hearings before the Subcommittee on Health of the Committee on Labor and Public Welfare, United States Senate, February 22–23, part 1, 92nd Cong., 1st sess. Washington, D.C.: U.S. Government Printing Office, p. 146.

Feldstein, M. S. 1971a. The high cost of hospitals—and what to do about it. *The Public Interest* 48 (Summer):40–54.

——— 1971b. Hospital cost inflation: a study of nonprofit price dynamics. *American Economic Review* 61 (December):853–872.

——— 1977. Quality change and the demand for hospital care. *Econometrica* 45 (October):1681–1702.

Foxman, B., R. B. Valdez, K. N. Lohr, et al. 1987. The effect of free care on the use of antibiotics: results from a population-based randomized controlled trial. *Journal of Chronic Disease* 40(5):429–437.

Goldsmith, J. 1984. Death of a paradigm: the challenge of competition. *Health Affairs* 3 (Fall):5–19.

Health Insurance Association of America. 1985 and 1987. Source Book of Health Insurance Data, 1984–1985 and 1986–1987. Washington, D.C.: The HIAA.

Helms, L. J., J. P. Newhouse, and C. E. Phelps. 1978. Copayments and demand for medical care: the California Medicaid experience. *Bell Journal of Economics* 9(1):192–208.

Hill, D. B., and J. E. Veney. 1970. Kansas Blue Cross/Blue Shield outpatient benefits experiment. *Medical Care* 8 (March-April):143–158.

Jones, S. B. 1989. Perspective: can multiple choice be managed? *Health Affairs* 8(3):51–59.

Keeler, E. B., E. M. Sloss, R. H. Brook, et al. 1987. Effects of cost sharing on physiological health, health practices, and worry. *Health Services Research* 22(3):279–306.

Lohr, K. N., R. H. Brook, G. A. Goldberg, et al. 1983 and subsequent. *Measurement of Physiologic Health for Children.* R-2898-HHS, vols. 1–6. Santa Monica, Calif.: The RAND Corporation.

Lohr, K. N., R. H. Brook, C. J. Kamberg, et al. 1986. Use of medical care in the RAND health insurance experiment: diagnosis- and service-specific analyses in a randomized controlled trial. *Medical Care* (Supplement) 24(9):S1-S87.

Luft, H. S. 1978. How do health maintenance organizations achieve their "savings"? *New England Journal of Medicine* 298(24):1336–43.

——— 1981. *Health Maintenance Organizations.* New York: John Wiley and Sons.

Lurie, N., N. B. Ward, M. F. Shapiro, et al. 1984. Termination from Medi-Cal: does it affect health? *New England Journal of Medicine* 311(7):480–484.

——— 1986. Termination of Medi-Cal benefits—a follow-up study one year later. *New England Journal of Medicine* 314(19):1266–68.

Manning, W. G., H. G. Bailit, B. Benjamin, et al. 1985. The demand for dental care: evidence from a randomized trial in health insurance. *Journal of the American Dental Association* 110:895–902.

Manning, W. G., J. P. Newhouse, N. Duan, et al. 1987. Health insurance and the demand for medical care: results from a randomized experiment. *American Economic Review* 77(3):251–277.

——— 1988. Health insurance and the demand for medical care: evidence from a randomized experiment. Santa Monica, Calif.: The RAND Corporation, R-3476-HHS.

Manning, W. G., K. B. Wells, N. Duan, et al. 1984. Cost sharing and the demand for ambulatory mental health services. *American Psychologist* 39 (October):1090-1100.

Marquis, M. S., and C. E. Phelps. 1985. Demand for supplementary health insurance. July (R-3285). Santa Monica, Calif.: The RAND Corporation.

Munnell, A., ed. 1986. Lessons from the income maintenance experiments. Conference Series no. 30. Boston: Federal Reserve Bank of Boston.

Newhouse, J. P. 1974. A design for a health insurance experiment. *Inquiry* 11(1):5–27. Reply to Hester and Leveson. *Inquiry* 11(3):236–241. Design reprinted in Lewis E. Weeks and Howard J. Berman, eds., *Economics in Health Care* (Germantown, Md.: Aspen Systems Corporation, 1977); Design and Reply reprinted in Lewis E. Weeks, Howard J. Berman, and Gerald E. Bisbee, Jr., eds., *Financing of Health Care* (Ann Arbor, Mich.: Health Administration Press, 1979).

Newhouse, J. P., W. G. Manning, N. Duan, et al. 1987. The findings of the RAND health insurance experiment—a response to Welch et al. *Medical Care* 25(2):157–79.

Newhouse, J. P., W. G. Manning, C. N. Morris, et al. 1981. Some interim results from a controlled trial of cost sharing in health insurance. *New England Journal of medicine* 305 (December 17):1501-7.

Newhouse, J. P., K. H. Marquis, C. N. Morris, et al. 1979. Design improvements in the second generation of social experiments: The health insurance study. *Journal of Econometrics* 11 (September):117–129.

Newhouse, J. P., and C. E. Phelps. 1974. Price and income elasticities for medical care services. In Shigeto Tsuru and Mark Perlman, eds., *The Economics of Health and Medical Care, Proceedings of a Conference of the International Economics Association.* London: Macmillan.

———— 1976. New estimates of price and income elasticities for medical care services. In Richard Rosett, ed., *The Impact of Health Insurance on the Health Services Sector.* New York: National Bureau of Economic Research.

Newhouse, J. P., C. E. Phelps, and W. B. Schwartz. 1974. Policy options and the impact of national health insurance. *New England Journal of Medicine* 290(24):1345–59. Reprinted in Richard Zeckhauser, ed., *Benefit-Cost and Policy Analysis, 1974* (Chicago: Aldine, 1975); also reprinted in Robert H. Haveman and Julius Margolis, eds., *Public Expenditure and Policy Analysis,* 2nd ed. (Chicago: Rand McNally, 1977).

Newhouse, J. P., J. E. Rolph, B. Mori, and M. Murphy. 1980. The effect of deductibles on the demand for medical care services. *Journal of the American Statistical Association* 75(371):525–533.

O'Grady, K. F., W. G. Manning, J. P. Newhouse, and R. H. Brook. 1985. The impact of cost sharing on emergency department use. *New England Journal of Medicine* 313 (August 22):484–490.

Perkoff, G. T., L. Kahn, and P. J. Haas. 1976. The effects of an experimental prepaid group practice on medical care utilization and cost. *Medical Care* 14:432–449.

Phelps, C. E., and J. P. Newhouse. 1972. Effects of coinsurance: a multivariate analysis. *Social Security Bulletin* 35 (June):20–29.

———— 1974. Coinsurance, the price of time, and the demand for medical services. *Review of Economics and Statistics* 56(3):334–342.

Price, J. R., J. W. Mays, and G. R. Trapnell. 1983. Stability in the federal employees health benefits program. *Journal of Health Economics* 2(3):207–223.

Roemer, M. I., C. E. Hopkins, L. Carr, and F. Gartside. 1975. Copayments for ambulatory care: penny-wise and pound foolish. *Medical Care* 13:457–466.

Rosett, R. N., and L. F. Huang. 1973. The effect of health insurance on the demand for medical care. *Journal of Political Economy* 81 (March/April):281–305.

Scitovsky, A. A., and N. M. Snyder. 1972. Effect of coinsurance on use of physician services. *Social Security Bulletin* 35 (June):3–19.

Siu, A. L., F. A. Sonnenberg, W. G. Manning, et al. 1986. Inappropriate use of hospitals in a randomized trial of health insurance plans. *New England Journal of Medicine* 315(20):1259–66.

Sloss, E. M., E. B. Keeler, and B. Operskalski. 1987. Effect of a health maintenance organization on physiologic health:results from a randomized trial. *Annuals of Internal Medicine* 106(1):130–138.

Tarlov, A. R., J. E. Ware, Jr., S. Greenfield, et al. 1989. The medical outcomes study: an application of methods for monitoring the results of medical care. *Journal of the American Medical Association* 272(7):925–930.

United States Bureau of the Census. 1988. Statistical Abstract of the United States, table 142.

Valdez, R. B. 1986. *The Effects of Cost Sharing on the Health of Children.* R-3270-HHS. Santa Monica, Calif.: The RAND Corporation.

Valdez, R. B., A. Leibowitz, J. E. Ware, Jr., et al. 1986. Health insurance, medical care, and children's health. *Pediatrics* 77 (January):124–128.

Ware, J. E., R. H. Brook, A. Davies-Avery, et al. 1980. *Conceptualization and Measurement of Health for Adults in the Health Insurance Study: Vol. I. Model of Health and Methodology.* R-1987/1-HEW, May. Santa Monica, Calif.: The RAND Corporation.

Ware, J. E., Jr., R. H. Brook, W. H. Rogers, et al. 1986. Comparison of health outcomes at a health maintenance organization with those of fee-for-service care. *The Lancet* 1(848):1017–22.

Ware, J. E., R. H. Brook, W. H. Rogers, et al. 1987. *Health Outcomes for Adults in Prepaid and Fee-for-Service Systems of Care: Results from the Health Insurance Experiment.* R-3459-HHS, October. Santa Monica, Calif.: The RAND Corporation.

Ware, J. E., A. Davies-Avery, and R. Brook. 1980. *Conceptualization and Measurement of Health for Adults in the Health Insurance Study: Vol. VI, Analysis of Relationships among Health Status Measures.* R-1987-6-HEW, November. Santa Monica, Calif.: The RAND Corporation.

8. Alternative Delivery Systems

Adamache, Killard W., and Louis F. Rossiter. 1986. The entry of HMOs into the Medicare market: implications for TEFRA's mandate. *Inquiry* 23(4):349–364.

American Medical Association. 1934. Minutes of the 8th Annual session, June 11–15, 1934. *Journal of the American Medical Association* 102:2200.

Appel, G., and D. Acquilina. 1982. Hospitals won't compete on price until spurred by buyers' shopping. *Modern Healthcare* 12(11):108–110.

Baldwin, M.F. 1987. HMO supporters praise HCFA's decision to terminate Medicare Contract with IMC. *Modern Healthcare* 17(11):11.

Bashshur, Rashid L., and Charles A. Metzner. 1967. Patterns of social differentiation between community health association and Blue Cross-Blue Shield. *Inquiry* 4:23–44.

Beebe, J., J. Lubitz, and P. Eggers. 1985. Using prior utilization to determine payments for Medicare enrollees in health maintenance organizations. *Health Care Financing Review* 6(3):27–38.

Berki, S., and M. Ashcraft. 1980. HMO enrollment: who joins what and why? A review of the literature. *Milbank Memorial Fund Quarterly/Health and Society* 58(4):588–632.

Blue Cross and Blue Shield Association. 1989. *Blue Cross and Blue Shield Consumer Exchange.* Chicago: Blue Cross and Blue Shield Association.

Buchanan, Joan L., and Shan Cretin. 1986. Risk selection of families electing HMO membership. *Medical Care* 24(1):39–51.

California Department of Health. 1975. Prepaid health plans: the California experience. In U.S. Senate, Committee on Government Operations, Permanent Subcommittee on Investigations, *Prepaid Health Plans.* Hearings, March 13–14, 1975, 94th Cong., 1st Sess. Washington, D.C.: U.S. Government Printing Office.

California State Legislative Analyst. 1973. A review of the regulation of prepaid health plans by the California Department of Health. Sacramento, Calif., November 15. Reprinted in U.S. Senate, Committee on Government Operations, *Prepaid Health Plans.* Hearings, March 13–14, 1975. Washington, D.C.: U.S. Government Printing Office, 1975.

Chavkin, D. F., and A. Treseder. 1977. California's prepaid health plan program: can the patient be saved? *Hastings Law Journal* 28 (January):685–760.

Davis, K. 1989. California may boost minimum net-worth level for HMOs. *Health Week* 3(7):5–6.

Densen, P. M. 1960. Prepaid medical care and hospital utilization in a dual choice situation. *American Journal of Public Health* 50(11):1710–26.

——— 1962. Prepaid medical care and hospital utilization: comparison of a group practice and a self-insurance situation. *Hospitals* 36 (November 16):62–68.

Densen, P. M., N. R. Deardorff, and E. Balamuth. 1958. Longitudinal analyses of four years of experience of a prepaid comprehensive medical care plan. *Milbank Memorial Fund Quarterly* 36(1):5–45.

Densen, P. M., S. Shapiro, and M. Einhorn. 1959. Concerning high and low utilizers of service in a medical care plan, and the persistence of utilization levels over a three year period. *Milbank Memorial Fund Quarterly* 37(3):217–250.

DesHarnais, Susan I. 1985. Enrollment in and disenrollment from health maintenance organizations by Medicaid recipients. *Health Care Financing Review* 6(3):39–50.

Donabedian, A. 1982, 1984. *The Definition of Quality and Approaches to Its Management.* Ann Arbor, Mich.: Health Administration Press.

——— 1988a. Quality assessment and assurance: unity of purpose, diversity of means. *Inquiry* 25:173–192.

——— 1988b. The quality of care: How can it be assessed? *Journal of the American Medical Association* 260:1743–48.

Dozier, Dave, et al. 1968. *Final Report of the Survey of Consumer Experience under the State of California's Employees' Hospital and Medical Care Act.* Sacramento, Calif.: State of California.

Enthoven, A. C. 1980. *Health Plan.* Menlo Park, Calif.: Addison-Wesley.

——— 1988. Managed competition: an agenda for action. *Health Affairs* 7:25–47.

Enthoven, A. C., and R. Kronick. 1989a. A consumer choice health plan for the 1990s: universal health insurance in a system designed to promote quality and economy. *New England Journal of Medicine,* Part 1: 320(1):29–37.

———— 1989b. A consumer choice health plan for the 1990s: universal health insurance in a system designed to promote quality and economy. *New England Journal of Medicine,* Part 2:320(2):94–101.

Epstein, A. M., and E. J. Cumella. 1988. Capitation payment: using predictors for medical utilization to adjust rates. *Health Care Financing Review* 10(1):51–69.

Fein, R. 1967. *The Doctor Shortage: An Economic Diagnosis.* Washington, D.C.: The Brookings Institution.

Feinson, M. C., S. Hansell, and D. Mechanic. 1988. Factors associated with Medicare beneficiaries' interest in HMOs. *Inquiry* 25 (Fall):364–373.

Feldman, R., J. Kralewski, and B. Dowd. 1989. Health maintenance organizations: the beginning or the end? *Health Services Research* 24(2):191–211.

Feldstein, Paul J., Thomas M. Wickizer, and John R. C. Wheeler. 1988. Private cost containment: the effects of utilization review programs on health care use and expenditures. *New England Journal of Medicine* 318(20):1310–14.

Freidson, Eliot. 1973. Prepaid group practice and the new demanding patient. *Milbank Memorial Fund Quarterly* 51(4):473–488.

Gabel, J., D. Ermann, T. Rice, and G. De Lissovoy. 1986. The emergence and future of PPOs. *Journal of Health Politics, Policy, and Law.* 11(2):305–322.

Gabel, J., C. Jachich-Toth, G. De Lissovoy, et al. 1988. The changing world of group health insurance. *Health Affairs* 7(3):48–65.

Galblum, T. W., and S. Trieger. 1982. Demonstrations of alternative delivery systems under Medicare and Medicaid. *Health Care Financing Review* 3(3):1–11.

Gardner, E. 1988a. Maxicare sues AMI over payments [news]. *Modern Healthcare* 18(14):6.

———— 1988b. Maxicare slapped with restraining order [news]. *Modern Healthcare* 18(29):4.

Garfield, S. R. 1970. The delivery of medical care. *Scientific American* 222(4):15–23.

Garfield, S. R., et al. 1976. Evaluation of an ambulatory medical-care delivery system. *New England Journal of Medicine* 294(8):426–431.

Goldberg, L. G., and W. Greenberg. 1981. The determinants of HMO enrollment and growth. *Health Services Research* 16 (Winter):421–438.

Goldberg, V. P. 1975. Some emerging problems of prepaid health plans in the Medi-Cal system. *Policy Analysis* 1(1):55–68.

Gray, Bradford H., ed. 1983. *The New Health Care for Profit.* Washington, D.C.: National Academy Press.

———— 1986. *For Profit Enterprise in Health Care.* Washington, D.C.: National Academy Press.

Greenberg, Jay, et al. 1988. The social HMO demonstration: early experience. *Health Affairs* 7(3):66–79.

Greenwald, Howard P. 1987. HMO membership, copayment, and initiation of care for cancer: a study of working adults. *American Journal of Public Health* 77(4):461–466.

Group Health Association of America (GHAA). 1989. The AAPCC explained. *Research Briefs* no. 8 (February). Washington, D.C.: Group Health Association of America.

Gruber, L. R., M. Shadle, and C. L. Polich. 1988. From movement to industry: the growth of HMOs. *Health Affairs* 7(3):197–208.

Gutterman, S., P. W. Eggers, G. Riley, T. F. Greene, and S. A. Terrell. 1988. The first 3 years of Medicare prospective payment: an overview. *Health Care Financing Review* 9(3):67–77.

Ham, Faith Lyman. 1989. Cost controls that didn't work. *Business and Health* 7(8):30.

Harrington, D.C. 1971. San Joaquin foundation for medical care. *Hospitals* 45(6):67–68.

Hastings, J. E. F., et al. 1970. An interim report on the Sault Ste. Marie study: a comparison of personal health services utilization. *Canadian Journal of Public Health* 61 (July–August):289–296.

Hay, J. W., and M. J. Leahy. 1987. Competition among health plans: some preliminary evidence. *Southern Economic Journal* 11 (January):831–846.

Hillman, Alan L. 1987. Financial incentives for physicians in HMOs: is there a conflict of interest? *New England Journal of Medicine* 317(27):1743–48.

Hillman, Alan L., Mark V. Pauly, and Joseph J. Kerstein. 1989. How do financial incentives affect physicians' clinical decisions and the financial performance of health maintenance organizations? *New England Journal of Medicine* 321 (2):86–92.

Hyman, David A., and Joel V. Williamson. 1989. Fraud and abuse: setting the limits on physicians' entrepreneurship. *New England Journal of Medicine* 320(19):1275–78.

Johns, Lucy, Robert A. Derzon, and Maren D. Anderson. 1985. Selective contracting in California: early effects and policy implications. *Inquiry* 22(1):24–32.

Kenkel, P. J. 1988a. S & P downgrades Maxicare debt to CCC [news]. *Modern Healthcare* 18(26):4.

——— 1988b. Maxicare troubles mount [news]. *Modern Healthcare* 18(13):5.

Kenkel, P. J., and K. S. Palm. 1988. Maxicare reports higher losses than expected [news]. *Modern Healthcare* 18(12):4.

Kralewski, J. E., D. Countryman, and D. Shatin. 1982. Patterns of interorganizational relationships between hospitals and HMOs. *Inquiry* 19(4):357–362.

Langwell, K., L. Rossiter, R. Brown, L. Nelson, S. Nelson, and K. Berman. 1987. Early experience of health maintenance organizations under Medicare competition demonstrations. *Health Care Financing Review* 8(3):37–55.

Larkin, H. 1989a. Maxicare fallout: will CA Blue Cross be next? *Hospitals* 63(9):49.

——— 1989b. Provider exodus, lawsuit prompted Maxicare filling. *Hospitals* 63(9):50.

Levinson, Douglas F. 1987. Toward full disclosure of referral restrictions and financial incentives by prepaid health plans. *New England Journal of Medicine* 317(27):1729–31.

Lohr, K. N., and R. H. Brook. 1984. Quality assurance in medicine. *American Behavioral Scientist* 27(5):583–607.

Luft, H. S. 1976. Benefit-cost analysis and public policy implementation: from normative to positive analysis. *Public Policy* 24(4):437–462.

——— 1978. Why do HMOs seem to provide more health maintenance services? *Milbank Memorial Fund Quarterly/Health and Society* 56(2):140–168.

——— 1981. *Health Maintenance Organizations: Dimensions of Performance.* New York: Wiley-Interscience.

——— 1986. Compensating for biased selection in health insurance. *Milbank Memorial Fund Quarterly* 64(4):566–591.

——— 1988. HMOs and the quality of care. *Inquiry* 25(1):147–156.

Luft, H. S., S. Maerki, and J. B. Trauner. 1986. The competitive effects of health maintenance organizations: another look at the evidence from Hawaii, Rochester and Minneapolis/St. Paul. *Journal of Health Politics, Policy, and Law* 10(4):625–658.

Luft, Harold S., and Robert H. Miller. 1988. Patient selection in a competitive health care system. *Health Affairs* 7(3):97–119.

Luft, Harold S., and Joan B. Trauner. 1985. Adverse selection in a large, multiple option health benefits program: a case study of the California public employees' retirement system. In Richard Scheffler and Louis Rossiter, eds., *Advances in Health Economics and Health Services Research,* vol. 6. Greenwich, Conn.: JAI Press, pp. 197–229.

Manning, Willard Jr., A. Liebowitz, G. A. Goldberg, et al. 1984. A controlled trial of the effect of a prepaid group practice on use of services. *New England Journal of Medicine* 310(23):1505–10.

McLaughlin, C. G. 1987. HMO growth and hospital expenses and use: a simultaneous-equation approach. *Health Services Research* 22(2):183–205.

——— 1988. The effect of HMOs on overall hospital expenses: is anything left after correcting for simultaneity and selectivity? *Health Services Research* 23(3):421–442.

——— 1989. Author response: HMO growth and Hospital expenses—will the "real" model please stand up? *Health Services Research* 24(3):414–425.

McLaughlin, Catherine G., Jeffrey C. Merrill, and Andrew J. Freed. 1984. The impact of HMO growth on hospital costs and utilization. In Richard Scheffler and Louis Rossiter, eds., *Advances in Health Economics and Health Services Research,* vol. 5. Greenwich, Conn.: JAI Press.

Newcomer, Robert J., Charlene Harrington, Cathleen Yordi, and Alan Friedlob. 1986. *Report to Congress: Evaluation of Social/Health Maintenance Organizations Demonstration.* HCFA Pub. no. 03283, USDHHS. Baltimore, Md.: Health Care Financing Administration.

Newhouse, Joseph P. 1974. A design for a health insurance experiment. *Inquiry* 11(1):5–27.

NICHMOD. National Industry Council for HMO Development. 1984. *The Health Maintenance Organization Industry Ten Year Report, 1973–1983.* Washington, D.C.: National Industry Council for HMO Development.

Numbers, R. L. 1978. The third party: health insurance in America. In Judith Walter Leavitt and Ronald L. Numbers, eds., *Sickness and Health in America: Read-*

ings in the History of Medicine and Public Health. Madison: University of Wisconsin Press, pp. 139–153.

Pauly, Mark V. 1970. Efficiency, incentives and reimbursement for health care. *Inquiry* 7(1):114–131.

Perrott, George S. 1971. *The Federal Employees Health Benefits Program.* Washington, D.C.: Office for Group Practice Development, U.S. Department of Health, Education and Welfare.

Relman, A. S. 1980. The new medical-industrial complex. *New England Journal of Medicine* 303(17):963–970.

Relman, Arnold. 1987. Doctors and the dispensing of drugs (editorial). *New England Journal of Medicine* 317(5):311–312.

Roemer, M. I. 1982. Sickness absenteeism in members of health maintenance organizations and open-market health insurance plans. *Medical Care* 20(11):1140–46.

Roos, Leslie L., Noralou P. Roos, and Sandra M. Sharp. 1987. Monitoring adverse outcomes of surgery using administrative data. *Health Care Financing Review* 7(Supplement):5–16.

Scheffler, Richard M., James O. Gibbs, and Dolores A. Gurnick. 1988. *The Impact of Medicare's Prospective Payment System and Private Sector Initiatives: Blue Cross Experience, 1980–1986.* Final Report to HCFA, HCFA Grant no. 15-C-98757/5-1, July. Berkeley, Calif.: University of California.

Schwartz, Harry. 1978. Conflicts of interest in fee for service and in HMOs. *New England Journal of Medicine* 299(19):1071–73.

Shapiro, S., L. Weiner, and P. Densen. 1958. Comparison of prematurity and perinatal mortality in a general population and in the population of a prepaid group practice medical care plan. *American Journal of Public Health* 48(2):170–185.

——— 1960. Further observations on prematurity and perinatal mortality in a general population and in the population of a prepaid group practice medical care plan. *American Journal of Public Health* 50(9):1304–17.

Thomas, J. W., and R. Lichtenstein. 1986. Functional health measure for adjusting health maintenance organization capitation rates. *Health Care Financing Review* 7(3):85–95.

Trauner, Joan B. 1977. From benevolence to negotiation: prepaid health care in San Francisco, 1850–1950. Ph.D. dissertation, Department of History of Health Sciences, June. University of California, San Francisco.

Trauner, Joan B., Harold S. Luft, and Sandra S. Hunt. 1986. A lifestyle decision: facing the reality of physician oversupply in the San Francisco Bay area. In Eli Ginzberg, ed., *From Physician Shortage to Patient Shortage.* Chapter 6. Boulder, Colo: Westview Press, pp. 119–147.

U.S. Congress. Office of Technology Assessment. 1988. *The Quality of Medical Care: Information for Consumers.* June. Washington, D.C.: Congress of the United States, Office of Technology Assessment.

U.S. General Accounting Office. 1986. *Medicare: Issues Raised by Florida Health Maintenance Organization Demonstrations.* July 16. Washington, D.C.: U.S. General Accounting Office.

U.S. Office of the White House Press Secretary. 1971. *Major Features of the Comprehensive Health Policy for the 70's.* February 18.

Ware, John E., et al. 1986. Comparison of health outcomes at a health maintenance organization with those of fee-for-service care. *The Lancet* 1(8488):1017–22.

Wilensky, Gail R., and Louis F. Rossiter. 1986. Patient self-selection in health maintenance organizations. *Health Affairs* 5(1):66–80.

Williamson, J. W. 1988. Future policy directions for quality assurance: lessons from the health accounting experience. *Inquiry* 25 (Spring):67–77.

Winslow, Constance M., David H. Solomon, Mark R. Chassin, et al. 1988. The appropriateness of carotid endarterectomy. *New England Journal of Medicine* 318(12):721–727.

Zellner, B. Bruce, and B. L. Wolfe. 1989. HMO growth and hospital expenses: a correction, research commentary. *Health Services Research* 24(3):409–413.

9. Health Manpower Forecasting

American College of Surgeons. 1989. *Statement of the College to the Council on Graduate Medical Education,* June 1. Chicago.

Auster, Richard, Irving Leveson, and Deborah Saracheck. 1969. The production of health: an exploratory study. *Journal of Human Resources* 4 (Fall):411–436.

Bane, Frank. 1959. U.S. Department of Health, Education and Welfare, *Physicians for a Growing America* (Bane Report). Report of the Surgeon General's consultant group on medical education. Washington, D.C.: U.S. Government Printing Office.

Bayne-Jones, Stanhope. 1958. *The Advancement of Medical Education and Research through the Department of Health, Education, and Welfare* (Bayne-Jones Report). Final report of the secretary's consultants on medical research and education. Washington, D.C.: U.S. Government Printing Office, June 1958.

Bazzioli, G. J. 1986. Does educational indebtedness affect physician specialty choice? *Journal of Health Economics* 5:1–19.

Berry, Charles B., Philip J. Held, Barbara Kehrer, and Uwe E. Reinhardt. 1978. *A Study of the Responses of Canadian Physicians to the Introduction of Universal Medical Care Insurance: The First Five Years in Quebec.* Princeton, N.J.: Mathematica Policy Research.

Blue Cross and Blue Shield Association. 1989. *Environmental Analysis 1989.* Chicago: Blue Cross and Blue Shield Association.

Blumberg, Mark S. 1971. *Trends and Projections of Physicians in the United States, 1967–2002.* A Technical Report Sponsored by the Carnegie Commission on Higher Education. New York: The Carnegie Foundation for the Advancement of Teaching.

Brook, Robert H., and Mary E. Vaiana. 1989. *Appropriateness of Care.* Washington, D.C.: The National Health Policy Forum of George Washington University, June.

Burstein, P. L., and J. Cromwell. 1985. Relative incomes and rates of return for U.S. physicians. *Journal of Health Economics* 4:63–78.

The Carnegie Commission on Higher Education. 1970. *Higher Education and the Nation's Health: Policies for Medical and Dental Education*. New York: McGraw-Hill, October.

Centre de Recherche pour l'Etude et l'Observation des Conditions de Vie (CREDOC). 1983. *Femmes Médecins: Démographie, Activité et Prescriptions en Médicine Libérale*. Paris: CREDOC, December.

Council on Graduate Medical Education. 1988. Bureau of Health Professions, U.S. Department of Health and Human Services. *First Report of the Council*, vols. 1 and 2, July 1. Rockville, Md.

Dickinson, Frank G. 1951. *Supply of Physicians' Services*. Chicago: American Medical Association, Bureau of Medical Economics Research.

Dowling, W. L. 1972. A linear programming approach to the analysis of hospital production. Ph.D. dissertation, University of Michigan, Ann Arbor.

Evans, Robert G. 1973. *Price Formation in the Market for Physician's Services in Canada, 1957–1969*. Study prepared for the Prices and Incomes Commission, Canada, 1972. Ottawa: Information Canada.

——— 1974. Supplier-induced demand: some empirical evidence and implications. In Mark Perlman, ed., *The Economics of Health and Medical Care*. London: Macmillan.

Ewing, O. W. 1948. *The Nation's Health, A Ten-Year Program: A Report to the President*. Washington, D.C.: U.S. Government Printing Office.

Farrell, M. J. 1957. The measurement of productive efficiency. *Journal of the Royal Statistical Association* 120 (Fall):253–282.

Fein, Rashi. 1967. *The Doctor Shortage: An Economic Diagnosis*. Washington, D.C.: The Brookings Institution.

Feldman, Roger, and Frank A. Sloan. 1988. Competition among physicians, revisited. *Journal of Health Politics, Policy, and Law* 13(2):239–261.

Flexner, Abraham. 1910. *Medical Education in the United States and Canada*. New York: The Carnegie Foundation for the Advancement of Teaching.

Fuchs, Victor R. 1974. *Who Shall Live?* New York: Basic Books.

Gerber, Alex. 1967. The medical manpower shortage. *Journal of Medical Education* 42 (April):306–319.

Ginzberg, Eli. 1960. A cautionary view of medical care. *New England Journal of Medicine* 262(7):367–368.

——— 1966. The physician shortage reconsidered. *New England Journal of Medicine* 275(2):85–87.

——— 1989. Physician supply in the year 2000. *Health Affairs* 8(2):84–90.

——— 1990. The politics of the U.S. physician supply. In *The Medical Triangle: Physicians, Politicians, and the Public*. Cambridge, Mass.: Harvard University Press.

Golladay, F. L., M. E. Manser, and K. E. Smith. 1974. Scale economies in the delivery of medical care: a mixed integer programming analysis of efficient manpower utilization. *Journal of Human Resources* 9(1):50–62.

Gorham, William B. 1967. *Medical Care Prices.* Report by the Department of Health, Education, and Welfare to the President. Washington, D.C.: U.S. Government Printing Office, February.

Graduate Medical Education National Advisory Committee (GMENAC). 1981. Department of Health and Human Services. *Summary Report,* vol. 1, September 1980. Washington, D.C.: U.S. Goverment Printing Office, GPO Publication no. 1980-0-721-748/266.

Hadley, Jack. 1977. An empirical model of medical specialty choice. *Inquiry* 14:384–400.

———— 1982. *More Medical Care, Better Health?* Washington, D.C.: The Urban Institute Press.

Harris, Jeffrey E. 1986. How many doctors are enough? *Health Affairs* 5(4):74–83.

Jacobsen, Steven J., and Alfred A. Rimm. 1987. The projected physician surplus reevaluated. *Health Affairs* 6(2):49–56.

Jussim, J., and C. Muller. 1975. Medical education for women: how good an investment? *Journal of Medical Education* 50:571–580.

Kehrer, Barbara H. 1976. Factors affecting the incomes of men and women physicians: an exploratory analysis. *Journal of Human Resources* 11(4):526–545.

Langwell, Katherine. 1982. Factors affecting the incomes of men and women physicians: further explorations. *Journal of Human Resources* 17(2):261–275.

Lee, Roger I., and Lewis Webster Jones. 1933. *The Fundamentals of Good Medical Care.* Chicago: University of Chicago Press.

Marder, William D., Phillip R. Kletke, Anne B. Silberger, and Richard J. Willke. 1988. *Physician Supply and Utilization by Specialty: Trends and Projections.* Chicago: American Medical Association.

McKinlay, John B., and Sonja B. McKinlay. 1977. The questionable contribution of medical measures to the decline of mortality in the United States in the twentieth century. *Milbank Memorial Fund Quarterly* 55 (Summer):405–429.

Mountin, Joseph W., Elliott H. Pennell, and Anne G. Berger. 1949. Health service areas: estimates of future physician requirements. Public Health Bulletin no. 305. Washington, D.C.: U.S. Government Printing Office.

Mulhausen, Robert, and Jeanne McGree. 1989. Physician need: an alternative projection from a study of large, prepaid group practices. *Journal of the American Medical Association* 261(13):1930–34.

National Advisory Commission on Health Manpower. 1967. *Report,* vols. 1 and 2. Washington, D.C.: U.S. Government Printing Office.

Pauly, Mark V. 1980. *Doctors and Their Workshops: Economic Models of Physician Behavior.* Chicago: University of Chicago Press.

———— 1988. Is medical care different? Old questions, new answers. *Journal of Health Politics, Policy, and Law* 13(2):227–237.

Peterson, Paul Q., and Maryland Y. Pennell. 1963. Physician population projections, 1961–75: their causes and implications. *American Journal of Public Health* 53 (February):163–172.

President's Commission on the Health Needs of the Nation. 1953. *Building America's Health: A Report to the President* (Magnuson Report), 5 vols. Washington, D.C.: U.S. Government Printing Office.

Reinhardt, Uwe E. 1972. A production function for physician services. *Review of Economics and Statistics* 54(1):55–66.

———— 1973. Manpower substitution and productivity in medical practice: review of research. *Health Services Research* 8(3):200–227.

———— 1974. Health manpower forecasting: current methodology and its impact on health manpower policy. In *Manpower for Health Care,* Papers of the Spring Meeting of the Institute of Medicine. Washington, D.C.: National Academy of Sciences.

———— 1975a. *Physician Productivity and the Demand for Health Manpower.* Cambridge, Mass.: Ballinger.

———— 1975b. Health manpower forecasting in a market context. In Norman T. J. Bailey and Mark Thompson, eds., *Systems Aspects of Health Planning,* Proceedings of the IIASA Conference, Baden, Austria, August 20–22, 1974. New York: North Holland.

———— 1978. Competition among physicians: comment. In Warren Greenberg, ed., *Competition in the Health Care Sector: Past, Present, and Future.* Germantown, Md.: Aspen Systems.

———— 1981. The GMENAC forecast: an alternative view. *American Journal of Public Health* 71(10):1149–57.

———— 1985a. On the economic implications of a physician surplus. *World Medical Journal* 32(1):2–14.

———— 1985b. The theory of physician-induced demand: reflections after a decade. *Journal of Health Economics* 4:187–193.

Rice, Thomas. 1984. Physician-induced demand for medical care: new evidence from the Medicare program. In Richard Scheffler, ed., *Advances in Health Economics and Health Services Research.* New York: JAI Press.

Riddick, Frank A., Jr. 1987. Statement of the American Medical Association to the Council on Graduate Medical Education. In U.S. Department of Health and Human Services, Bureau of Health Professions, Council on Graduate Medical Education. *Public Hearing,* HRP-0907157. Bethesda, Md., November 19–20, pp. 138–173.

Rossiter, Louis F., and Gail R. Wilensky. 1987. Health economist-induced demand for theories of physician-induced demand. *Journal of Human Resources* 22 (Fall):624–627.

Schloss, Ernest P. Beyond GMENAC—another physician shortage from 2010 to 2030? *New England Journal of Medicine* 318(14):920–922.

Schroeder, Steven A. 1984. Western European responses to physician oversupply. *Journal of the American Medical Association* 252 (July 20):373–384.

Schwartz, William B., Frank A. Sloan, and Daniel N. Mendelson. 1988. Why there will be little or no physician surplus between now and the year 2000. *New England Journal of Medicine* 318(14):892–897.

Silver, Morris. 1972. An econometric analysis of spatial variations in mortality rates. In Victor R. Fuchs, ed., *Essays in the Economics of Health.* New York: National Bureau of Economic Research.

Sloan, Frank A. 1970. Lifetime earnings and the physicians' choice of specialty. *Industrial and Labor Relations Review* 24:47–56.

————— 1971. The demand for medical education: a study of medical school application behavior. *Journal of Human Resources* 6(4):466–489.

————— 1984. *Affidavit in re American Medical Association vs. Margaret M. Heckler.* Cause no. IP84-1317C, U.S. District Court for the Southern District of Indiana, Indianapolis Division, December 12.

Sloan, Frank A., and Roger Feldman. 1978. Competition among physicians. In Warren Greenberg, ed., *Competition in the Health Care Sector: Past, Present, and Future.* Germantown, Md.: Aspen Systems.

Smith, Kenneth R., Marianne Miller, and Frederick L. Golladay. 1972. An analysis of the optimal use of inputs in the production of medical services. *Journal of Human Resources* 7(2):208–255.

Steinwachs, Donald M., J. P. Weiner, Sam Shapiro, P. Batalden, K. L. Cotlin, and F. A. Wasserman. 1986. A comparison of the requirements for primary care physicians in HMOs with projections made by the GMENAC. *New England Journal of Medicine* 314:217–222.

Tarlov, Alvin R. 1986. HMO enrollment growth and physicians: the third compartment. *Health Affairs* 5(1):23–35.

U.S. Bureau of Health Professions, U.S. Department of Health and Human Services. 1988a. *Sixth Report to the President and Congress on the Status of Health Personnel in the United States.* Rockville, Md.: Bureau of Health Professions, HRP-0907200, June.

————— 1988b. An assessment of the W. B. Schwartz, F. A. Sloan and D. N. Mendelson Study, *Why There Will Be Little or No Physician Surplus Between Now and the Year 2000.* Rockville, Md.: Bureau of Health Professions, Office of Data Analysis and Management, ODAM Report no. 7-88, July.

U.S. Congress, House of Representatives. 1963. *Health Professions Educational Assistance, Hearing before the Committee on Interstate and Foreign Commerce.* 88th Cong., 1st Sess., February 6. Washington, D.C.: U.S. Government Printing Office.

————— 1967. *Medical Care Prices.* A Report to the President. (Also referred to as the "Gorham Report.") Washington, D.C.: U.S. Government Printing Office, February.

U.S. Department of Labor, Bureau of Labor Statistics. 1967. A study of requirements and supply. In *Health Manpower 1966–75.* Washington, D.C.: U.S. Government Printing Office.

U.S. Department of Labor, Manpower Administration. 1970. *Manpower Report of the President: A Report on Manpower Requirements, Resources, Utilization, and Training.* Washington, D.C.: U.S. Government Printing Office.

————— 1972. *Manpower Report of the President: A Report on Manpower Requirements, Resources, Utilization, and Training.* Washington, D.C.: U.S. Government Printing Office.

U.S. National Advisory Commission on Health Manpower. 1967. *Report of the Commission.* 2 vols. Washington, D.C.: U.S. Government Printing Office.

U.S. Public Health Service, Department of Health, Education and Welfare. 1967. *Health Manpower Perspectives: 1967.* Washington, D.C.: U.S. Government Printing Office.

U.S. Surgeon General's Consultant Group on Medical Education. 1959. *Physicians for a Growing America.* U.S. Public Service Publication no. 709. Washington, D.C.: U.S. Government Printing Office.

Yett, Donald E., John L. Drabek, Michael D. Intriligator, and Larry J. Kimbal. 1971. The use of an econometric model to analyze selected features of national health insurance plans. Mimeo. Los Angeles: Human Resources Research Center, University of Southern California.

10. Maintaining Quality of Care

American Psychiatric Association. 1987. *Diagnostic and Statistical Manual of Mental Disorders* (3rd ed., rev.). Washington, D.C.: American Psychiatric Association.

Avorn, J., et al. 1988. Reduction of incorrect antibiotic dosing through a structured educational order form. *Archives of Internal Medicine* 148:1720–24.

Bergner, J., R. M. Kaplan, and J. E. Ware. 1987. Measuring overall health: an evaluation of three important approaches. *Journal of Chronic Diseases* 40 (Supplement 1):23S–26S.

Bergner, M. 1985. Measurement of health status. *Medical Care* 23(5):696–704.

Bergner, M., R. A. Bobbitt, et al. 1981. The sickness impact profile: development and final revision of a health status measure. *Medical Care* 19(8):787–805.

Bernstein, L. R., S. L. Barriere, et al. 1982. Utilization of antibiotics: analysis of appropriateness of care. *Annals of Emergency Medicine* 11:400–403.

Brand, D. B., et al. 1983. Adequacy of antitetanus prophylaxis in six hospital emergency rooms. *New England Journal of Medicine* 309:636–640.

Brook, R. H., C. J. Kamberg, A. Mayer-Oakes, et al. 1989. *Appropriateness of Acute Medical Care for the Elderly: An Analysis of the Literature.* Santa Monica, Calif.: The RAND Corporation, R-3717, September.

Chassin, M. R., R. H. Brook, R. E. Park, et al. 1986a. Variations in the use of medical and surgical services by the Medicare population. *New England Journal of Medicine* 314:285–290.

Chassin, M. R., A. Fink, S. Rauchman, et al. 1986b. *Indications for Selected Medical and Surgical Procedures: A Literature Review and Ratings of Appropriateness: Coronary Angiography.* Santa Monica, Calif.: The RAND Corporation, R-3204/1.

Chassin, M. R., R. E. Park, A. Fink, et al. 1986c. *Indications for Selected Medical and Surgical Procedures: A Literature Review and Ratings of Appropriateness: Coronary Artery Bypass Graft Surgery.* Santa Monica, Calif.: The RAND Corporation, R-3204/2.

Chassin, M. R., J. Kosecoff, D. H. Solomon, and R. H. Brook. 1987a. How coronary angiography is used: clinical determinants of appropriateness. *Journal of the American Medical Association* 258(18):2543–47.

Chassin, M. R., J. Kosecoff, R. E. Park, et al. 1987b. Does inappropriate use explain geographic variations in the use of health services? A study of three procedures. *Journal of the American Medical Association* 258(18):2533–37.

Chassin, M. R., R. E. Park, K. N. Lohr, et al. 1989. Differences among hospitals in Medicare patient mortality. *Health Services Research* 24(1):1–31.

Cochrane, A. L., et al. 1978. Health service "input" and mortality "output" in developed countries. *Journal of Epidemiology and Community Health* 32:200.

Codman, E. A. 1914. The product of a hospital. *Surgery, Gynecology, and Obstetrics* 18(4):491–494.

Crossley, K. B. 1984. Antibiotic prophylaxis in surgery: improvement after a multi-hospital education program. *Southern Medical Journal* 77:864–867.

Daley, J., S. Jencks, D. Draper, et al. 1988. Predicting hospital-associated mortality for Medicare patients: a method for patients with stroke, pneumonia, acute myocardial infarction, and congestive heart failure. *Journal of the American Medical Association* 260(24):3617–24.

Deming, W. E. 1986. *Out of the Crisis*. Cambridge, Mass.: MIT Center for Advanced Engineering Study.

Dubois, R. W., and R. H. Brook. 1988. Preventable deaths: who, how often, and why? *Annals of Internal Medicine* 109:582–589.

Dubois, R. W., R. H. Brook, and W. H. Rogers. 1987. Adjusted hospital death rates: a potential screen for quality of medical care. *American Journal of Public Health* 77(9):1152–55.

Dubois, R. W., W. H. Rogers, J. H. Moxley, et al. 1987. Hospital inpatient mortality: is it a predictor of quality? *New England Journal of Medicine* 317(26):1674–80.

Duncan, A. J., and A. J. Campbell. 1988. Antidepressant drugs in the elderly: are the indications as long term as the treatment? *British Medical Journal* 296:1230–32.

Eddy, D. M., et al. 1987. Screening for colorectal cancer in a high-risk population: results of a mathematical model. *Gastroenterology* 92:682.

Eddy, D. M., and J. Billings. 1988. The quality of medical evidence: implications for quality of care. *Health Affairs* 7(4):19–32.

Elliott, R. V., K. A. Kahn, and R. Kaye. 1981. Physicians measure up. *Journal of the American Medical Association* 245:595–600.

Fink, A., R. H. Brook, and J. Kosecoff. 1987. The sufficiency of the clinical literature for learning about the appropriate uses of six medical and surgical procedures. *Western Journal of Medicine* 147(5):609–615.

Friedman, L. M., R. P. Byington, and the Beta-Blocker Heart Attack Trial Research Group. 1985. Assessment of angina pectoris after myocardial infarction: comparison of the Rose questionnaire with physician judgment in the beta-blocker heart attack trial. *American Journal of Epidemiology* 121:555–562.

Fuchs, V. 1974. *Who Shall Live?* New York: Basic Books.

Gosney, M., and R. Tallis. 1984. Prescription of contraindicated and interacting drugs in elderly patients admitted to hospital. *Lancet* 2:564–567.

Greenfield, S., H. U. Aronow, R. M. Elashoff, and D. Watanabe. 1988. Flaws in mortality data: the hazards of ignoring comorbid disease. *Journal of the American Medical Association* 260(15):2253–55.

Greenfield, S., D. M. Blanco, R. M. Elashoff, et al. 1987. Patterns of care related to age of breast cancer patients. *Journal of the American Medical Association* 257:2766–70.

Greenspan, A. M., H. R. Kay, B. C. Berger, et al. 1988. Incidence of unwarranted implantation of permanent cardiac pacemakers in a large medical population. *New England Journal of Medicine* 318:158–163.

Groves, E. W. 1908. A plea for a uniform registration of operation results. *British Medical Journal* 2:1008–9.

Heller, T. A., E. B. Larson, and J. P. LoGerfo. 1984. Quality of ambulatory care of the elderly: an analysis of five conditions. *Journal of the American Geriatric Society* 32:782–788.

Helling, D. K., G. J. Norwood, and J. D. Donner. 1982. An assessment of prescribing using drug utilization review criteria. *Drug Intelligence and Clinical Pharmacy* 16:930–934.

Jencks, S. F., J. Daley, D. Draper, et al. 1988a. Interpreting hospital mortality data: the role of clinical risk adjustment. *Journal of the American Medical Association* 260(24):3611–16.

Jencks, S. F., D. K. Williams, and T. L. Kay. 1988b. Assessing hospital-associated deaths from discharge data: the role of length of stay and comorbidities. *Journal of the American Medical Association* 260(15):2240–46.

Jewesson, P. J., et al. 1983. Auditing antibiotic use in a teaching hospital: focus on cefoxitin. *Canadian Medical Association Journal* 309:636–640.

Kahn, K. L., J. Kosecoff, M. R. Chassin, et al. 1988. Measuring the clinical appropriateness of the use of a procedure: can we do it? *Medical Care* 26(4):415–422.

Kahn, K. L., C. P. Roth, A. Fink, et al. 1986. *Indications for Selected Medical and Surgical Procedures: A Literature Review and Ratings of Appropriateness: Colonoscopy.* Santa Monica, Calif.: The RAND Corporation, R-3204/5.

Kahn, K. L., C. P. Roth, J. Kosecoff, et al. 1986. *Indications for Selected Medical and Surgical Procedures: A Literature Review and Ratings of Appropriateness: Diagnostic Upper Gastrointestinal Endoscopy.* Santa Monica, Calif.: The RAND Corporation, R-3204/4.

Kaplan, E. B., L. B. Sheiner, A. J. Boeckmann, et al. 1985. The usefulness of preoperative laboratory screening. *Journal of the American Medical Association* 253:3576–81.

Kaplan, R. M., and J. W. Bush. 1982. Health-related quality of life measurement for evaluation research and policy analysis. *Health Psychology* 1(1):61–80.

Kennedy, J. W., G. C. Kaiser, L. D. Fisher, et al. 1980. Multivariate discriminant analysis of the clinical and angiographic predictors of mortality from the collaborative study in coronary artery surgery (CASS). *Journal of Thoracic and Cardiovascular Surgery* 6:876–877.

Kosecoff, J., M. R. Chassin, A. Fink, et al. 1987. Obtaining clinical data on the appropriateness of medical care in community practice. *Journal of the American Medical Association* 258(18):2538–42.

Kosecoff, J., A. Fink, R. H. Brook, and M. R. Chassin. 1987. The appropriateness of using a medical procedure: is information in the medical record valid? *Medical Care* 25(3):196–201.

Kostrzewski, J. 1979. The interface of health and social services. In W. W. Holland, J. Ipsen, and J. Kostrzewski, eds., *Measurement of Levels of Health.* Copenhagen: World Health Organization (Regional Office for Europe).

Laporte, J. R., M. Porta, and D. Capella. 1983. Drug utilization studies: a tool for determining the effectiveness of drug use. *British Journal of Clinical Pharmacy* 16:301–304.

Lohr, K. N., R. H. Brook, C. Kamberg, et al. 1986. Use of medical care in the RAND health insurance experiment: diagnosis-and service-specific analyses in a randomized controlled trial. *Medical Care* 24(9):Supplement.

Lohr, K. N., and J. E. Ware, eds. 1987. Proceedings of the advances in health assessment conference. *Journal of Chronic Diseases* 40 (Supplement 1):1S-191S.

Lurie, N., N. B. Ward, M. F. Shapiro, and R. H. Brook. 1984. Termination from Medi-Cal: does it affect health? *New England Journal of Medicine* 311:480–484.

Mas, X., J. R. Laporte, et al. 1983. Drug prescribing and use among elderly people in Spain. *Drug Intelligence and Clinical Pharmacy* 17:378–381.

McGlynn, E. A., and J. P Newhouse. 1985. Medi-Cal and indigent health care. In J. J. Kirlin and D. R. Winkler, eds., *California Policy Choices*, vol. 2. Los Angeles: University of Southern California School of Public Administration.

Melton, L. J., R. N. Stauffer, E. Y. Chao, et al. 1982. Rates of total hip arthroplasty. *New England Journal of Medicine* 307:1242–45.

Merrick, N. J., R. H. Brook, A. Fink, et al. 1986. Use of carotid endarterectomy in five California Veterans Administration medical centers. *Journal of the American Medical Association* 256:2531–35.

Merrick, N. J., A. Fink, R. H. Brook, et al. 1986. *Indications for Selected Medical and Surgical Procedures: A Literature Review and Ratings of Appropriateness: Carotid Endarterectomy.* Santa Monica, Calif.: The RAND Corporation, R-3204/6.

Merrick, N. J., A. Fink, R. E. Park, et al. 1987. Derivation of clinical indications for carotid endarterectomy by an expert panel. *American Journal of Public Health* 77(2):187–190.

Mizrahi, A., A. Mizrahi, and S. Sandier. 1983. *Medical Care, Morbidity and Costs: Graphic Presentations of Health Statistics.* New York: Pergamon Press.

Mullooly, J. P. 1984. Tetanus immunization of adult members of an HMO. *American Journal of Public Health* 74:841–842.

Mushlin, A. I., and F. A. Appel. 1980. Testing an outcome-based quality assurance strategy in primary care. *Medical Care* 18 (Supplement 5):1–100.

Newhouse, J. P. 1974. A design for a health insurance experiment. *Inquiry* 11:5–27.

——— 1987. Cross national differences in health expenditures: what do they mean? *Journal of Health Economics* 6:159–162.

Nightingale, F. 1858. Mortality of the British army at home and abroad and during the Russian war as compared with the mortality of the civil population in England. Reprinted from Report of the Commission Appointed to Inquire into the Regulations Affecting the Sanitary State of the Army. London: Harrison and Sons.

——— 1862. *Hospital Statistics and Hospital Plans.* London: Emily and Faithfull.

——— 1863. *Proposal for Improved Statistics of Surgical Operations.* London: Savill and Edwards.

Park, R. E., A. Fink, R. H. Brook, et al. 1986. Physician ratings of appropriate indications for six medical and surgical procedures. *American Journal of Public Health* 76(7):766–771.

Phibbs, B., and H. J. Marriott. 1985. Complications of permanent intravenous pacing. *New England Journal of Medicine* 312:1428–32.

Ray, W. A., C. F. Federspiel, and W. Schaffner. 1980. A study of antipsychotic drug use in nursing homes: epidemiologic evidence suggesting misuse. *American Journal of Public Health* 70:485–491.

Restuccia, J. D., P. M. Gertman, S. J. Dayno, et al. 1984. A comparative analysis of appropriateness of hospital use. *Health Affairs* 3:130–138.

Rubenstein, L. V., R. H. Brook, et al. 1989. Improving patient function: a randomized trial of functional disability screening. *Annals of Internal Medicine* 111:836–842.

Setia, U., I. Serventi, and P. Lorenz. 1985. Factors affecting the use of influenza vaccine in the institutionalized elderly. *Journal of the American Geriatric Society* 33:856–858.

Shapiro, M., T. R. Townsend, et al. 1979. Use of antimicrobial drugs in general hospital. *New England Journal of Medicine* 301:351–355.

Sisk, J. E., and R. K. Riegelman. 1986. Cost effectiveness of vaccination against pneumococcal pneumonia: an update. *Annals of Internal Medicine* 104:79–86.

Siu, A. L., A. Leibowitz, R. H. Brook, et al. 1988. Use of the hospital in a randomized trial of prepaid care. *Journal of the American Medical Association* 259:1343–46.

Siu, A. L., F. A. Sonnenberg, W. G. Manning, et al. 1986. Inappropriate use of hospitals in randomized trial of health insurance plans. *New England Journal of Medicine* 315:1259–66.

Solomon, D. H., R. H. Brook, A. Fink, et al. 1986. *Indications for Selected Medical and Surgical Procedures: A Literature Review and Ratings of Appropriateness: Cholecystectomy.* Santa Monica, Calif.: The RAND Corporation, R-3204/3.

Stander, P. E., and G. R. Yates. 1988. Modifying physician prescribing patterns of h2 receptor antagonists in an ambulatory setting. *Quality Review Bulletin* 14:206–209.

Stewart, A. L., S. Greenfield, R. D. Hays, et al. 1989. Functional status and well-being of patients with chronic conditions. *Journal of the American Medical Association* 262(7):907–913.

Studnicki, J., and C. E. Stevens. 1984. The impact of a cybernetic control system on inappropriate admissions. *Quality Review Bulletin* 10:304–311.

Ulaszek, K. M., K. D. Seabloom, et al. 1984. Appropriateness of long term cimetidine prescribing. *Drug Intelligence and Clinical Pharmacy* 18:623–625.

U.S. Department of Health and Human Services. 1987. *Medicare Hospital Mortality Information 1986.* Washington, D.C.: U.S. Government Printing Office.

——— 1988. *Medicare Hospital Mortality Information 1987.* Washington, D.C.: U.S. Government Printing Office.

Vuori, H. V. 1982. *Quality Assurance of Health Services.* Copenhagen: World Health Organization (Regional Office for Europe).

Ware, J. E., R. H. Brook, K. N. Williams, et al. 1978. *Conceptualization and Mea-*

surement of Health for Adults in the Health Insurance Study. Model of Health and Methodology, vol. 1, R-1987/1-HEW. Santa Monica, Calif.: The RAND Corporation.

Ware, J. E., A. Davies-Avery, and C. A. Donald. 1978. *Conceptualization and Measurement of Health for Adults in the Health Insurance Study. General Health Perceptions,* vol. 5, R-1987/5-HEW. Santa Monica, Calif.: The RAND Corporation.

Wells, K. B., G. Goldberg, and R. H. Brook. 1988. Management of patients on psychotropic drugs in primary care clinics. *Medical Care* 26:645–657.

Wells, K. B., A. Stewart, R. D. Hays, et al. 1989. The functioning and well-being of depressed patients. *Journal of the American Medical Association* 262(7):914–919.

Wennberg, J. E., and A. Gittlesohn. 1973. Small area variations in health care delivery. *Science* 182:1102–8.

Wennberg, J. E., A. Gittlesohn, and N. Shapiro. 1975. Health care delivery in Maine, III: evaluating the level of hospital performance. *Journal of the Maine Medical Association* 66(11):298–306.

Wilcosky, T., R. Harris, and L. Weissfeld. 1987. The prevalence and correlates of Rose questionnaire angina among women and men in the lipid research clinics program prevalence study population. *American Journal of Epidemiology* 125:400–409.

Winslow, C. M., J. B. Kosecoff, M. R. Chassin, et al. 1988. The appropriateness of performing coronary artery bypass surgery. *Journal of the American Medical Association* 260:505–509.

Winslow, C. M., D. H. Solomon, M. R. Chassin, et al. 1988. The appropriateness of carotid endarterectomy. *New England Journal of Medicine* 318:721–727.

World Health Organization. 1948. Constitution of the World Health Organization. In *Basic Documents,* 15th ed. Geneva: World Health Organization.

——— 1981. *Health Services in Europe.* Vol. 1, Regional Analysis. Copenhagen: World Health Organization (Regional Office for Europe).

Acknowledgments

4. Physician Payment

The authors are grateful to Thomas Rice and Eli Ginzberg for their helpful comments on earlier drafts.

5. Financing Health Care for the Poor

The authors wish to thank Paula Grant for research assistance. The views expressed are our own and not necessarily those of the institutions with which we are affiliated or of the Commonwealth Fund.

6. Financing Health Care for Elderly Americans

The author wishes to thank Barbara Lyons and Alina Salganicoff for research and editorial assistance and the Brookdale Foundation for its continued support. The views expressed are my own and not necessarily those of the institutions with which I am affiliated or of the Commonwealth Fund.

Index